COMMUNITY
DENTAL HEALTH

In Memoriam

Professor Anthony Westwater Jong, D.D.S., M.P.H., D.Sc., of Bolton, Mass., associate dean of the Boston University, Henry M. Goldman School of Graduate Dentistry and chairman of the School's department of dental care management, died at home on July 22, 1992, after a lengthy battle with cancer. He was 53.

Dr. Jong was nationally recognized for his preeminence in the field of public health dentistry. His development of the Goldman School's Master of Science in Dental Public Health Program for dental hygienists was the first of its kind in the country.

Dr. Jong was previously assistant dean for student affairs at the Harvard School of Dental Medicine, the director of dental services at the Dimock Community Health Center in Roxbury, Mass., and head of the Child and Youth Project of Boston, a $3 million program to assess and address the health needs of the city's youth.

"Dr. Jong brought to all his work the same vigor and sense of purpose that distinguished his 19-year tenure at the school," said Spencer N. Frankl, dean of the Goldman School. "His passion for providing community service and improving the health status of the underserved was an inspiration. The dental profession has lost a leader, and the community, a valued friend."

"As associate dean for academic affairs at the Goldman School, Professor Jong set and maintained the highest possible standards," said John Silber, Boston University's president. "He worked constantly to improve the quality of training offered to our dental students so that they, in turn, would provide excellent care to their patients. He has been a stalwart member of our faculty, a tireless administrator, and a good friend to Boston University."

A native of New York City, Dr. Jong graduated from the City College of New York in 1960 and the New York University College of Dentistry in 1964. He served an internship at the Jewish Me-

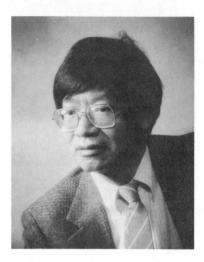

morial Hospital in New York City in 1965, earned a Master of Public Health degree from the Harvard School of Public Health in 1966, and received a postdoctoral certificate from Harvard's dental school in 1968. In 1976 he earned his Doctor of Science degree from the Goldman School.

A diplomate of the American Board of Dental Public Health, Dr. Jong had been a consultant to the U.S. Department of Health and Human Services, the U.S. Department of Health, Education and Welfare, the National Institutes of Health, Boston's Headstart health program, and the Bridge Over Troubled Waters free dental clinic in Boston. He had held numerous offices with the American Association of Dental Schools and the American Public Health Association, was active in the Massachusetts Dental Society and held a faculty appointment at the Harvard School of Dental Medicine.

In 1991 Dr. Jong was the recipient of the Massachusetts Public Health Association's James M. Dunning Award for achievement in the field of dental public health.

COMMUNITY DENTAL HEALTH

Edited by

Anthony W. Jong, D.D.S., M.P.H., D.Sc.

Professor and Chairperson, Department of Dental Care Management,
Associate Dean, Goldman School of Graduate Dentistry, Boston University;
Associate Professor, Department of Socio-Medical Sciences and
Community Medicine, School of Medicine, Boston University Medical Center;
Lecturer, Department of Dental Care Administration, School of Dental Medicine,
Harvard University, Boston, Massachusetts

THIRD EDITION

with 48 illustrations

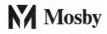 Mosby

St. Louis Baltimore Boston Chicago London Philadelphia Sydney Toronto

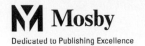
Mosby
Dedicated to Publishing Excellence

Editor: Robert W. Reinhardt
Developmental Editor: Leslie Fenton
Production Editor: Ross Goldberg
Designer: Julie Taugner

THIRD EDITION
Copyright © 1993 by Mosby–Year Book, Inc.

Previous editions copyrighted 1981, 1988

Printed in the United States of America

Mosby–Year Book, Inc.
11830 Westline Industrial Drive
St. Louis, Missouri 63146

Library of Congress Cataloging in Publication Data
Community dental health / edited by Anthony W. Jong.—3rd ed.
    p.   cm.
    Includes bibliographical references and index.
    ISBN 0-8016-6387-3
    1. Dental public health. 2. Community dental services. 3. Dental
public health—United States. I. Jong, Anthony.
    [DNLM: 1. Community Dentistry—United States. WU 113 C734]
  RK52.C665 1993
  362.1'976'00973—dc20
  DNLM/DLC   92-48273
  for Library of Congress   CIP

93 94 95 96 97 CL/DC 9 8 7 6 5 4 3 2 1

Contributors

Helene Bednarsh, B.S., R.D.H., M.P.H.

Program Manager, HIV Dental Ombudsperson Program, Bureau of Community Dental Programs, Boston Department of Health and Hospitals, Boston, Massachusetts

Lester E. Block, D.D.S., M.P.H.

Associate Professor, Division of Health and Management Policy, School of Public Health, and former Director, Program in Dental Public Health, University of Minnesota, Minneapolis, Minnesota

Joseph Boffa, D.D.S., M.P.H.

Associate Professor, Department of Dental Care Management, Boston University Medical Center, Goldman School of Graduate Dentistry, Boston, Massachusetts

David O. Born, Ph.D.

Professor, Division of Health Ecology, Department of Preventive Sciences, School of Dentistry, University of Minnesota, Minneapolis, Minnesota

Mitchell Burek, M.Ed., Ph.D.

Associate Professor, Department of Dental Care Management, Boston University Medical Center, Goldman School of Graduate Dentistry, Boston, Massachusetts

Virginia A. Callanen, M.S., M.P.H.

Washington, D.C.

Marianne B. DeSouza, R.D.H., B.A., M.S.

Assistant Professor and Coordinator, Advanced Standing Program, Department of Dental Care Management, Boston University Medical Center, Goldman School of Graduate Dentistry, Boston, Massachusetts

Jean Marie Doherty-Greenberg, D.M.D., M.P.H., D.Sc.

Assistant Professor, Department of Health Resources Management, University of Illinois at Chicago School of Public Health; Chief, Geriatric Dentistry Section, Department of Dental Service, Veterans Affairs West Side Medical Center, Chicago, Illinois

Paula K. Friedman, D.D.S., M.S.D.

Professor, Department of Dental Care Management, Associate Dean for Administration, Boston University Medical Center, Goldman School of Graduate Dentistry; Assistant Attending Dental Surgeon, Beth Israel Hospital, Boston, Massachusetts

George M. Gluck, D.D.S., M.P.H.

Associate Professor, Division of Comprehensive Care and Applied Practice Administration and Behavioral Sciences, Kriser Dental Center, New York University, New York, New York; Division Director of Public Health, Department of Dentistry, Newark Beth Israel Medical Center, Newark, New Jersey

Gary S. Leske, D.D.S., M.P.H., M.Sc.Hyg.

Professor, Department of Children's Dentistry, State University of New York at Stony Brook, Stony Brook, New York

Dennis H. Leverett, D.D.S., M.P.H.

Professor and Chair, Department of Community Dentistry, Eastman Dental Center; Rochester, New York

Madalyn L. Mann, R.D.H., M.S.

Associate Professor, Department of Dental Care Management, Boston University Medical Center, Goldman School of Graduate Dentistry, Boston, Massachusetts

Jane B. Moosbruker, Ph.D.

Organization Development Consultant, Bolton, Massachusetts; Former Lecturer, Department of Dental Administration, Harvard School of Dental Medicine, Boston, Massachusetts

Julia A. Oberweis, R.D.H., M.S.

Instructor of Dental Hygiene, Forsyth School for Dental Hygienists, Boston, Massachusetts

Maxine Peck, C.D.A., M.S.

Director, Auxiliary Programs, Department of Dental Care Management, Boston University Medical Center, Goldman School of Graduate Dentistry, Boston, Massachusetts

Burton R. Pollack, D.D.S., M.P.H., J.D.

Dean, School of Dental Medicine, State University of New York at Stony Brook, Stony Brook, New York

Louis W. Ripa, D.D.S., M.S.

Professor and Chairman, Department of Children's Dentistry, School of Dental Medicine, State University of New York at Stony Brook, Stony Brook, New York

Lynda Rose, B.A.

Instructor, Department of Dental Care Management, Boston University Medical Center, Goldman School of Graduate Dentistry, Boston, Massachusetts

To my mother
Lily Jong Chin
for the love that has provided me with inspiration
throughout my life

To my wife
Patricia Westwater-Jong
for the understanding and love that has given me peace of mind

To my daughter
Jessica Westwater Jong
for bringing out the adult in me

To my son
Alexander Robert Westwater Jong
for always being the bright little boy in my heart

Foreword

Dr. Anthony Jong, one of the progenitors of the Organization of Teachers of Dental Practice Administration, recognized the inseparable relationship of dental public health (and its commitment to the underserved) and private practice in the delivery of dental care. During the past 12 years, when public health activities of all sorts were eroding, private practice took on an even more important role in the provision of dentistry at all levels. It was out of this notion that the theme of this book developed. The goal of this text became, therefore, to provide the reader with the basic precepts of dental public health and to discuss issues that impact on both public health and the private practice of dentistry.

The authors of the various chapters read like a "who's who" in dental community health. Born discusses program evaluation, Leske reviews the latest concepts of prevention, and Friedman and Bednarsh, in their chapter on private practice, describe the impact of AIDS. Boffa enumerates issues in the financing of dental care and Leverett relates public health research to the understanding of dental care delivery. There are two new chapters, one on international health and the other, by Pollack, on risk management and related legal issues. Mann, Peck and DeSouza discuss the roles of auxiliaries and the importance of dental health education (and how it is delivered). There are chapters on public health, epidemiology, geriatric dentistry and Jong's chapter on professional ethics.

The titles of the chapters could serve as topics in a dental community health course, and they are also significant to anyone interested in the delivery of dental services in the United States. The discussion of health care during the 1992 election campaign and the acknowledgment of the need for change requires a closer look at the contemporary and salient issues. These issues are discussed in Jong's text.

Born in 1938 among the apartment dwellers of uptown New York City Dr. Jong emerged as one of dental education's finest thinkers. The development of this book is part of his legacy. The authors of the various chapters have expressed their respect and affection for the editor by crafting their chapters. Dentistry has lost one of its most respected contributors.

George M. Gluck, D.D.S., M.P.H.

It is a privilege to pay tribute to Dr. Anthony Jong, whose professional goal was to advance the cause of dental public health. Tony Jong championed quality care delivery at both the microscopic and macroscopic level. While he was concerned with educating individuals to maximize their potential within the profession, he was equally concerned with developing systems for improving and maintaining oral health on a larger scale. Since its inception, *Community Dental Health* has been a vehicle for effecting change. It was Tony Jong's wish that his book help you, his readers, develop the skills that would enable you to lead the next generation of dental healthcare providers. It was his hope that you would become the movers and the shakers, the policymakers, who would champion the cause of public health dentistry world-wide.

Ellen Wolfe, M.A.T.
Assistant to Dr. Jong

Preface

The dental health professional faces in the 1990s a world far different from that of the last decade. Growing up in the United States in the 1970s, the emerging professional prepared for a practice in a country that was short of dentists and dental auxiliaries. Labor statistics emphasized the need for more health professionals in a nation with a population explosion and a growing economy. Today the picture is not so clear: Are there too many dentists? Are there too many dental hygienists? How does the budding professional cope with the present environment? Can we now eliminate dental disease? These are questions we face whether we are involved in private practice or in public health. This book focuses on the role of the dental professional in the evolving socially conscious health field.

In this text we introduce essential concepts in the study of dental care and disease prevention, being ever mindful of the social matrix in which we exist. We cannot talk about sophisticated and expensive restorative dentistry without considering the economic impact on the patient and the community. To the public, health care has become a "right." The Senate Committee on Labor and Public Welfare in 1975 reaffirmed that the availability of high-quality health care to all Americans was a national goal. Although the federal government has been moving inexorably toward the achievement of this goal, progress has been slow and painful. Congressional polemic concerning national health insurance legislation has been raging for many years, and to the weary health professional it seems we are no closer to an equitable solution. Thus the public's expectations of access to high-quality health care do not necessarily coincide with the practical realities of the nation's economy.

In other countries such as the United Kingdom, New Zealand, and Sweden, access to health care has been guaranteed by government. However, regardless of the actual implementation of a national program in this country, the new social ethic of responsibility for all has been firmly established. The norms that many health care providers have accepted during their education—that every individual is directly responsible for his or her own personal health care and that professionals determine the needs of society and provide the necessary services—are now being questioned by professionals and consumers.

As the role of the dentist changes in society from an isolated purveyor of essentially rehabilitative clinical services to an integrated member of a health team concerned with preventive and early diagnostic services, dental education must be modified to provide the student with additional relevant information and skills. The role of consumer groups, the proliferation of third-party payment programs, and the emergence of independently practicing dental auxiliaries are affecting the practice of dentistry, and dentistry must respond to these forces. As the prevalence of dental caries decreases in this country, dental public health professionals can direct their efforts toward special population groups that are still in need of their services. The elderly and disabled continue to receive inadequate dental care.

This book, through the contributions of professionals involved in health care delivery, responds to specific need areas such as community dental health education, prevention of dental disease, ethical concerns in dental health care, and so on. The book would not have been possible without the efforts of all the contributors—professionals who are active in teaching and practicing, yet who took the time to write a practical chapter on their field. I would like to thank these contributors and the staff of my department for their interest and help.

A special note of appreciation goes to Ellen Wolfe, who edited every chapter and organized my efforts to produce this third edition.

The editor of a book has the rare opportunity to reach a large audience and to put on paper thoughts that for most people must remain as thoughts, never to be seen or heard. I would like to take advantage of this opportunity to thank James M. Dunning, D.D.S., M.P.H., for having guided me on this path of dental public health, a path that over the past 25 years has been rewarding and ever-stimulating. For those readers who find meaning in the words in this book and seek careers in dental public health, my best wishes for a successful career. Not many have trod this path, but those who did have moved the profession a little closer to improving the dental health of the whole community and the society in which we live.

Anthony W. Jong

Contents

SECTION ONE
PROVIDERS OF DENTAL SERVICES

1   **Dental Public Health—An Overview,** 3
    Lester E. Block, D.D.S., M.P.H.

2   **Factors Affecting the Practice of
    Dentistry,** 20
    Paula K. Friedman, D.D.S., M.S.D.
    Helene Bednarsh, B.S., R.D.H., M.P.H.

3   **Role of Auxiliaries in Dental Care,** 63
    Maxine Peck, C.D.A., M.S.

SECTION TWO
**SOCIAL AND FINANCIAL ASPECTS
OF DENTAL CARE**

4   **International Dental Health,** 79
    Julia A. Oberweis, R.D.H., M.S.

5   **Geriatric Dental Health,** 105
    George M. Gluck, D.D.S., M.P.H.

6   **Financing Dental Care,** 121
    Joseph Boffa, D.D.S., M.P.H.

SECTION THREE
**DENTAL DISEASE—PREVALENCE
AND PREVENTION**

7   **Epidemiology of Dental Disease,** 141
    Jean Marie Doherty-Greenberg, D.M.D.,
    M.P.H., D.Sc.

8   **Prevention of Dental Disease,** 156
    Gary S. Leske, D.D.S., M.P.H., M.Sc.Hyg.
    Louis W. Ripa, D.D.S., M.S.
    Virginia A. Callanen, M.S., M.P.H.

SECTION FOUR
COMMUNITY DENTAL PROGRAMS

9   **Dental Health Education,** 197
    Marianne B. DeSouza, R.D.H., B.A., M.S.

10 **Planning for Community Dental
    Programs,** 225
    Madalyn L. Mann, R.D.H., M.S.

SECTION FIVE
**RESEARCH AND EVALUATION
IN DENTAL CARE**

11 **Introduction to Biostatistics,** 245
    Lynda Rose, B.A.
    Mitchell Burek, M.Ed., Ph.D.

12 **Program Evaluation in Health Care,** 257
    David O. Born, Ph.D.
    Mitchell Burek, M.Ed., Ph.D.

13 **Research in Community Dental
    Health,** 268
    Dennis H. Leverett, D.D.S., M.P.H.

SECTION SIX
**MANAGEMENT AND ETHICS IN DENTAL
CARE**

14 **Team Management in Dental
    Practice,** 285
    Jane B. Moosbruker, Ph.D.

15 **Ethical Issues in Dental Care,** 299
    Anthony W. Jong, D.D.S., M.P.H., D.Sc.

16 **Risk Management in Dental Practice,** 307
    Burton R. Pollack, D.D.S., M.P.H., J.D.

SECTION ONE

Providers of Dental Services

Section one introduces the concept of the dental care delivery system in the United States. It focuses on the providers of dental care—the dentist, the dental hygienist, the dental assistant—and their roles in a rapidly changing environment. The way in which we as providers of services integrate ourselves into a system of dental care to promote the health of our patients is the challenge facing members of our profession today. As Dr. Lester Block so aptly states in Chapter 1, "dental public health is a concern for and activity directed toward the improvement and promotion of the dental health of the population as a whole, as well as of individuals within that population."

The methods that government agencies use to address the problems of dental disease are treated in this first chapter. Dr. Paula Friedman and Ms. Helene Bednarsh, in Chapter 2, discuss the forces that are currently affecting the practice of dentistry, including the impact of acquired immunodeficiency syndrome and also present alternatives to the traditional one-dentist private practice. In Chapter 3, Ms. Maxine Peck attempts to forecast the future for dental auxiliaries in health care delivery by examining the history and current trends in auxiliary education and practice.

Section One will give the student insight into the ecological milieu in which that person will be practicing in the near future and hopefully will reduce the future shock that recent graduates have incurred. The practice of dentistry is rapidly changing, and the goals and models we had as students may not be achievable in today's world. The greatly accelerated rate of change in society has brought on a dizzying disorientation for many people, health professionals included. The attempt to maintain the status quo will prove futile under the ever-increasing forces of change. As Alvin Toffler cautioned in his timely book *Future Shock,* "Future shock will not be found in *Index Medicus* or in any listing of psychological abnormalities. Yet, unless intelligent steps are taken to combat it, millions of human beings will find themselves increasingly disoriented, progressively incompetent to deal rationally with their environments."

1 Dental Public Health—An Overview

The dental profession has primary responsibility for the oral health care of the public and, through the state dental practice acts, has essentially exclusive jurisdiction over the provision of this care. Although the public might not think of the major dental diseases—dental caries and periodontal disease—as particularly serious ones, the magnitude of the problem as evidenced by the universality of the diseases and the extensive levels of untreated pathology results in a public health problem of major proportions. Each dentist, dental hygienist, dental assistant, and dental laboratory technician is, in fact, a health worker combating diseases that jeopardize the health of the public.

Dental public health is simultaneously a field of study within the broader field of public health and one of dentistry's eight specialties. Although dental public health evolved from organized dentistry, its philosophy and substance have been more reflective of that of public health. This difference arose in part because the focus of the dental practitioner is the individual patient, whereas the focus of the dental public health practitioner is the community. In today's complex society, however, dental health issues cannot be the exclusive concern of any one aspect of dentistry. In view of current economic, political, and social factors influencing the health services delivery system in the United States, dental public health and organized dentistry will find it mutually beneficial to work more closely together.

The current emphasis in the dental public health field is on the total dental care delivery system and its impact on oral health status. This increasing focus on the delivery of dental care has been due to the development of alternative delivery systems (e.g., dental health maintenance organizations, independent practice associations, preferred provider organizations), the increased role of third-party payers (e.g., insurance companies), the in-creasing role of government in the payment for care (e.g., Medicaid), an overall increasing emphasis on cost control, and an increased concern about the quality of care.

WHAT IS PUBLIC HEALTH?

In defining *public health*, it is first helpful to define health. The traditional dictionary definition is being free from disease or pain.[67] This limited definition has proved to be insufficient to address issues of public health concern, and the World Health Organization (WHO) in its constitution created a more encompassing definition. WHO defines *health* as "a state of complete physical, mental and social well-being and not merely the absence of disease or infirmity."[64] A problem with the WHO definition is that it is impossible to quantify, and the criteria of freedom from disease, stress, frustration, and disability are actually incompatible with the process of living and aging. As Dubos[64] has stated, "complete and lasting freedom from disease is but a dream remembered from imaginings of a Garden of Eden designed for the welfare of man." Thus Pickett and Hanlon[64] suggest considering health as a continuum under which a disease or injury may lead to an impairment, which may lead to a disability, which may lead to a dependency requiring external resources or aids to carry out activities of daily living. Health in this continuum then can be defined as "the absence of a disability."[64]

Knutson[48] defined *public* as "of or pertaining to the people of a community, state, or a nation," and he offered a simple yet comprehensive definition of public health:

Public health is people's health. It is concerned with the aggregate health of a group, a community, a state, or a nation. Public health in accordance with this broad definition is not limited to the health of poor folks, or to rendering health services or to the nature of the health problems. Nor is it defined by the method of payment for health services, or by the type of agency responsible for supplying those services. It is simply a concern for and activity directed toward the improvement and protection of the health of a population group in the aggregate.

A more widely used definition of public health was developed by Winslow[86] in 1920.

The science and art of preventing disease, prolonging life, and promoting physical and mental efficiency through organized community effort for the sanitation of the environment, the control of communicable infections, the education of the individual in personal hygiene, the organization of medical and nursing services for the early diagnosis and preventive treatment of disease, and the development of the social machinery to insure everyone a standard of living adequate for the maintenance of health, so organizing these benefits as to enable every citizen to realize his birthright of health and longevity.

This definition shows great understanding in that Winslow recognized the impact of social, educational, and economic factors on health. Winslow,[64] however, did not include either medical care or mental health in his definitions, two areas that have more recently come to be of public health concern.

Public health work has expanded from its original focus on asepsis to, in sequence, sanitary engineering, preventive physical medical science, preventive mental medical science, the positive or promotive as well as social behavioral aspects of personal and community medicine, and more recently the promotion and assurance of comprehensive health services for all.[64]

In general, public health is concerned with four broad areas: (1) life-style and behavior, (2) the environment, (3) human biology, and (4) the organization of health programs and systems.[64] Public health, then, is concerned with keeping people as healthy as possible and controlling or limiting factors that impede health and is the organization and application of public resources to prevent dependency that would otherwise result from disease or injury.[64]

Future of public health report

The most current overview of public health, *The Future of Public Health,* was published in 1988. The report details the findings of a blue-ribbon committee appointed by the Institute of Medicine to study the public health field. Among the areas the report addresses is the complex issue of the definition of public health. The report defines the mission of public health as the fulfillment of society's interest in assuring the conditions in which people can be healthy[43] and states that the substance of public health–organized community efforts–should be aimed at the prevention of disease and promotion of health. In addition, the report states that public health links many disciplines and rests upon the scientific core of epidemiology.[43] Public health practitioners share the belief that the public's health "can be improved by altering conditions—behavior, the environment, biological interactions, and the organization of services—that might otherwise, at a future time have an adverse impact on health."[64]

The organizational framework of public health encompasses "both activities undertaken within the formal structure of government and the associated efforts of private and voluntary organizations." The history of dental public health as well as of public health has been one of "identifying health problems, developing knowledge and expertise to solve problems, and rallying political and social support around solutions."[43]

What is dental public health?

The American Board of Dental Public Health[3] modified the Winslow definition of public health and defined *dental public health* as

. . . the science and art of preventing and controlling dental disease and promoting dental health through organized community efforts. It is that form of dental practice which serves the community as a patient rather than the individual. It is concerned with the dental health education of the public, with research and the application of the findings of research, with the administration of programs of dental care for groups, and with the prevention and control of dental disease through a community approach."

A problem with these presently accepted definitions is that they imply that dental public health is concerned only with organized community efforts and only with the dental health of aggregate populations. Now is a good time to reevaluate these definitions and to amend them so that they more accurately reflect current public health activities and interests. A suggested modification of Knutson's definition is dental public health is a concern for and activity directed toward the improvement and promotion of the dental health of the population as a whole, as well as of individuals within that population.

Dental public health practitioners

It is generally agreed that those people who are interested in careers and leadership roles in dental public health or community dentistry should be knowledgeable in both oral health practice and dental public health.

Most dental public health practitioners are initially educated as dentists or as dental hygienists and then go on to graduate-level training in dental public health. Dental public health training programs are offered primarily at schools of public health and at schools of dentistry. Competency objectives for dental public health specialists were recently revised by a committee established by the American Board of Dental Health. Although these objectives will be specifically applied to the education and qualifications of dentists desiring to become dental public health specialists (at this time there are no specialties in dental hygiene), they certainly can be applied to all dental public health educational programs. The objectives fall within four overall categories: (1) health policy and program management and administration, (2) research methods in dental public health, (3) oral health promotion and disease, and (4) oral health services delivery system.[4,68,69]

The specific areas of knowledge and expertise aside from those in oral health include planning, implementation, operation, and evaluation of dental public health programs; policy process; regulation; management information systems; human resources management; financial management; marketing; communications; quality assurance; and risk management.[4,69]

Community health and public health

The term *community health* came into popular use in the late 1960s and early 1970s. Some view community health as focusing on personal health care provided in the local community, others use the term to mean environmental health activity, and still others have in mind the totality of personal health services for the whole community. Cecil Sheps[74] suggests that the term community health is comparable and synonymous with public health and "encompasses the full range of health services, environmental and personal, including other major activities such as health education of the public and the social context of life as it affects the community, the latter referring to a total population. And this is not limited to governmental efforts." Thus both public health and community health could be seen as "the effort that is organized by society to protect, promote, and restore the health and quality of life of the people." Specific activities within public health change as the "needs and demands of the society which they are serving undergo change."

The same confusion has arisen with regard to the meaning of the terms dental public health, previously called public health dentistry, and community dentistry or community dental health, which, of course, is the title of this book. As with the terms public health and community health, for all practical purposes, dental public health and community dental health can be considered as equivalent terms.

The multidisciplinary character of dental public health is important to understand. Many professional disciplines, which are discussed in later chapters in this book, are involved. The more important ones are epidemiology and biostatistics; health economics, political and other social and behavioral sciences; biological and physical sciences; health education, health administration, and nutrition.

The dental profession has recently been focusing more on dental public health–related interests in its dual attempt to increase the strength and effectiveness of the profession and to improve the oral health of the population. The major reason for this increased interest is the perception on the part of organized dentistry that it is facing critical issues, such as the rising cost of dental education, the declining pool of dental school applicants, the increased indebtedness of students, the perceived oversupply of dental personnel, the increasing number of alternative forms of developing services, deregulation, and a highly competitive marketplace.[6]

To address the future problems confronting the dental profession, the American Dental Association (ADA) established the Special Committee on the Future of Dentistry,[6] which produced a report in which a series of issues and their implications were raised and discussed. Although this document is a decade old, its concern that the future will bring to the dental profession a more complex and challenging set of problems that will need to be addressed, using the knowledge and skills of the dental public health field, is still current.

The closer alignment of dental public health and organized dentistry also applies to medicine. A visitor to the American Medical Association's House of Delegates meeting thought he was at a public health meeting. He suggested that medicine now needs the association with public health because a concern for public health makes medicine more complete. Public health should welcome this interest by organized medicine and dentistry in that public health alone does not have the resources to accomplish its goals and it requires the help of others. Public health is the health of all people and therefore is everyone's business.[29]

Dental public health programs

The definition of dental public health leaves the specific objectives of a dental public health program to be developed. Dunning[26] has raised a number of important questions that must be addressed if a program is to be planned effectively:

1. What are the dental needs of the community or population?
2. How extensive is the demand for dental treatment in the population?
3. What dental personnel are available to serve the population, and what is the political climate in regard to the type of staffing that can be used?
4. What is the prevailing philosophy of the people regarding the extent of health care they expect to receive and the manner in which they are willing to receive it?
5. To what extent will prevention of disease obviate the need for treatment? If in fact preventive measures could accomplish this, would they be acceptable for a particular society or segment of society?
6. What scope of service will be offered in a public program, who will receive the service, and in what manner will the service be delivered?

7. How can the service be adjusted to the mores of the population?

Implementation and evaluation of programs

The WHO Expert Committee on Dental Health[87,88] made recommendations regarding the implementation of dental public health programs. It suggested that a dental health problem should be examined in the context of the prevailing health problems and the overall situation of the country, region, or community. Six phases of planning have been identified that should follow in this sequence: (1) collection of preliminary information, (2) establishment of priorities, (3) selection of targets and objectives, (4) consultation and coordination, (5) drafting of the plan, and (6) periodic assessment and readjustment.

Program evaluation is important if one is to know what the program has accomplished, whether the objectives have been achieved, and what the extent of the program's contribution is to the improvement of the dental health of the community. Therefore information regarding conditions that existed before the program began (baseline information) is essential.[25]

The main criteria for evaluation of dental health programs include:

1. Effectiveness: Has the stated objective been attained?
2. Efficiency: How much has the attainment of the stated objective cost, and how did that cost compare with what had been anticipated?
3. Appropriateness: Has the priority been given to the most useful strategy for the attainment of the stated objectives, and is the strategy acceptable?
4. Adequacy: Has the program covered the total health problem it was aimed at or just part of it? What are the levels of availability to the various sections of the population?

Schonfeld[71] has suggested that four levels be used to evaluate the quality of dental care programs: the first would evaluate the individual restoration, procedure, or service; the second would evaluate the mouth, that is, the relationship of one dental procedure to another; the third would consider the patient's total oral health and the influence that dental care has had on the attitude toward dentistry and on dentally related behavior; and the fourth would look at the family and community, evaluate the dental services provided for groups and communities, and determine the number of and social distribution of persons receiving adequate dental care.

A regular system of evaluation can indicate:
1. Whether the prevalence of dental disease is changing
2. Whether existing disease is being treated at a greater or lesser rate than new disease is occurring
3. If any groups in the community are not receiving the services they should be receiving
4. If providers of services are performing at acceptable levels
5. Whether preventive or educational measures being conducted are effective in reducing needs or promoting demands for treatment.[19]

DENTAL DISEASE

For better understanding of the public health impact of dental disease, one should keep in mind that dental diseases are not reversible and are not self-curing. Although preventive procedures are highly successful in reducing the major dental diseases (caries and periodontal disease), they have not been able to eliminate them. Therefore, in addition to a preventive component, a treatment component is an essential element of any dental public health program.[89]

At least three unique characteristics of the two most common dental diseases of the mouth—dental caries and periodontal disease—are important to consider: (1) They are of universal prevalence; (2) they do not undergo remission or termination if left untreated but accumulate a backlog of unmet needs; and (3) they usually require technically demanding, expensive, and time-consuming professional treatment. The importance of these characteristics is often underestimated by clinicians and nondental public health practitioners.[89]

Almost all individuals are subject to continually recurring attacks of dental disease. For this reason most people experience a periodic need for services from the time their teeth erupt. Failure to detect and treat infectious diseases has little impact on total physician labor requirements because

most of those affected either die or recover spontaneously. Dental disease, however, if left untreated, continues to develop and accumulates a backlog of needs almost always requiring surgical excising of hard or soft tissues and the replacement of diseased, defective, or missing tissues.[89]

Epidemiology of dental disease

One of the pillars upon which public health is built is the field of epidemiology, which is "the study of health of human populations." Its functions are to discover the agent, host, and environmental factors that affect health; determine the relative importance of causes of illness, disability, and death; identify groups in the population that are at the greatest risk from causes of ill health; and evaluate the effectiveness of health programs and services.[79]

Studies of the prevalence of dental disease in recent decades have placed problems of dental health in a position of major importance with regard to health needs of the nations.[35] That does not negate the success—of which the practicing community of dentists, dental hygienists, dental assistants, and dental public health practitioners can be proud—of the continued improvement in the nation's dental health status. For example, the dental health of schoolchildren has been steadily improving, as shown by a 1986-1987 National Institute for Dental Research (NIDR) national survey. The survey found that half of schoolchildren have no tooth decay, they have 36% fewer dental caries as compared with the early 1980s, and they had an average of three decayed, missing, or filled surfaces on permanent teeth as compared to five in 1980.[82]

Preliminary data from a survey on employed adults and older Americans found that "the dental health of most younger Americans is improving steadily, that employed adults are retaining their teeth at significantly higher rates than their parents, and that more people are benefiting from the services of the dental profession than ever before."[82]

The substantial decreases in the prevalence of dental caries in children could give a false impression that dental disease is no longer a major public health problem. The reality is that significant dental disease, as well as treatment needs, continues to exist. The reporting of continued improvement in oral health status has created a perception in the mind of health policymakers that all is well with oral health, thus negating the need for continued support of dental programs. Niessen[61] has referred to these numbers as dental "myths." In looking at the data indicating that 50% of children are caries-free, Niessen points to the comparative data between the 1979-1980 and 1986-1987 NIDR children's surveys that show a steady decline in caries from ages 5-17. However, half of that aggregate total is composed of caries-free children who do not have a full complement of 28 permanent teeth. In fact, Niessen shows that if only the children with a full complement of 28 teeth were examined, the percentage of caries-free children drops to 20% or less in 16- to 17-year-olds, a far cry from the 50% figure that has been publicized.[61]

So even with our successes, the magnitude of the problem that confronts dental public health is still great. For example, 84% of 17-year-olds have experienced dental decay; 41% of the population aged 65 and older and more than one quarter of those older than age 45 are edentulous; about 50% of the population experiences gingival infection at any point in time; and 30,000 new cases of oral cancer occur annually, with 8,600 individuals dying each year from that disease.[10]

ROLE OF FEDERAL AND STATE GOVERNMENT IN PUBLIC HEALTH

Although the focus in this chapter is on government-related activities, it should be clear from the previous discussion of the meaning of public and community health that neither is exclusively in the domain of government. However, the more formal public health programs and activities are generally under the aegis of government.

Although there is no constitutionally defined role for the federal government in the maintenance of public health, and such activities have traditionally been the province of the states, nonetheless, over the years there has been a continuing gradual development of a federal presence in the health field. This has come about primarily because of (1) responsibility for special population groups, such as merchant seamen, members of the armed forces, veterans, and Native Americans; (2) the constitutional power to regulate interstate commerce, from which most of the regulatory power

of the federal government in health is derived; (3) grants-in-aid to states and institutions for a wide variety of activities; and (4) sponsorship and financial participation in the payment for health services (for example, Medicaid and Medicare).[84]

Department of health and human services

The federal government's role in focusing on dental health–related concerns has been primarily within the Department of Health and Human Services (DHHS). This role has been significantly reduced in recent years from what formerly was an identifiable organizational presence to one that was found by the Interim Study Group on dental activities to be

fragmented, lacking and uncoordinated, preventing the Department of Health and Human Services from effectively carrying out its responsibilities. Most importantly, the Study Group was unable to identify within the Department either a discernible oral health policy or a mechanism whereby oral health perspectives are assured of receiving appropriate consideration in the development of health policies.[44]

An inventory of resources and activities devoted to dental and oral health completed in 1988 revealed that the oral health activities of the DHHS as well as the resources devoted to those activities "have been disaggregated, dispersed, reduced drastically, or altogether eliminated since 1972." The inventory also found that the emphasis on decentralization over the past years caused the various department programs that share the same goal of improving oral health to be severely fragmented, leading to decreased interagency communication, limited collaboration, duplication of efforts, and uncoordinated programs lacking direction or purpose. In addition, communication lines between federal and nonfederal sectors of the oral health care community, including state and local programs and other oral health organizations, have decreased.[32,44]

The inventory pointed out that it was difficult to find any central unit in DHHS that has dental health policy as its mission and that there was no discernible oral health policy. This current situation is a far cry from department activities in the 1960s and 1970s, when there was a strong, coordinated oral health focus.[32]

The DHHS budget is second only to that of the Department of Defense.[33,84] The department consists of seven primary operating agencies[1]:

1. The Public Health Service (PHS), which is under the direction of the assistant secretary of health, with the surgeon general as the principal deputy.
2. Health Care Financing Administration (HCFA)
3. Social Security Administration (SSA)
4. Health Resources and Services Administration (HRSA)
5. National Institutes of Health (NIH)
6. Agency for Toxic Substances and Disease Registry
7. Agency for Health Care Policy and Research

With the passage of the Omnibus Budget Reconciliation Act of 1989, the National Center for Health Services Research and Policy was replaced by the Agency for Health Care Policy and Research. The expectation is that this new agency will enhance the quality, appropriateness, and effectiveness of health care services and improve access to that care. Within the agency are the Offices of Planning and Resources Management, Science and Data Development, Forum for Quality and Effectiveness in Health Care, Health Technology Assessment, and the Centers for Medical Effectiveness Research, General Health Services Intramural Research, General Health Services Extramural Research, and Research Dissemination and Liaison.[1,2]

FEDERAL GOVERNMENT DENTAL ACTIVITIES

Dental activities undertaken by the federal government can be placed in two categories and are distributed among the several agencies of the department, which allocates approximately 1.25% of its budget for these activities.[33]

The first group of dental activities consists of programs that seek to improve the nation's capability to provide better oral health protection. They include biologic research, disease prevention and control, planning and development programs in dental labor, education and services research, and regulation and compliance functions such as quality assessment. These programs account for about 40% of the department's dental budget. The other

60% is assigned to the second group, which includes those programs concerned with the provision of dental services.[33]

Activities related to dental care in the PHS can be found primarily in the (1) Centers for Disease Control, in the Center for Prevention Services, and Center for Health Promotion and Education; (2) Health Resources and Services Administration, in the Bureau of Health Professions, Division of Associated and Dental Health Professions; (3) National Institutes of Health, National Institute of Dental Research (NIDR), which carries out support programs of basic and clinical dental research; and (4) Agency for Health Care Policy and Research.[1,5,30,84]

The HCFA is responsible for the Medicare and Medicaid programs, including quality and utilization control. The SSA administers the "social security" program of Old Age, Survivors, and Disability Insurance (OASDI); the program of Supplemental Security Income for the Aged, Blind, and Disabled (SSI); and the federal-state public assistance program of Aid to Families with Dependent Children (AFDC). The Office of Human Development Services (HDS) contains the Administration on Aging, the Administration on Developmental Disabilities, the Administration for Native Americans, and the Administration for Children, Youth, and Families, which oversees the Head Start program with its important dental component.[84]

The PHS provides dental services to specific groups of beneficiaries, with the care usually, but not always, provided by members of the PHS Commissioned Dental Corps. One of the direct care programs is the care provided to the Alaskan Natives and American Indians through the Indian Health Service.[33] Other beneficiaries of dental care by PHS commissioned officers are prisoners in federal penitentiaries, personnel of the Coast Guard, and personnel of the U.S. Merchant Marines. These direct service programs are based on federal responsibility resulting either from treaties, as with the Native Americans, or from historical commitments.[33]

Funding for dental activities

Fiscal year 1988. The total fiscal year (FY) 1988 expenditures for federally funded dental activities was $579,824,835, of which $256,573,835

was for programs of the PHS. Approximate allocations by type of PHS program are 52% or $135 million for dental research–related activities, 42% for direct provision of dental services, 4% for education and training–related activities, and 2% for technical assistance and support activities.[32] Table 1-1 shows the distribution of DHHS dental expenditures by agency. For a detailed analysis of federal expenditures, see Ginsburg and Schmidt.[32]

Healthy People 2000. *Healthy People 2000* is a publication of the DHHS. It lists 297 different health objectives to be achieved by the year 2000. Among these are 16 oral health objectives, which address reductions in dental caries, periodontal disease, oral cancer, and dental trauma from accidents, as well as improvement in use of oral health services, dental sealants, and fluorides.[13]

Healthy People 2000 follows the previously published 1979 *Healthy People,* which established goals and objectives for 1990. *Healthy People 2000* has been developed hand in hand with the revision of *Healthy Communities 2000: Model Standards,* the workbook for applying the objectives in *Healthy People* to individual community needs.[55]

Nursing homes

With the passage of the Omnibus Budget Reconciliation Act of 1990, new regulations were developed regarding dental care for nursing home residents. To participate in either Medicare or Medicaid, *skilled nursing facilities,* a term for Medicare participating nursing homes (serving people 65 and over), and *nursing facilities,* the new term for nursing homes under Medicaid, must provide or obtain dental care from outside resources for their residents. If qualified personnel are not available on site, the nursing home must have a written agreement with an outside provider stating that the nursing home assumes responsibility that the dental services meet professional standards. Coverage must be for emergency and routine dental services.[52]

Maternal and child health services. Since 1935, state health services for women of childbearing age and children to age 21 have been provided federal support through Title V of the Social Security Act. The Maternal and Child Health (MCH) program was responsible for extending and improving health care services for mothers and children through formula grants to state maternal and child health agencies. The grants supported the following activities with dental components: (1) Maternity and Infant Care Projects, (2) Children and Youth Projects, (3) Dental Health Projects for Children, and (4) Crippled Children Services.[39]

The Maternity and Infant Care Projects, through grants to projects serving particular target populations or to areas identifying high-risk mothers, provided necessary health care for prospective mothers and for infants in their first year of life. Emergency dental services were provided at all centers, but only a few offered comprehensive dental care.[37] By 1972 the Children and Youth Projects, started in 1966, provided comprehensive care to about 500,000 children in low-income areas. A program of preventive dental health services, and dental care was an essential component of comprehensive child health services, and its inclusion was a statutory requirement.[36]

Table 1-1 Fiscal year 1988 Department of Health and Human Services dental expenditures

Agency	Percentage of total	Amount ($)
Health Care Financing Administration	54	312,351,000
National Institutes of Health	23	133,418,090
Health Resources and Services Administration	12	68,611,961
Indian Health Service	8	47,900,705
Head Start	2	10,900,000
Other Public Health Service	1	6,643,079
TOTAL	100	$579,824,835

From Ginsburg S and Schmidt RE: An inventory of resources and activities devoted to dental and oral health in the Department of Health and Human Services, Bethesda, MD, 1989, Richard Schmidt Associated Ltd, pp. 1-6B.

The Child Health Act of 1967 authorized Special Project Grants for Dental Health of Children in essentially low-income areas for school and preschool children. The projects were first funded in 1971, when seven grants were made. By the end of 1974, 19 projects were in operation. By July 1, 1975, each state's maternal and child health plan had to include at least one of the following projects: maternal and infant care, children and youth, family planning, or dental care.[37]

A major shift in U.S. health policy occurred with the passage of the Omnibus Budget Reconciliation Act of 1981, which included the Maternal and Child Health Block Grant Act. The amendments consolidated seven grant programs from Title V of the Social Security Act and from the Public Health Service Act into a block grant under a new Title V: Maternal and Child Health Services Block Grant. The consolidated programs are the maternal and child health and crippled children programs, genetic disease research, adolescent pregnancy services, sudden infant death syndrome research, hemophilia research, Supplemental Security Income payments to crippled children, and lead-based poisoning research. Dental health is no longer a separate mandatory program under Title V.[81,84]

It is not yet clear what the impact of this major change in maternal and child health policy will be, but to date total funding is not yet back to the levels before block grants, and in many states cuts have resulted in the closing of maternal and child health clinics. At the same time, increased applications for services, because of loss of insurance coverage as a result of unemployment, has increased the need.[34,84]

The Reagan administration's philosophy of turning social programs back to the states has caused the loss of needed services with the substitution of block grants for categorical grants. When funds are lumped together to be used at a state's discretion, dentistry is likely to suffer and, in fact, appears to be doing so now. The immediate future for traditional public health programs does not look optimistic, although philosophies may well change when large numbers of people are shown to be unable to get needed care.[20] Thus the Maternal and Child Health Block Grant program suffered from dramatic funding cuts in the early 1980s, was subject to across-the-board cuts, and was open to each state's discretion regarding the allocation of funds for specific priorities within the MCH programs. Although some improvement has more recently occurred in overall MCH funding, the oral health component has not benefited. In fact, little emphasis has been placed on oral health.[46]

It is difficult to provide an accurate figure for the number of public dollars allocated for oral health programs for the maternal and child health population because of the number and diversity of programs and the various levels of government and jurisdictions involved, as well as a lack of accurate reporting.[46]

What was previously called Crippled Children Services and is now Children with Special Health Care Needs provides funds that enable states to offer medical, surgical, corrective, and additional services and care to children who are handicapped or who are suffering from conditions that lead to handicapping.[22a] Children may be defined as handicapped because of a dental disability or disfiguring condition, for example, cleft lip, cleft palate, or other oral disfigurement.[75] Unfortunately, public financing for the dental care of those with other handicapping conditions, such as cerebral palsy and mental retardation, has not been readily available. Although some states do have reasonable programs for the treatment of children with handicapping conditions, few have any kind of financing available for the treatment of these persons when they become adults.[20] Minnesota, among the first states to recognize the term *crippled children* as anachronistic and unacceptable, led the way by changing the name of its program to Services for Children with Handicaps.[56] The federal government later adopted its new name and philosophy of family-centered, community-based, coordinated care.

Community and migrant health centers. The Community Health Center program, as authorized by Section 330 of the Public Health Service Act, provides grants to support the planning, development, and operation of primary care projects in rural and urban underserved areas.

The Migrant Centers Program is intended to provide comprehensive primary care for migratory farm workers and their families. There are approximately 600 community and migrant health centers with approximately only half providing dental services.[32,46]

Head Start. In 1965 Head Start programs were launched by the Office of Economic Opportunity under the provisions of the Economic Opportunity Act of 1964 to provide educational health and social services to preschool children of the needy so that the children would enter school on an equal basis with their more affluent peers. Each Head Start program is required to provide dental services to enrolled children.[80] Total basic dental services for every enrolled child is the objective of the program, but available funds and lack of dental personnel have been constraints.[22,65]

There is evidence that Head Start early education programs are effective. It was demonstrated in Michigan that children who were assigned to an experimental early education group for 1 year maintained remarkable gains over the control group for 15 years, with half the number of arrests, school dropouts, and teenage pregnancies.[34] In another follow-up, a 20-year longitudinal study of former Head Start children, it was found that they had a higher employment rate, performed better in school, and rated higher in terms of self-esteem and sense of control of their lives than did control children of similar disadvantaged backgrounds who did not attend Head Start programs.[47]

Head Start has been one of the few federal programs to receive increased funding. For FY 1991, $1.95 billion was appropriated for Head Start, an increase of $399 million. However, the additional money is still not enough to accomplish the administration's goals of boosting overall enrollment and maintaining the quality of programs.[77] The increase proposed for 1992 barely covered inflation and allowed the program to reach only one third of eligible children. The Children's Defense Fund also has claimed that it will take nearly 180 years for Head Start to reach all eligible children. The Children's Defense Fund also determined that a dollar spent on Head Start saves nearly five times that amount in future social costs.[78]

In 1989 approximately 454,000 children were served by 1,200 grantees with an estimated dental services budget of $10,900,000 for children not enrolled in Medicaid or other reimbursement programs.[32]

Medicaid and Early Periodic Screening, Diagnosis, and Treatment (EPSDT). Medicaid (Title XIX of the Social Security Act) was authorized by the Social Security Amendments of 1965 to provide medical assistance to specified groups of needy people. Dental care is an optional benefit under Medicaid.[80] It is mandated under the EPSDT portion of Medicaid that covers children, but this program has never been enforced.[20]

Since 1973 the EPSDT program has been more or less operational in all states with Medicaid programs. It offers all Medicaid beneficiaries under 21 years of age the services in its title: a periodic screening for health defects, followed by any necessary diagnosis and treatment.[33,76] The EPSDT program was slow to get off the ground, and in 1975 only 4% of the 13 million needy children that it was intended to benefit had actually been screened, let alone treated. Children in the EPSDT age group who were eligible for the program appeared to have a more urgent need for dental care than for medical care. Treated children in the middle 1970s required an average of $90 per child for dental care compared with $35 per child for medical care.[20] Unfortunately, funds have not been available recently to provide the treatment needed for eligible children. All Medicaid programs are required to provide an EPSDT program to receive federal funds, and dental services are mandated for persons under age 21. Under the EPSDT program, state or local agencies must screen all eligible children under age 21, assess the need for health services, and refer those in need to follow-up treatment.[33,76] As part of the Medicaid program, one of the largest sources of funding for health care of poor children, EPSDT has had limited success in many states. Many children are not covered, and there has often been a separation of the diagnostic from the therapeutic, resulting in low rates of flow-through from screening to treatment of conditions found during screening. An amendment to EPSDT regulations added in 1983 now encourages continuity of care by allowing EPSDT money to be used for payment for treatment as well as screening when an eligible child is under the care of private health care providers or a health center.[34]

EPSDT, which was heralded in 1967 as the most

important legislation for low-income children, has resulted in only 31% of eligible children being screened and only 13% of those over 5 years of age having been screened. Many states fail to cover under their Medicaid programs all the services needed to achieve full use of the program.

Amendments to Title XIX of the Social Security Act (Medicaid) passed by the 101st Congress through the passage of the Omnibus Reconciliation Act of 1989 (OBRA 89), which went into effect in April 1990, include sweeping changes in EPSDT. OBRA 89 raised the eligibility level for Medicaid coverage from 100% to 133% of the federal poverty line for pregnant women, infants, and children under age 6. This means more women and children are eligible for Medicaid. Also, reimbursement rates to providers must be sufficient to enlist enough of them to participate in the Medicaid program. For EPSDT the law now requires states to provide any medically necessary allowable follow-up service, even if not covered under the state plan. For example, dental sealants should now be provided in the 28 states that have not allowed their provision under their state Medicaid programs.[40]

Additional Medicaid amendments were passed within the Omnibus Budget Reconciliation Act of 1990 (OBRA 90). States no longer have the option of discontinuing a pregnant woman's eligibility for Medicaid through her pregnancy, even if her income increases and she would have been no longer eligible for that program. A similar provision applies to infants under age 1. Congress also expanded the number of poor children covered under Medicaid.[59] OBRA 90 requires that, by the year 2002, Medicaid coverage is mandated for children age 18 and under in families earning up to 100% of the federal poverty level.[41]

Many states offer only a limited number of oral health services through their Medicaid programs, and only about one third of Medicaid-eligible persons receive dental care under the program. Less than half of private-practice dentists report treating Medicaid or other government-assisted patients.[62]

Medicaid spending for dental services declined nearly 40% from 1979 to 1986, at the same time that spending in most other health care categories increased.[23] Medicaid spends less than 1% of its payments on dental care.[18]

In 1987, 23.1 million persons were estimated to be recipients of Medicaid services, with 5.1 million receiving oral health care. About half the Medicaid recipients are children. Fewer than half of an estimated 33 million Americans with poverty-level incomes are enrolled in Medicaid and of these users of Medicaid, only one third are users of dental services. Medicaid dental benefits are not available to adults in eight states and the District of Columbia, and many other states provide only emergency care for adults. In 1981, payments of $543 million were made for 5,173,000 dental Medicaid recipients. In 1987, $541 million was spent for 5,120,000 recipients, the largest percentage loss in any Medicaid service category. Payments for dental services under the Medicaid program have progressively been representing a smaller percentage of total Medicaid expenditures, as well as of total national dental expenditures. Another problem with the Medicaid program has been the low rates of reimbursement to providers, which has discouraged many dentists from accepting Medicaid patients.[68]

The Medicaid program cost the federal government approximately $65 billion in FY 1992, up from $49 billion in FY 1991. In the last 4 years there has been a steady increase in the number of people using the program: from 22 million to 28 million.[40]

Medicare. Medicare (Title XVIII of the Social Security Act) was authorized by the Social Security Amendments of 1965 and covers persons aged 65 and over and certain disabled persons. Its purpose is to provide insurance protection against the costs of health care.

Part 1 of Medicare is a basic plan for hospital and related care. Payment to dentists for routine dental services is specifically excluded. Services by dental interns or residents in training, where services are ordinarily furnished by a hospital to its inpatients, are covered. The dental coverage of Medicare is limited to those services requiring hospitalization, usually for surgical treatment for fractures and cancer, and thus constitutes a negligible proportion of the program.[11,20]

Part 2 is a voluntary supplementary plan for

physicians' services and other medical and health services. Routine dental care is not covered, and dental procedures are specifically excluded. The need for dental care is great for the population over 65 years of age, and the ability to pay for those services is greatly diminished at that age level. Medicare does virtually nothing to help the elderly with their dental health problems.[21]

In regard to having dental care covered under Medicare, the ADA has argued before Congress the necessity of a supplemental dental benefits program under Medicare because there are fundamental barriers to dental services for this population. In its testimony the ADA said, "By the end of this decade our population will have increased by one-third over what it was when Medicare started. That population will live longer and increasingly be in need of health services. It is time the public at large faced this fact and supported an effective initiative to meet the needs of our citizens."[7,48]

Medicare expenditures for dental services in 1984 were $7.2 million, an increase of $600,000 from the previous year.[32]

National Health Service Corps. The National Health Service Corps (NHSC) is a federal health labor deployment program established by Public Law 91-623, the Emergency Health Personnel Act of 1970. It authorizes the assignment of commissioned officers and civil service personnel of the PHS to areas where health services are inadequate because of critical shortages of health personnel. Physicians, dentists, and nurses, as well as supporting health personnel, may be assigned for 2 years to critical shortage areas designated by the secretary of Health and Human Services.[60] In 1974 the corps had 551 health professionals in 268 communities: 325 physicians, 80 dentists, and the balance were physician assistants, nurse practitioners, and other types of physician extenders. In 1977 there were 97 dentists.[54] In 1986 a total of 1,109 health practitioners, whose training was supported by NHSC scholarships, were assigned to shortage areas in all 50 states and several other U.S. jurisdictions. Of this number 1,068 were physicians and 24 were dentists. This 1986 total marks a decrease in the placement figure that peaked at 1,440 in 1985. The decrease reflects a reduction in the number of scholarships awarded in recent years.[12]

NHSC 1988 expenditures for dentistry were about 10% of the total NHSC dollars or $5.2 million. This represents a yearly decrease in program funds and in dental activity. There is also a loan program associated with placement of health providers, but no support for dentistry was provided in 1988.[32]

The Bureau of Health Professions defines and designates health personnel shortage areas that are eligible for assignment of NHSC personnel.[84] Except in unusual cases, state and district dental societies must certify the area's need for a dentist. Patients pay prevailing prices, and the dentist is encouraged to stay in the community once the tour of duty is over. Some states have been looking at the problem of labor distribution and are trying to find their own solutions. Some local dental societies have chosen to argue against federal involvement at the expense of the dental needs of the community and the public image of the dental profession.[33]

Veterans Administration. The Veterans Administration (VA) was established as an independent agency in 1930 for the purpose of consolidating and coordinating federal agencies created for or concerned with administration of laws providing benefits to veterans. In March 1989 legislation elevated the VA to cabinet-level status as the Department of Veterans' Affairs.[63]

The difference between the Department of Defense (DOD) and the VA is that the DOD primarily serves current and retired members of the armed forces, whereas the VA serves those with some service-connected disability who have honorably left the service.[84]

The VA provides some dental care to eligible patients through its system of hospitals and absorbed 12% of all public expenditures for dental care in 1977. In 1980 the VA spent $6.2 billion on medical care.[20] In 1990 $12.6 billion was spent on medical care, with $138 million of that amount expended on dental care.[24,28]

ACTIVITIES OF STATE PUBLIC HEALTH AGENCIES

Of the 50 state health departments, plus the District of Columbia, American Samoa, Guam, Puerto Rico, Trust Territory, and the Virgin Islands, the following states or locations had no reported dental budget: Alaska, Connecticut, Maryland,

Mississippi, Nevada, North Dakota, South Dakota, Wisconsin, Trust Territory, and the Virgin Islands. The remainder of the states reported a total of $54,390,000 expended on dentally related activities. Twenty-five states and the District of Columbia reported having spent a portion of the Maternal and Child Health Services Block Grant on dentally related services. Twenty-five states reported expending a portion of their Prevention Block Grant on dentally related services. Few state health agencies reported expending more than a limited portion of their budget on dentally related services.[66]

USE AND DELIVERY OF DENTAL SERVICES

Several important distinctions, especially in regard to dental care, exist among the need for care, the demand for care, and the actual use of services. A dental need is considered to exist when an individual has dental disease, although the patient may not perceive this need. A demand for care exists when an individual believes there is a need for care and is able to translate that need into actively presenting for care. Sheiham[73] believes that a demand for care exists when the individual perceives a need and wishes to receive care, although that person may not actually use the service. Use occurs only when the individual actually receives care.[73] Sheiham's concept considers that one may perceive a need, may desire that the need be treated, and then, in an attempt to make a demand upon the delivery system, find the system unable or unwilling to provide treatment. For example, the individual may not be able to afford care, there may not be an available source of care, or the source might not accept the individual for care.

As stated previously, a major concern of public health is the issue of access to care and the fact that access to health services is not equitably distributed among population groups in this country. This has been especially true in regard to the delivery of dental services. Access to even basic medical and dental care for all our citizens is still not a reality. The uneven distribution of health services hits the poor and minorities hardest, with substantial numbers of underserved people "who are different ethnically from the controlling group." The United States, along with South Af-

rica, is still the only developed country with no national policy ensuring that all citizens have access to health care. The term *rationing* has recently come into usage in regard to limiting the distribution and allocation of health services. When individuals or population groups do not get the care that is needed, in that there is currently no official policy to ration care the term *de facto rationing* is being used to describe situations in which care is denied or not provided because of economic or social factors that are brought about by the nature of our health care system.[53] Whereas the term rationing has to date been applied primarily to medical services, it should not be long before it begins appearing in the dentally related literature.

Forms of dental health services

Historically, dental health services in the United States have been classified into three groups:

1. Services provided by dentists and dental auxiliaries and financed by the patient or a source other than the government
2. Services provided by nongovernment dentists and dental auxiliaries partly or entirely remunerated by the government
3. Services provided by dentists and dental auxiliaries employed by the government, such as military personnel

The prevailing philosophy in the United States continues to place the prime responsibility for health and the acquisition of health services on the individual and not on society, even though there has been increased involvement for payment by the federal, state, and local governments. In the 1940s the ADA established the Council on Dental Health. One of the fundamental principles formulated by a Council subcommittee was that the responsibility for the health of the people of the United States is first that of the individual, then the community, then the state, and lastly the nation.[85] This attitude that the individual has the first responsibility contrasts with an attitude in European countries that suggests that society as a whole is responsible. By the 1970s national state-operated social programs were the norm in Europe. It has been suggested that the catastrophic events that befell Europe, primarily the effects of two wars in the first half of the twentieth century, hastened the development of social welfare programs in European countries. The United States, it must be remembered, largely escaped the physical and social devastation of those wars.[20,83]

Use of dental services

Although the National Health Interview Survey conducted by the National Center for Health Statistics showed an increase in the use of dental services between 1964 and 1986, there are still significant numbers of people who do not use dental services. Forty-two percent of the population had visited a dentist in 1964, whereas in 1986 55% had visited a dentist, certainly a welcome increase but still leaving almost half the population without a yearly dental visit. The percentage of the population who had never visited a dentist was decreased from 16.6% to 10.1%. That is certainly an improvement, but still 10% of the population has never visited a dentist.[32]

An important fact to keep in mind is that the use of dental services is not evenly distributed among population groupings. Whereas 40% of Caucasians had never visited a dentist, 56% of African-Americans and 60% of Mexican-Americans had never visited a dentist. Of the 130 million people without dental insurance, 50% did not visit a dentist. Of the 32 million people in this country in families with incomes below $10,000, 59% had not visited a dentist.[82]

So, despite improvements that have been made, this country is far from meeting the dental needs of its citizens. Unlike general medical services, which are heavily supported by government and insurance funds, "dental services are funded primarily on an out-of-pocket basis with the result that dental care has not been available for many segments of the population."[82]

Expenditures for dental care

Health care spending has continued to command a larger proportion of the nation's resources, rising from 5.3% of the gross national product in 1960 to 11.6% in 1989.[49] This accelerated spending on health care has produced what many are calling a health care crisis. If the overall economy had continued to increase at previous rates, the increase in health services spending would not look as significant as it now does, but between the multibillion dollar deficit and the weakened economy, what has actually been a real increase in health

care spending has become a problem of major concern. Expenditures for dental services exhibited the slowest growth among all of the personal health care categories between 1988 and 1989, 6.7%, as compared with 10% for hospitals and 11.9% for physicians. Total health expenditures in 1989 rose to $604.1 billion. As mentioned previously, a major reason for an increasing interest in the cost of health care, especially on the part of government, is that the government-financed portions of the expended health care dollar has greatly increased between 1960 (24.5%) and 1989 (41.9%). In 1985, United States citizens spent $425 billion on health care, including $27.1 billion for dentists' services. Private-sector payments accounted for all but $600 million of dental expenditures. Patients paid $17.2 billion directly to dentists, with private insurance paying for $9.3 billion worth of dental care. Of the $600 million spent by the federal, state, and local governments for dental care, approximately $500 million was spent on Medicaid, and the rest was spent on dental care in community and migrant health centers and other programs.[49] The estimated $500 million spent on Medicaid dental services in 1984 represented less than 2% of the $39.8 billion spent by Medicaid on health care for needy persons.[9,14] In 1976, of the total amount of $8.6 billion dollars spent for dental care in the United States, the government spent $469 million, or 5%.[31] In 1985 the $600 million governmental agencies spent on dental care was 2.2% of the total dental expenditures, a percentage that has been decreasing from 5.6% in 1975 to 2.9% in 1982.[9,14] The actual drop in 1989 was down to 2%,[49] and it has been projected that by the year 2000, government expenditures for dental services will decrease to 1.5%.[82]

In 1989, expenditures for dental services were $31.4 billion. Most of the financing for dental care, as in previous years, came from private sources, with 54.9% coming from out-of-pocket or personal payments, 42.7% from private health insurance, and only 2.4% from public spending. Medicare and Medicaid paid for more than one fourth of health expenditures. Increases in government revenue have not kept up with increases in government spending for health.[66]

It is clear that public support for dental health care has been limited to (1) direct services for selected beneficiaries (for example, military personnel), residents of dental shortage areas, and Native Americans; (2) dental research; (3) grants for services to special populations (for example, programs for low-income pregnant women, Services for Children with Handicaps, and Head Start programs); and (4) payment for services for certain low-income populations, such as Medicaid.

CODA

Harold Hillenbrand, former executive director of the ADA, stated in 1977[42]:

The United States is the only industrially developed country in the world without a coherent, identifiable national health program and has only now reached the stage of making a statement of intent . . . the delivery of dental health care is not now, if it ever was, solely a problem for the dental profession. Real solutions must be found in the unselfish collaboration of dentists, the other health professions, the dental auxiliaries, social and behavioral scientists, epidemiologists, educators, statisticians, government and public health officials, consumers, and a whole host of others. There are enough problems to challenge and plague us all.[42]

Since then, little has changed, and Hillenbrand's words are as appropriate in 1993 as they were in 1977. There is still much for dental professionals and dental public health to accomplish to meet the dental needs of the people in the United States, and "enough problems to challenge and plague us all."

Waldman and Niessen, as previously mentioned, point out that during the 1980s much of what appeared in the public media about dentistry focused on the improvement in oral health, the increase in access to care, and the improved ratio of dentists to patients.[61,82] As a result of this "positive" coverage, the perception on the part of state and national policymakers has been that all is well with dental health and there is no longer a need to expend public dollars on dentally related programs. Although the dental profession can be proud of the progress that has been made, there is still a long way to go before the oral health status of U.S. citizens is at an acceptable level. As an analogy, one could think of someone who has received a 50% increase in salary from $4 to $6 per hour. That would certainly be a significant increase, but trying to support a family in the United States in 1993 on $6 per hour is virtually impossible. The fact that the percentage of caries-free children increased by more than 10 percentage

points between 1979 and 1986—from 36.6% to 49.9%—still leaves more than 50% of the population not caries-free.[61] To help ensure that dental health receives a fair share of third-party and public funds, a continued emphasis on, as newscaster Paul Harvey says, "the rest of the story" is necessary. Once a perception becomes planted in the public mind, it is difficult to change. Although there have been major accomplishments in dental public health, there is still much to be done and much to be publicized before the goal of dental health for all can be in sight.[82]

REFERENCES

1. Agency For Health Care Policy and Research (1): *AHCPR purpose and programs*. Public Health Service No OM90-0096, Rockville, Md, 1990, United States Department of Health and Human Services.
2. Agency for Health Care Policy and Research (2): *Omnibus budget reconciliation act of 1989—section 6103* (PL 101-239). Public Health Service No. OM90-0084, Rockville, Md, 1990, United States Department of Health and Human Services.
3. American Board of Dental Public Health: *Guidelines for graduate education in dental public health,* Ann Arbor, Mich, 1970, American Board of Dental Public Health.
4. American Board of Dental Public Health: Competency objectives for dental public health, *J Public Health Dent* 50:338, 1990.
5. American Dental Association: No denture care coverage in 24 states, *ADA News* 10(13):7, 1979.
6. American Dental Association: *Strategic plan report of the American Dental Association's special committee on the future of dentistry: issue papers on dental research, manpower education, practice and public and professional concerns,* Chicago, 1983, American Dental Association.
7. American Dental Association: ADA argues for Medicare dental plan, adult care under Medicaid termed "inadequate," *ADA News* 17(16):2 1986.
8. American Dental Association: Committee ok's $116.3 million for NIDR, *ADA News* 17(5):1, 1986.
9. American Dental Association: U.S. dental spending reaches $27.1 billion, *ADA News* 17(17):11, 1986.
10. American Dental Association: *Oral health facts and indicators of oral health problems in the U.S.,* Chicago, 1989, American Dental Association.
11. American Dental Association: Medicare to include oral surgery, *ADA News* (June 4, 1990) p. 1.
12. American Medical Association: 1,109 NHSC aided practitioners placed in U.S. shortage areas, *Am Med News* 29(36):14, 1986.
13. American Public Health Association, Professional Affairs Division: *Summary of Healthy people 2000,* Washington, DC, American Public Health Association.
14. Arnett RH and others: Projections of health care spending to 1990, *Health Care Financing Rev* 7(3):1, 1986.
15. Association of State and Territorial Health Officials Foun-

dation: *Public health agencies 1980, A report on their expenditures and activities,* Pub No 61, Washington, DC, 1981, Association of State and Territorial Health Officials.

16. Association of State and Territorial Health Officials Foundation: *Public health agencies 1983, vol 2, Services and activities,* Pub No 80, Washington, DC, 1985, Association of State and Territorial Health Officials.

17. Association of State and Territorial Health Officials Foundation: *Public health agencies 1983, vol 4, An inventory of programs and block grants,* Pub No 82, Washington, DC, 1985, Association of State and Territorial Health Officials.

18. Bonner P: Medicaid—a program under fire, *Dentistry Today,* December 1990, p 19.

19. Burt BA: *Administration of public dental treatment programs.* In Slack GL, editor: *Dental public health,* Bristol, Eng, 1974, John Wright and Sons.

20. Burt BA: *Financing for dental care services.* In Striffler DF, Young WO, Burt BA, editors: *Dentistry, dental practice and the community,* ed 3, Philadelphia, 1983, WB Saunders.

21. Campbell EM, Hayden CH, Van Burskirk H: *Summaries of recent legislation affecting dentistry,* Bethesda, Md, 1968, Public Health Service, Division of Dental Health.

22. Clark JP, Goforth V: *Organizing dental programs for Head Start preschool groups,* Washington, DC, US Department of Health, Education and Welfare, Office of Child Development.

22a. Consolidated omnibus budget reconciliation of act 1985, PL 99-272, April 7, 1986, *US statutes at large,* vol 100, pp 82-93.

23. Dentistry Today: Medicaid spending has dropped 40%, *Dentistry Today,* June/July 1989, p 20.

24. Deputy Assistant Secretary for Planning and Management Analysis: *Geographic distribution of VA expenditures fiscal year 1990 state, county, and congressional district.* Washington, DC, 1991, Department of Veterans' Affairs.

25. Dunning JM: A word of warning in incremental dental care, *NYJ Dent* 38:56, 1968.

26. Dunning JM: *Dental needs, resources, and objectives.* In Dunning JM, editor: *Principles of dental public health,* ed 2, Cambridge, Mass, 1970, Harvard University Press.

27. Editorial, *J Public Health Policy* 6(4):435, 1985.

28. Floyd, D, Director of Dental Policy and Planning, Department of Veterans Affairs, Washington, DC: Personal communication, July 10, 1991.

29. Foege W: On AMA's interest in public health, *Am Med News* 29(36):4, 1986.

30. *Forward plan for health, FY 1977-1981,* DHEW Pub No (05) 76-50024, Washington, DC, 1975, US Department of Health, Education and Welfare.

31. Gibson RM, Mueller MS: National health expenditures, FY 1976, *Soc Secur Bull* 40(3):22, 1977.

32. Ginsburg S, Schmidt RE: *An inventory of resources and activities devoted to dental and oral health in the Department of Health and Human Services,* Bethesda, Md, 1989, Richard Schmidt Associated Ltd.

33. Greene JC: Federal programs and the profession, *J Am Dent Assoc* 92:689, 1976.

34. Haggerty RJ, Darney PD: *Maternal and child health services.* In Last JM, editor: *Maxcy-Rosenau public health and preventive medicine,* Norwalk, Conn, 1986, Appleton-Century-Crofts.

35. Hanlon JJ, Pickett GE: *Public health administration and practice,* ed 8, St Louis, 1984, Mosby–Year Book.

36. Health Services Administration: *The children and young projects,* DHEW Pub No (HSM) 72-5006, Washington, DC, 1972, Public Health Service.

37. Health Services Administration: *The maternity and infant care projects,* DHEW Pub No (HSM) 75-5012, Washington, DC, 1975, Public Health Service.

38. Reference deleted in proofs.

39. Health Services Administration: *Promoting community health,* DHEW Pub No (HSA) 77-5000, Washington, DC, 1976, Public Health Service.

40. Hilts P: U.S. to study big rise in Medicaid costs, *New York Times,* p A15, May 1, 1991.

41. Holahan J, Zedlewski S: Expanding Medicaid to cover insured Americans, *Health Aff (Millwood),* Spring 1991, pp 45-61.

42. Ingle J, Blair P, editors: *International dental care delivery systems,* Cambridge, Mass, 1978, Ballinger.

43. Institute of Medicine Committee for the Study of the Future of Public Health, Division of Health Care Services: *A vision of public health in America: an attainable ideal.* In *The future of public health,* Washington, DC, 1988, National Academy Press.

44. Interim Study Group on Dental Activities: *Improving the oral health of the American people opportunity for action: a study of the oral health activities of the Department of Health and Human Services,* Rockville, Md, 1989, Department of Health and Human Services.

45. Jack SS: *Use of dental services: United States, 1983,* Charlottesville, Va, 1986, Medical Benefits.

46. Johnson K, Siegal M: Resources for improving the oral health of maternal and child populations, *J Public Health Dent* 50:418, 1990.

47. Jordheim AE: Welfare kids: outlook bleak, *Med Tribune* 27:3, 1986.

48. Knutson JW: *What is public health?* In Pelton WJ, Wisan JM, editors: *Dentistry in public health,* ed 2, Philadelphia, 1955, WB Saunders.

49. Lazenby HC, Letsch S: National health expenditures 1989, *Health Care Financing Rev* 12(2):1, 1990.

50. Leske GS and others: *Dental public health.* In Last JM, editor: *Maxcy-Rosenau public health and preventive medicine,* Norwalk, Conn, 1986, Appleton-Century-Crofts.

51. Levit K and others: National health care spending 1989, *Health Aff (Millwood)* Spring 1991, pp 116-130.

52. Litch S: Medicare and Medicaid dental requirements for nursing homes, Washington, DC, 1990, American Association of Dental Schools.

53. Lundberg GD: National health care reform: an aura of inevitability is upon us, *JAMA* 265:2566, 1991.

54. Manpower Analysis Branch, Division of Dentistry: *Dental manpower fact sheet,* Bethesda, Md, 1977, Public Health Service.

55. McGinnis MJ: Healthy people: public health macroview 3:4, Washington, DC, 1990, Public Health Foundation.

56. Minnesota Department of Health: *Services for children*

with handicaps, SCH-706, Minneapolis, 1984, Minnesota Department of Health.

57. National Caries Program, National Institute of Dental Research: *The prevalence of dental caries in United States children, 1979-80.* NIH Pub No 82-2245, 1981, US Department of Health and Human Services.

58. National Center for Health Statistics: *Decayed, missing and filled teeth among persons 1-74 years, United States,* Pub No (PHS) 81-1673, 1981, US Department of Health and Human Services.

59. National Health Law Program: *The omnibus budget reconciliation act of 1990: an analysis of health related provisions, Health Advocate* (Los Angeles) 167:1, 1991.

60. National Health Service Corps rules and regulations, *Federal Register* 40:34080, 1975.

61. Niessen L: Some myths in dentistry and their implications for public health, Communique. *American Association of Public Health Dentistry* 8(3):1, 1989.

62. Office of Disease Prevention and Health Promotion: *Oral diseases in adults: a prevalent problem. Prevention report,* Washington, DC, 1990, Department of Health and Human Services, Public Health Service.

63. Office of Inspector General: *Inspector General semiannual report Oct 1, 1989-March 31, 1990,* No RC550-0568, Washington, DC, 1990, Department of Veteran Affairs.

64. Pickett G, Hanlon JJ: *Philosophy and purpose of public health. In Public health administration and practice,* ed 9, St Louis, 1990, Mosby–Year Book.

65. *Project Head Start dental services,* Washington, DC, US Department of Health, Education and Welfare, Office of Child Development.

66. Public Health Foundation: *Public health agencies 1990: an inventory of programs and block grant expenditures,* Washington DC, 1990, Public Health Foundation.

67. *The Random House College Dictionary,* rev ed, New York, 1988, Random House.

68. Rozier GR: New opportunities for dental public health, Communique. *American Association of Public Health Dentistry,* Richmond, Va, 9(3):1, 1990.

69. Rozier GR: Proceedings: workshop to develop competency objectives in dental public health, *J Public Health Dent* 50:330, 1990.

70. Schoen MH, Freed JR: Prevention of dental disease, *Annu Rev Public Health* 2:71, 1981.

71. Schonfeld HK: Peer review of quality of dental care, *J Am Dent Assoc* 79:1376, 1969.

72. *Services, expenditures, and programs of state and territorial health agencies, 1974,* Washington, DC, 1976, Association of State and Territorial Health Officials, Health Program Reporting System.

73. Sheiham A: *Planning for manpower requirements in dental public health.* In Slack GL, editor: *Dental public health,* Bristol, Eng, 1974, John Wright and Sons.

74. Sheps CG: *Higher education for public health: progress and potential,* Delta Omega lecture, New Orleans, October 22, 1974.

75. Smith DC: *Organization of maternal and child health services.* In Wallace H and others, editors: *Maternal and child health practices, problems, resources, and methods of delivery,* Springfield, IL, 1973, Charles C Thomas.

76. *Social and rehabilitative statistics from Medicaid statistics, FY 1976,* DHEW Pub No SRS077-03154, Washington, DC, 1977, US Department of Health, Education and Welfare.

77. *Star Tribune:* Some fear Bush goal to extend Head Start's reach stretches too far, Minneapolis, April 28, 1991, p 21A.

78. *Star Tribune:* Full funding for Head Start (editorial), Minneapolis, May 15, 1991, p 16A.

79. Terris M: Epidemiology and the public health movement, *J Public Health Policy* 8(3):315, 1987.

80. US Department of Health and Human Services: *Head Start program performance standards* (45-CFR-1304), DHHS Pub No (OHDS) 84-31131, Washington, DC, 1984.

81. US House of Representatives: *Opportunities for success: cost-effective programs for children,* staff report of the Select Committee on Children, Youth, and Families, Washington, DC, 1985, US Government Printing Office.

82. Waldman HB: The future of dentistry: we need to tell the whole story, *J Am Coll Dent* 57:46, 1990.

83. Willcocks AJ: *Dental health and the changing society.* In Slack GL, editor: *Dental public health,* Bristol, Eng, 1981, John Wright and Sons.

84. Wilson FA, Neuhauser D: *Health services in the United States,* ed 2, Cambridge, Mass, 1985, Ballinger.

85. Wilson WA: The future role of government in dental practice and education, *J Am Coll Dent* 40:111, 1973.

86. Winslow CEA: The untilled field of public health, *Mod Med* 2:183, 1920.

87. World Health Organization Expert Committee on Dental Health: *Organization of dental public health services report,* WHO technical report series no 298, Geneva, 1965, World Health Organization.

88. World Health Organization Expert Committee on Dental Health: *Planning and evaluation of public dental health services report,* WHO technical report series no 589, Geneva, 1976, World Health Organization.

89. Young WO: Dentistry looks toward the twenty-first century. In Brown WE, editor: *Oral health dentistry and the American public,* Norman, Okla, 1974, University of Oklahoma Press.

2 Factors Affecting the Practice of Dentistry

As we approach the turn of the century, the role of the dental professional is changing. Some of the changes are a function of advances in technology. Others are the result of increased and improved education, of both patients and dentists. However, some are the result of the changes in society and the socioeconomic structure of which dentistry is a part. People and systems over which dentists have limited control are affecting the way dentistry is practiced today. The purpose of this chapter is to explore some important issues in dentistry and to discuss implications for the profession. The issues selected for discussion are those that most significantly affect the profession, for example, demographics, financial considerations, and the medically compromised patient.

DEMOGRAPHICS

Several factors have been operating concurrently over recent years to change the characteristics of the population that the dental profession serves and the characteristics of the dental profession itself.

The post–World War II baby-boom cohort is choosing to have fewer children than its historical predecessors. Moreover, women who have begun careers or are in the educational process in pursuit of careers are delaying the start of their families so that the average age of college-educated mothers has risen to the early thirties. Therefore there are relatively fewer pediatric dental patients, and, among them, the incidence and prevalence of dental caries have declined.

Introduction of fluoride

In spite of overwhelming evidence in its favor, fluoridation of public water supplies is still a hotly contested issue in some areas. Antifluoridationists campaign vigorously and vociferously to prevent fluoridation of community water supplies. Their attacks are based on political or ideological issues or simply misinformation. Presently about 80 million individuals using public water supplies do not have community fluoridation. Despite the irrefutable evidence about the efficacy of fluoridation, almost 40% of public tap water remains unfluoridated or does not have enough fluoride to combat caries effectively. Dr. Harold Loe, director of the National Institute of Dental Research, attributes this to lack of public funding. Because fluoridation of public water supplies is determined locally and is often determined by referenda, the implementation of this dental public health policy is subject to local political action groups. Misguided antifluoridation activists, some of whom claim that fluoride promotes cancer, sickle cell anemia, and acquired immunodeficiency syndrome (AIDS), have succeeded in persuading local government agencies and voters in many areas to reject fluoridation.

Increased dental health education through school systems and professional offices, as well as the generalized increase in nutritional education of the public, has also had a positive impact on decreasing dental caries. However, a decrease in dental caries does not necessarily mean a decrease in dental disease or a lessening of demand for dental care. Lower incidence of caries and loss of teeth resulting from caries at a young age means that, at adulthood, more teeth have been retained. This fact, in conjunction with another demographic trend, the increase in the number of elderly in the population, has created a different dental need.

THE ELDERLY

The over-65 age group is the fastest-growing segment of our society. By the end of the century, it is expected that the U.S. population over 65 years of age will increase from the present 11% of the population to 13%, and by the year 2030 will reach 20%. In 1981, according to U.S. census figures, 48.2 million people were in the 55-plus segment of the population. By 2010 the number will soar to

74 million. The population doubled from 1950 to 1980 and will nearly double again by 2030 to 98.6 million people over 55 years of age (Table 2-1).

In Table 2-2 it can be seen that by 2000, 22% of the U.S. population will be 55 years of age or older. By 2010, 26.4%, over one quarter of the same population, will be 55 or older.[42] Table 2-3 shows that in 1970 approximately 38.5 million people were 55 years of age or older; in 1989, more than 52 million people were in that age bracket. Clearly the percentage and numbers of aging U.S. residents are increasing rapidly.

At a conference on geriatric education for health professionals in 1985, Dr. Lawrence Kerr, past president of the American Dental Association (ADA), discussed the state of oral health of the elderly and identified the following group of dental diseases requiring treatment:

1. Mobile and brittle teeth
2. Periodontal disease
3. Fractured crowns of teeth with sharp edges
4. Recession of gingival tissue
5. Root caries
6. Ill-fitting bridges and dentures, full and partial
7. Malaligned jaws with temporomandibular joint diseases
8. Higher incidence of caries
9. Neglect of oral hygiene
10. Edentulousness
11. Xerostomia, salivary gland impairment
12. Changes in the oral mucosa
13. Tissue changes in the tongue
14. Bone changes
15. Changes in tooth structure

The impact of this increase in the elderly population on dental practice will be significant. Historically, use of dental services by the elderly has been less than significant. According to a report issued by the ADA in 1983:

Except for children under six years, the percentage of elderly persons who visit a dentist is lowest compared to other age groups. Lower income is a further barrier to receiving care. About one of five among the poorest elderly (under $5000) visit the dentist in a year's time. The percent rises to one-third of the elderly with incomes of $5000 to $10,000; 41 percent in the $10,000 to $15,000; and 48 to 56 percent for the elderly with incomes of $15,000 or more. For those utilizing dental services, number of visits per person is highest in the lowest income group. This indicates the impact of Medicaid and access for the elderly programs, combines with the large amount of care needed by the oldest and poorest, which is being converted to demand.

Use of dental services by the elderly is changing. The elderly of today, and certainly of tomorrow, will be healthier, wealthier, and wiser (or at least better educated) than the elderly of yesterday. Table 2-4 shows the number of dental visits by patient characteristics from 1970 to 1988. The number of dental visits per person has increased in every category in the range of years examined. The increment is largest (1.4 visits in 1980 to 2.1 visits in 1986) for the 65-and-over age group. The elderly group is now the third-highest user of dental services, following only those 6 to 16 years old and those 45 to 64 years old. This is evidence that dental offices will become even busier in the future.

That existing need will be translated into de-

Table 2-1 Elderly population estimate, 1980-2000 (in millions)

Age group	1980	1990	2000	Annual rate of change	
				1980-90	1990-2000
65-69	8,780.8	10,006.3	9,110.2	1.3%	−0.9%
70-74	6,796.7	8,048.0	8,582.8	1.7%	0.6%
75-79	4,792.6	6,223.7	7,242.2	2.6%	1.5%
80-84	2,934.2	4,060.1	4,964.6	3.3%	2.0%
85+	2,239.7	3,460.9	5,136.3	4.4%	4.0%
TOTAL	25,544.0	31,799.0	35,036.1	2.2%	1.0%

From U.S. Bureau of the Census: *Population estimates and projections,* Series P-25, No 937, 1983.

Table 2-2 Projections of the total population by age, sex, and race: 1995 to 2010*

Age, sex, and race	Population (1,000)				Percent distribution		Percent change	
	1995	2000	2005	2010	2000	2010	1990-2000	2000-2010
TOTAL	**260,138**	**268,266**	**275,604**	**282,575**	**100.0**	**100.0**	**7.1**	**5.3**
Under 5 years old	17,799	16,898	16,611	16,899	6.3	6.0	−8.2	(Z)
5-17 years old	48,374	48,815	47,471	45,747	18.2	16.2	7.0	6.3
18-24 years old	24,281	25,231	26,918	27,155	9.4	9.6	−3.5	7.6
25-34 years old	40,962	37,149	35,997	37,572	13.8	13.3	−15.4	1.1
35-44 years old	42,336	43,911	40,951	37,202	16.4	13.2	15.9	15.3
45-54 years old	31,297	37,223	41,619	43,207	13.9	15.3	46.0	16.1
55-64 years old	21,325	24,158	29,762	35,430	9.0	12.5	13.1	46.7
65-74 years old	18,930	18,243	18,410	21,039	6.8	7.4	−0.7	15.3
75 years old and over	14,834	16,639	17,864	18,323	6.2	6.5	26.2	10.1
16 years old and over	201,018	210,134	219,301	227,390	78.3	80.5	8.9	8.2
Male, total	**127,123**	**131,191**	**134,858**	**138,333**	**100.0**	**100.0**	**7.3**	**5.4**
Under 5 years old	9,118	8,661	8,517	8,668	6.6	6.3	−8.1	0.1
5-17 years old	24,787	25,027	24,350	23,473	19.1	17.0	7.1	−6.2
18-24 years old	12,290	12,770	13,628	13,752	9.7	9.9	−3.4	7.7
25-34 years old	20,579	18,662	18,091	18,878	14.2	13.6	−15.5	1.2
35-44 years old	21,104	21,945	20,458	18,586	16.7	13.4	16.8	15.3
45-54 years old	15,292	18,296	20,585	21,432	13.9	15.5	47.5	17.1
55-64 years old	10,149	11,557	14,321	17,173	8.8	12.4	14.4	48.6
65-74 years old	8,476	8,242	8,407	9,691	6.3	7.0	0.9	17.6
75 years old and over	5,326	6,032	6,501	6,681	4.6	4.8	28.9	10.8
16 years old and over	96,834	101,392	105,984	110,024	77.3	79.5	9.2	8.5
Female, total	**133,016**	**137,076**	**140,746**	**144,241**	**100.0**	**100.0**	**7.0**	**5.2**
Under 5 years old	8,681	8,237	8,094	8,231	6.0	5.7	−8.3	−0.1
5-17 years old	23,587	23,788	23,121	22,274	17.4	15.4	6.9	−6.4
18-24 years old	11,991	12,461	13,290	13,402	9.1	9.3	−3.6	7.6
25-34 years old	20,384	18,487	17,906	18,694	13.5	13.0	−15.4	1.1
35-44 years old	21,233	21,966	20,493	18,616	16.0	12.9	14.9	−15.3
45-54 years old	16,005	18,927	21,034	21,775	13.8	15.1	44.7	15.0
55-64 years old	11,175	12,601	15,441	18,257	9.2	12.7	11.9	44.9
65-74 years old	10,454	10,001	10,004	11,348	7.3	7.9	−2.0	13.5
75 years old and over	9,507	10,607	11,364	11,642	7.7	8.1	24.7	9.8
16 years old and over	104,184	108,742	113,317	117,366	79.3	81.4	8.6	7.9

*As of July 1. Includes Armed Forces overseas. Data are for middle series. Minus sign (−) indicates decrease.
Z, Less than .05 percent.
Data from: U.S. Bureau of the Census: *Current Population Reports,* series P-25, No. 1018.

mand is substantiated by the following information from Robert J. Forbes,[17] a staff member of the American Association of Retired Persons:

Myth 1: Older people have limited needs and limited dollars

In part this is true. People in retirement no longer have children at home or in college, and some economists estimate that because of smaller household size, lower taxes, no regular commuting costs, and limited wardrobe purchases, older households need only 80 percent of their former income to maintain their lifestyles.

Myth 2: Most older people are in institutions

A 1982 study by the U.S. Census Bureau states that fewer than 5 percent of people 65-74 are institutionalized. . . . In fact, 70% of all older Americans own their own homes and the majority of mortgages are paid in full.

Table 2-2 Projections of the total population by age, sex, and race: 1995 to 2010*—cont'd

Age, sex, and race	Population (1,000)				Percent distribution		Percent change	
	1995	2000	2005	2010	2000	2010	1990-2000	2000-2010
White, total	**216,820**	**221,514**	**225,424**	**228,978**	**100.0**	**100.0**	**5.2**	**3.4**
Under 5 years old	14,251	13,324	12,936	13,084	6.0	5.7	−10.5	−1.8
5-17 years old	38,493	38,569	37,118	35,258	17.4	15.4	5.6	−8.6
18-24 years old	19,452	19,998	21,188	21,298	9.0	9.3	−6.2	6.5
25-34 years old	33,680	29,988	28,603	29,585	13.5	12.9	−18.1	−1.3
35-44 years old	35,635	36,574	33,639	29,997	16.5	13.1	13.2	−18.0
45-54 years old	26,879	31,618	34,911	35,860	14.3	15.7	44.0	13.4
55-64 years old	18,327	20,667	25,407	29,913	9.3	13.1	10.9	44.7
65-74 years old	16,681	15,811	15,708	17,875	7.1	7.8	−3.5	13.1
75 years old and over	13,421	14,965	15,914	16,108	6.8	7.0	25.1	7.6
16 years old and over	169,665	175,579	181,478	186,417	79.3	81.4	6.8	6.2
Male	106,365	108,774	110,785	112,610	49.1	49.2	5.4	3.5
Female	110,455	112,739	114,639	116,368	50.9	50.8	4.9	3.2
Black, total	**33,199**	**35,129**	**37,003**	**38,833**	**100.0**	**100.0**	**12.8**	**10.6**
Under 5 years old	2,790	2,748	2,764	2,820	7.8	7.3	−2.3	2.6
5-17 years old	7,697	7,895	7,889	7,809	22.5	20.1	10.1	−1.1
18-24 years old	3,703	3,924	4,198	4,314	11.2	11.1	2.9	9.9
25-34 years old	5,534	5,264	5,299	5,590	15.0	14.4	−7.4	6.2
35-44 years old	5,041	5,481	5,332	5,076	15.6	13.1	30.2	−7.4
45-54 years old	3,261	4,106	4,928	5,369	11.7	13.8	52.9	30.8
55-64 years old	2,288	2,578	3,155	3,995	7.3	10.3	19.6	55.0
65-74 years old	1,762	1,848	1,994	2,277	5.3	5.9	14.9	23.2
75 years old and over	1,122	1,283	1,445	1,584	3.7	4.1	27.7	23.5
16 years old and over	23,860	25,708	27,638	29,467	73.2	75.9	15.7	14.6
Male	15,840	16,787	17,707	18,602	47.8	47.9	13.2	10.8
Female	17,359	18,342	19,296	20,231	52.2	52.1	12.4	10.3
Other races, total	**10,119**	**11,624**	**13,177**	**14,764**	**100.0**	**100.0**	**34.5**	**27.0**
Under 5 years old	758	826	911	995	7.1	6.7	17.8	20.4
5-17 years old	2,184	2,350	2,464	2,680	20.2	18.2	22.2	14.1
18-24 years old	1,126	1,309	1,532	1,542	11.3	10.4	31.1	17.9
25-34 years old	1,748	1,897	2,095	2,396	16.3	16.2	17.1	26.3
35-44 years old	1,660	1,856	1,980	2,129	16.0	14.4	34.5	14.7
45-54 years old	1,156	1,500	1,780	1,979	12.9	13.4	76.2	32.0
55-64 years old	711	912	1,200	1,523	7.8	10.3	59.9	67.1
65-74 years old	487	584	708	886	5.0	6.0	51.9	51.8
75 years old and over	290	391	506	632	3.4	4.3	79.3	61.8
16 years old and over	7,493	8,847	10,186	11,506	76.1	77.9	40.5	30.1
Male	4,918	5,629	6,366	7,122	48.4	48.2	33.3	26.5
Female	5,202	5,995	6,811	7,642	51.6	51.8	35.6	27.5

Myth 3: Most older people are in poor health and inactive

A recent survey of retirees found that 70 percent stated that they were in good health and were enjoying active lives in their families and communities.

Other supporting information is found in mar-

keting journals. *Madison Avenue* in 1984 published an article called "The Invisible Consumer," which discussed the senior market. The author states that the 1981 household per capita income for those ages 55 to 64 was $9,874, 34% higher than the national average. This age group com-

Table 2-3 Resident population by age, sex, and race: 1970 to 1989*

Year, sex, and race	Total, all years	Under 5 years	5 to 9 years	10 to 14 years	15 to 19 years	20 to 24 years	25 to 29 years	30 to 34 years	35 to 39 years	40 to 44 years
1970, TOTAL[†,‡]	**203,235**	**17,163**	**19,969**	**20,804**	**19,064**	**16,383**	**13,486**	**11,437**	**11,113**	**11,988**
Male	98,928	8,750	10,175	10,598	9,641	7,925	6,626	5,599	5,416	5,823
Female	104,309	8,413	9,794	10,206	9,443	8,458	6,859	5,838	5,697	6,166
White	178,098	14,464	16,941	17,724	16,412	14,327	11,850	10,000	9,749	10,633
Black	22,581	2,434	2,749	2,812	2,425	1,816	1,429	1,254	1,196	1,199
1980, TOTAL	**226,546**	**16,348**	**16,700**	**18,242**	**21,168**	**21,319**	**19,521**	**17,561**	**13,965**	**11,669**
Male	110,053	8,362	8,539	9,316	10,755	10,663	9,705	8,677	6,862	5,706
Female	116,493	7,986	8,161	8,926	10,413	10,655	9,816	8,884	7,104	5,961
White§	194,713	13,414	13,717	15,095	17,681	18,072	16,658	15,157	12,122	10,110
Black§	26,683	2,459	2,509	2,691	3,007	2,749	2,342	1,904	1,469	1,260
Other races§	5,150	475	474	456	480	498	521	500	375	299
1964, total	236,477	17,830	16,464	17,511	18,786	21,328	21,535	19,696	16,932	13,614
1965, total	238,736	18,004	16,822	17,101	18,552	21,000	21,758	20,269	17,708	14,056
1966, total	241,107	18,154	17,295	18,565	18,610	20,411	22,005	20,773	18,722	14,348
1967, total	243,427	18,267	17,662	16,485	18,459	19,791	21,979	21,333	18,737	15,570
1968, total	245,785	18,432	18,027	16,626	18,214	19,182	21,873	21,796	19,140	16,125
1989, TOTAL	**248,239**	**18,752**	**18,212**	**16,950**	**17,812**	**18,702**	**21,699**	**22,135**	**19,621**	**16,882**
Male	120,982	9,598	9,321	8,689	9,091	9,368	10,865	11,078	9,731	8,294
Female	127,258	9,155	8,891	8,260	8,721	9,334	10,834	11,058	9,690	8,588
White	208,961	15,050	14,628	13,574	14,343	15,359	18,103	18,567	16,625	14,550
Male	102,223	7,716	7,504	6,973	7,327	7,731	9,142	9,385	8,342	7,229
Female	106,738	7,335	7,124	6,601	7,015	7,628	8,960	9,182	8,283	7,321
Black	30,660	2,890	2,802	2,679	2,758	2,651	2,827	2,744	2,260	1,726
Male	14,545	1,469	1,423	1,382	1,394	1,279	1,342	1,289	1,035	782
Female	16,115	1,421	1,378	1,318	1,365	1,372	1,485	1,455	1,225	945
Other races	8,618	813	782	696	711	692	769	824	736	605
Male	4,213	414	394	355	371	357	381	404	354	283
Female	4,404	399	389	342	341	335	389	420	382	322
Percent:										
1970	100.0	8.4	9.8	10.2	9.4	8.1	6.6	5.6	5.5	5.9
1980	100.0	7.2	7.4	8.1	9.3	9.4	8.6	7.8	6.2	5.2
1989, total	100.0	7.6	7.3	6.8	7.2	7.5	8.7	8.9	7.9	6.8
Male	100.0	7.9	7.7	7.2	7.5	7.7	9.0	9.2	8.0	6.9
Female	100.0	7.2	7.0	6.5	6.9	7.3	8.5	8.7	7.8	6.7
White	100.0	7.2	7.0	6.5	6.9	7.4	8.7	8.9	8.0	7.0
Black	100.0	9.4	9.1	8.7	9.0	8.6	9.2	8.9	7.4	5.6
Other races	100.0	9.4	9.1	8.1	8.3	8.0	8.9	9.6	8.5	7.0

*In thousands, except as indicated. 1970 and 1990 based on enumerated population as of April 1; other years based on estimated population as of July 1. Excludes Armed Forces overseas.
X, Not applicable.
†Includes other races, not shown separately.
‡Official count. The revised 1970 resident population count is 203,302,031; the difference of 66,733 is due to errors found after release of the official series.
§The race data shown for April 1, 1980 have been modified.
Data from: U.S. Bureau of the Census, *Current Population Reports,* series P-25, Nos. 917, 1045, and 1067.

Table 2-3 Resident population by age, sex, and race: 1970 to 1989—cont'd

45 to 49 years	50 to 54 years	55 to 59 years	60 to 64 years	65 to 74 years	75 years and over	5 to 13 years	14 to 17 years	18 to 24 years	16 years and over	65 years and over	Median age (yr)
12,124	**11,111**	**9,979**	**8,623**	**12,443**	**7,530**	**36,675**	**15,851**	**23,714**	**141,268**	**19,972**	**28.0**
5,855	5,351	4,769	4,030	5,440	2,927	18,687	8,069	11,583	67,347	8,367	26.8
6,269	5,759	5,210	4,593	7,002	4,603	17,987	7,782	12,131	73,920	11,605	29.3
10,868	10,019	9,021	7,818	11,300	6,972	31,171	13,579	20,655	125,520	18,272	28.9
1,124	990	874	734	1,043	501	5,009	2,073	2,271	14,053	1,544	22.4
11,090	**11,710**	**11,615**	**10,088**	**15,581**	**9,969**	**31,159**	**16,247**	**30,022**	**171,196**	**25,549**	**30.0**
5,386	5,621	5,482	4,670	6,757	3,548	15,923	8,298	15,054	81,766	10,305	28.8
5,702	6,089	6,133	5,418	8,824	6,420	15,237	7,950	14,969	89,429	15,245	31.3
9,693	10,360	10,394	9,078	14,045	9,117	25,691	13,492	25,381	149,121	23,182	30.9
1,150	1,135	1,041	874	1,344	748	4,629	2,380	3,948	18,425	2,092	24.9
246	215	180	135	191	104	839	376	693	3,650	295	26.8
11,463	11,032	11,444	10,872	16,740	11,231	30,238	14,704	29,146	180,991	27,971	31.1
11,645	10,944	11,342	10,995	17,009	11,531	30,110	14,865	28,500	183,040	28,540	31.4
11,926	10,889	11,273	10,962	17,334	11,840	30,351	14,797	27,733	185,248	29,174	31.8
12,350	10,927	11,126	10,899	17,674	12,167	30,824	14,468	27,106	187,474	29,841	32.1
13,026	11,138	10,896	10,934	17,906	12,468	31,405	13,983	26,661	189,345	30,374	32.4
13,521	**11,375**	**10,726**	**10,867**	**18,182**	**12,802**	**31,834**	**13,496**	**26,346**	**191,047**	**30,984**	**32.7**
6,601	5,509	5,121	5,079	8,095	4,541	16,302	6,922	13,246	91,693	12,636	31.6
6,920	5,866	5,605	5,788	10,087	8,261	15,532	6,574	13,100	99,354	18,348	33.8
11,672	9,789	9,310	9,569	16,222	11,600	25,534	10,790	21,579	163,091	27,822	33.6
5,758	4,791	4,480	4,498	7,250	4,098	13,105	5,541	10,890	78,686	11,347	32.5
5,915	4,998	4,830	5,071	8,972	7,502	12,429	5,250	10,689	84,404	16,475	34.7
1,395	1,223	1,116	1,035	1,577	978	4,960	2,145	3,786	21,770	2,555	27.7
626	544	508	467	676	349	2,520	1,091	1,847	10,027	1,025	26.3
769	679	608	567	901	628	2,440	1,054	1,939	11,743	1,529	29.1
454	363	300	264	383	225	1,341	560	960	6,187	607	29.0
217	174	133	113	169	94	678	290	509	2,979	264	27.8
237	189	167	150	213	131	663	270	472	3,208	344	30.1
6.0	5.5	4.9	4.2	6.1	3.7	18.0	7.8	11.7	69.5	9.8	(X)
4.9	5.2	5.1	4.5	6.9	4.4	13.8	7.2	13.3	75.6	11.3	(X)
5.4	4.6	4.3	4.4	7.3	5.2	12.8	5.4	10.6	77.0	12.5	(X)
5.5	4.6	4.2	4.2	6.7	3.8	13.5	5.7	10.9	75.8	10.4	(X)
5.4	4.6	4.4	4.5	7.9	6.5	12.2	5.2	10.3	78.1	14.4	(X)
5.6	4.7	4.5	4.6	7.8	5.6	12.2	5.2	10.3	78.1	13.3	(X)
4.5	4.0	3.6	3.4	5.1	3.2	16.2	7.0	12.3	71.0	8.3	(X)
5.3	4.2	3.5	3.1	4.4	2.6	15.6	6.5	11.4	71.8	7.0	(X)

Table 2-4 Physician and dental visits, by patient characteristics: 1970 to 1988

Type of visit and year	Total visits (million)				Visits per person									
	Sex		Race		Sex		Race		Age (years)					
	Male	Female	White	Black	Male	Female	White	Black	Under 6	6 to 16	17 to 24	25 to 44	45 to 64	65 and over
Physicians: 1970	396	531	832	87	4.1	5.1	4.8	3.9	5.9	2.9	4.6	4.6	5.2	6.3
1980	426	610	903	115	4.0	5.4	4.8	4.5	6.7	3.2	4.0	4.6	5.1	6.4
1985	498	733	1,074	132	4.4	6.1	5.4	4.7	6.3	3.1	4.2	4.9	6.1	8.3
1986	515	756	1,110	131	4.5	6.2	5.5	4.6	*6.3	†3.3	‡4.2	4.7	6.6	9.1
1987	523	765	1,118	140	4.5	6.2	5.5	4.9	*6.7	†3.3	‡4.4	4.8	6.4	8.9
1988	530	774	1,139	136	4.5	6.2	5.6	4.6	*7.0	†3.4	‡3.8	5.1	6.1	8.7
Dentists: 1970	133	171	283	17	1.4	1.7	1.6	0.8	0.5	1.9	1.8	1.7	1.5	1.1
1980	158	207	333	26	1.5	1.8	1.8	1.0	0.5	2.3	1.6	1.7	1.8	1.4
1983	183	239	382	31	1.6	2.0	1.9	1.1	0.5	2.6	1.6	1.9	2.0	1.5
1986	210	256	416	37	1.9	2.2	2.1	1.4	*0.7	†2.4	‡1.7	2.0	2.2	2.1

*Under 5.
†5 to 17.
‡18 to 24.
Data from: U.S. National Center for Health Statistics, *Vital and Health Statistics,* series 10, and unpublished data.

prises a third of all buying power in the U.S. marketplace. The author further suggests that those who perceive the elderly as being in their vital years or freedom years will have more success in reaching them than those who perceive them as the gray market. The suggestion seems appropriate for those in the practice of dentistry as well, especially in that many retirees will carry dental benefits they held while employed with them into retirement. (More detailed information on geriatric dentistry can be found in Chapter 5.)

STATUS OF DENTAL PERSONNEL IN THE UNITED STATES

The educational system for dental professionals has experienced major changes over the past 10 years.* First-year enrollment (FYE) in dental schools peaked at 5,498 in 1982† and declined to a low of 3,979 in 1989. First-year enrollment increased in each of the succeeding two years: 1990

*For more comprehensive data on the issues discussed here, the reader is referred to the American Dental Association's *Council on Dental Education Supplement 2* to the *1991/92 Annual Report on Dental Education,* January 1992.
†The highest first-year enrollment for dental students was recorded in 1978, with 6,301 entering.

(4,001) and 1991 (4,047). The number of applications increased 15.15% from 1990-91 (23,099) to 1991-92 (26,599). The number of applications submitted by women increased 12.43% from 1990-91 (8,377) to 1991-92 (9,418). The ratio of applicants to first-year enrollment has increased from 1988 (1.2) to 1991 (1.39) to a level virtually identical with 1982 (1.4). The FYE for women (1,468) accounts for 36.27% of the total 1991-92 FYE. The FYE for minority students (1,255) reflects 31.01% of the total FYE for 1991-92. The FYE for minority students has increased 13.84% during the 10 years between 1982-83 (17.17%) to 1991-92 (31.01%). The mean of first-year tuition and fees at dental schools has more than doubled between 1984-85 ($6,970) and 1991-92 ($15,902).

Although the cost of dental education has increased significantly, the return on investment (ROI) is substantial, even in an economy with recessionary characteristics. *Money* magazine conducted an analysis of 100 representative occupations.[25] They surveyed 220 subscribers from various occupations to determine a ranking of occupations based on response to questions regarding pay, satisfaction, prestige, and security. Dentistry was ranked 18 and dental hygiene ranked 32. For purposes of comparison, physician ranked number 3; clergy member ranked number 34; TV news reporter ranked number 57; and stockbroker ranked number 87. In assessing each occupation's earnings potential, the study estimated the earnings of the top 10% of earners in each field from data provided by professional organizations and other sources. For the sample professions cited, the top 10% annual earnings in each field are listed as follows:

Physician	$315,000
Dentist	116,550
Dental hygienist	43,001
Clergy member	44,733
TV news reporter	58,188
Stockbroker	106,493

The prestige perceived to be associated with their profession by dentists was "excellent," whereas dental hygienists reported "average" prestige.

The high prestige and income earned by dentists results, among many variables, from the years of education and training invested in establishing professional credentials. Additional years of training and education are elected by those who choose to pursue advanced educational programs in dentistry, including advanced education in general dentistry (AEGD) programs, general practice residency (GPR) programs, and the dental specialties. The number of first-year positions available for postgraduate programs in dental school and nondental school settings has increased by 17% between 1982 and 1991, from 2,158 to 2,528. As seen in Tables 2-5 and 2-6, the largest increase has occurred in a nonspecialty AEGD programs (from 74 first-year positions in 1982 to 366 in 1991); GPR program enrollment declined slightly during the same period (from 914 first-year positions in 1982 to 903 in 1991).

Some dental educators have proposed a mandatory fifth year of dental education for all. At the 1992 American Association of Dental Schools (AADS) House of Delegates meeting, the following resolution was considered:[28]

Resolution on II:

c. The AADS should encourage the further development of postdoctoral positions in general dentistry, including nontraditional and innovative models, so that by the year 2000 all graduates of U.S. dental schools will be able to enroll in one year of postdoctoral training. Further, the AADS, in cooperation with appropriate associations and agencies, should examine the current status of PGY-1 (a year of postgraduate study) and the financial implications of the expansion to students, schools, and the public.

The number of women enrolled in first-year dental classes has increased from 2.1% in 1970-71 to 27.1% in 1984-85. Table 2-7 shows the significant increase in number of women dental graduates since 1970. Their number as first-year enrollees and graduates is expected to increase through the year 1995 and then level off, although the number of active female dentists is projected to increase through the year 2000. Women may soon comprise the majority of entering first-year dental students.[24] For the 1991 entering class of 4,047 first-year students, 1,468 were women. In two dental schools, women were the majority of the first-year class, one school had 50% women in the first-year class, and the national average was 35% women in the 1991 entering class. Of the 26,599 applications submitted to dental schools in 1991, 9,418 were submitted by women. The increased number of women entering dental school and the profession has revealed several interesting dilemmas these women face as they progress. One is the paucity of women in leadership positions within dental education and within organized dentistry.[12,24,26,27] Dolan reports that approximately 6% to 8% of practicing dentists are female, and that by the year 2000 the number will rise to approximately 15%.[12] In 1991, Dr. Geraldine Morrow became the first woman president of the ADA. However, there are only five female members of the ADA House of Delegates, and the male-female ratio on the board of trustees is 20:1. Solomon reported that of 117 dean-level positions in dental schools, only eight were held by women; and that of 281 department chair positions in dental schools, only 20 were held by women.[38] However, some positive changes appear to be occurring. In fact, to borrow the title from Alvin Toffler's most recent book, a "powershift" may be underway. In 1992, Ms. Linda Rubenstein-Devore was elected as the third woman president of the AADS, and Dr. Jean Sinkford was appointed as assistant to the executive director of AADS for Women and Minority Affairs. Unfortunately, there are still very few role models to serve as mentors for women entering the profession, and

Table 2-5 Advanced education in dental and nondental institutions, 1982-1991: dental school programs

Advanced program	1982	1983	1984	1985	1986	1987	1988	1989	1990	1991
First-year enrollment										
Dental public health	16	8	10	9	12	15	7	9	5	5
Endodontics	102	116	102	113	105	114	126	128	140	141
Oral pathology	22	17	19	17	7	10	14	7	8	11
Oral-maxillofacial surgery	98	102	98	95	101	100	103	97	97	95
Orthodontics	262	271	259	263	266	265	261	252	243	249
Pediatric dentistry	118	109	124	119	112	130	120	125	118	131
Periodontics	155	159	150	153	172	173	181	178	179	169
Prosthodontics	117	122	132	139	143	127	136	142	142	143
Orthodontics/pediatric dentistry	1	1	3	1	2	1	1	2	2	2
Orthodontic/periodontics	0	0	1	0	0	0	1	0	1	1
Endodontics/periodontics	0	0	0	0	0	0	0	0	0	0
Specialty TOTAL	891	905	898	909	920	935	950	940	935	947
General practice residency	108	123	126	129	138	145	150	135	132	117
General dentistry	5	17	25	32	65	110	127	137	164	183
Nonspecialty TOTAL	113	140	151	161	203	255	277	272	296	300
Total enrollment										
Dental public health	29	17	20	22	27	27	14	20	21	20
Endodontics	223	230	222	235	230	237	248	263	280	301
Oral pathology	52	47	46	46	35	35	38	31	28	31
Oral-maxillofacial surgery	321	329	333	331	341	349	360	368	375	397
Orthodontics	541	542	542	561	557	578	576	539	549	554
Pediatric dentistry	254	235	237	267	255	252	256	267	260	256
Periodontics	343	341	334	361	375	380	397	401	413	422
Prosthodontics	234	258	263	307	306	296	296	316	320	326

some of the issues facing women dentists are different than those facing men dentists, so women mentors would be able to provide a special expertise. What issues are different? Combining a professional life with child-rearing is still unique to the woman dentist. Dolan reports that women dentists have fewer children (0.94) than male dentists (2.24).[12] Female dentists are less likely to be married than their male colleagues: 17% of females and 6% of males had never been married in the ADA study she cites. Women tend to work slightly fewer hours per week (41.3 for women, 43.8 for men) and about the same number of weeks per year. Women dentists tended to spend slightly longer with their patients (44.9 minutes per appointment for women, 42.2 minutes for men). One of the more dramatic differences reported was the gender wage gap: Women dentist specialists earned 57.5% of their male counterparts' earnings on average. On average, women dentists earned 75.4% of male pretax income from the private-practice, administration, or teaching of dentistry, with a mean annual difference of almost $10,000.[12]

As a cautionary note to those who might view the gender wage gap as of little concern to male practitioners, in a competitive hiring environment, market forces tend to equalize disparities toward the mean or even the lower end of the scale. It will ultimately be in the entire profession's interest to

Table 2-5 Advanced education in dental and nondental institutions, 1982-1991: dental school programs—cont'd

Advanced program	1982	1983	1984	1985	1986	1987	1988	1989	1990	1991
Total enrollment										
Orthodontic/pediatric dentistry	7	6	6	4	5	4	4	4	5	6
Orthodontics/periodontics	1	1	2	0	0	0	1	1	2	1
Endodontics/periodontics	0	0	0	0	0	0	0	0	0	0
Specialty TOTAL	2,005	2,006	2,005	2,134	2,131	2,162	2,190	2,210	2,253	2,314
General practice residency	118	136	141	145	152	161	166	155	155	134
General dentistry	5	17	25	32	67	113	131	142	168	200
Nonspecialty TOTAL	123	153	166	177	219	274	297	297	323	334
Graduates										
Dental public health	15	14	7	7	11	6	10	3	5	8
Endodontics	114	119	106	109	116	105	115	103	121	120
Oral pathology	23	34	17	14	16	10	11	6	10	8
Oral-max surgery	100	101	89	97	95	90	93	82	99	78
Orthodontics	266	261	269	251	259	250	252	267	217	235
Pediatric dentistry	122	130	119	112	119	107	102	133	104	116
Periodontics	164	171	162	150	152	158	151	150	154	164
Prosthodontics	109	135	138	122	128	122	132	130	122	143
Orthodontic/pediatric dentistry	0	3	3	2	1	2	1	2	1	1
Orthodontics/periodontics	0	0	0	1	0	0	0	0	0	1
Endodontics/periodontics	0	0	0	0	0	0	0	0	0	0
Specialty TOTAL	913	968	910	865	897	850	867	856	833	874
General practice residency	102	109	119	126	133	136	137	141	143	124
General dentistry	0	16	17	24	37	63	92	115	117	168
Nonspecialty TOTAL	102	125	136	150	170	199	229	256	260	292

minimize wage disparities and inequalities between genders. There appears to be a strong consensus among the authors referenced here that men and women who currently hold positions of power, leadership, and authority need to facilitate the development of the growing numbers of women in the profession to similar positions of responsibility.

Of concern to practicing dentists is the number of active dentists per 100,000 total population because this number represents the relative proportion of the dental market each practitioner holds. In 1984 there were 58 dentists per 100,000 people. Regardless of the methodology used for future projections (that is, low or high), this number

will remain fairly stable through the year 2000. Table 2-8 shows that in 1989, there were 58 dentists per 100,000 people, although regionally there were wide variations, from a high of 94 per 100,000 in Washington, D.C., to a low of 37 per 100,000 in Mississippi. The national mean (58) is lower than that projected for 1990 (60) by the Bureau of Health Professions in 1984. This may be due to six dental schools closing since 1984: Oral Roberts, Emory, Georgetown, Washington University, Fairleigh Dickinson, and Loyolas.

Other data describing the dental profession concern the nature of the dental practice itself. In 1988 approximately 58% of dental offices had one to

Table 2-6 Advanced education in dental and nondental institutions, 1982-1991: nondental school programs

Advanced program	1982	1983	1984	1985	1986	1987	1988	1989	1990	1991
First year enrollment										
Dental public health	18	12	9	12	12	10	13	13	9	15
Endodontics	21	23	21	18	21	16	19	15	16	15
Oral pathology	4	2	3	3	4	1	3	7	4	5
Oral-maxillofacial surgery	118	114	117	116	112	112	112	111	115	120
Orthodontics	22	26	22	31	35	37	33	43	37	36
Pediatric dentistry	39	40	40	38	40	35	42	43	43	46
Periodontics	18	24	23	26	24	22	25	30	26	26
Prosthodontics	38	56	51	56	50	51	48	49	51	49
Orthodontic/pediatric dentistry	0	0	0	0	0	0	0	0	0	0
Orthodontics/periodontics	0	0	0	0	0	0	0	0	0	0
Endodontics/periodontics	0	0	0	0	0	0	0	0	0	0
Specialty TOTAL	279	297	286	300	298	284	295	311	301	312
General practice residency	806	794	816	814	773	758	762	742	744	786
General dentistry	69	81	90	88	113	133	121	160	183	183
Nonspecialty TOTAL	875	875	906	902	886	891	883	902	927	969
Total enrollment										
Dental public health	26	22	14	16	19	13	18	17	17	22
Endodontics	46	45	44	37	39	37	35	34	31	31
Oral pathology	6	5	6	6	6	3	5	12	12	14
Oral-maxillofacial surgery	367	363	373	378	383	389	397	397	389	414
Orthodontics	49	53	50	59	69	78	73	85	78	78
Pediatric dentistry	81	78	80	77	76	73	79	85	87	93
Periodontics	48	53	53	52	52	52	54	71	65	60
Prosthodontics	91	105	103	104	102	97	96	101	103	95
Orthodontic/pediatric dentistry	0	0	0	0	0	0	0	0	0	0

four employees on the payroll, and 43% had between 5 and 19 employees (Table 2-9). The number of employees reported includes part-time as well as full-time employees. The aggregate annual receipts by all dental offices increased from $20 million in 1985 to $27.6 million in 1989 (Table 2-10), a 40% increase in 5 years. The increase in gross receipts occurred despite an essentially flat Medicaid reimbursement level during the same time period (Table 2-11), with a significant drop between 1988 to 1989 ($577 million to $498 million). The profile of the practicing dentist has expanded to include increased numbers of females, African-Americans, and Hispanics (Table 2-12).

The numbers of dental auxiliary students and practicing auxiliaries is important to examine because they are critical to the success of any practicing dentist. These are discussed in Chapter 3.

MALPRACTICE

The issue of malpractice insurance is one of growing concern to health care providers. Insurance rates have soared nationally, with regional differences driving practitioners to make a choice:

Table 2-6 Advanced education in dental and nondental institutions, 1982-1991: nondental school programs—cont'd

Advanced program	1982	1983	1984	1985	1986	1987	1988	1989	1990	1991
Total enrollment										
Orthodontics/periodontics	0	0	0	0	0	0	0	0	0	0
Endodontics/periodontics	0	0	0	0	0	0	0	0	0	0
Specialty TOTAL	714	724	723	729	746	742	757	802	782	807
General practice residency	866	849	881	880	835	809	818	797	803	800
General dentistry	86	98	113	110	150	182	172	210	241	243
Nonspecialty TOTAL	972	947	994	990	985	991	990	1007	1044	1043
Graduates										
Dental public health	10	7	9	6	7	7	7	8	7	4
Endodontics	25	26	21	23	19	18	20	16	19	15
Oral pathology	2	3	3	3	2	2	0	3	2	3
Oral-maxillofacial surgery	124	106	111	108	105	110	102	114	98	89
Orthodontics	17	20	20	21	30	28	39	36	40	35
Pediatric dentistry	49	38	38	36	39	34	34	34	38	43
Periodontics	25	27	20	25	21	23	22	24	29	28
Prosthodontics	47	49	50	61	49	52	44	53	52	50
Orthodontic/pediatric dentistry	0	0	0	0	0	0	0	0	0	0
Orthodontics/periodontics	0	0	0	0	0	0	0	0	0	0
Endodontics/periodontics	0	0	0	0	0	0	0	0	0	0
Specialty TOTAL	299	276	272	283	272	274	268	288	285	267
General practice residency	792	789	771	804	778	772	740	781	732	744
General dentistry	42	75	82	89	119	121	135	126	175	192
Nonspecialty TOTAL	834	864	853	893	897	893	875	907	907	936

(1) to relocate; (2) to become employees of health maintenance organizations (HMOs) in which malpractice insurance is paid for by the organization, not the individual; (3) to join the armed services, for similar reasons; or (4) to leave the practice of medicine altogether through early retirement or change in careers. In Massachusetts the rates for private practitioners in general dentistry over the past 3 years were as follows:

1984-85	$368	
1985-86	$1,940	427% increase
1986-87	$2,400	23.7% increase plus $50 additional for each dental assistant and hygienist employed

The implications of the increasing cost of malpractice insurance are great for two reasons:

1. The out-of-pocket expense is large; even though payment may be made in installments, this expenditure is in addition to other personal and professional cost-of-living items such as salaries, rent (office, home), mortgage payments, and so on.
2. Insurance companies such as Blue Cross/ Blue Shield place limits on annual profile increases, which may not exceed either the annual consumer price index increase in a given geographic area or an amount determined as the maximum by Blue Cross/Blue Shield for each annual update of allowable

Table 2-7 Degrees conferred in selected professions: 1960 to 1988

Type of degree and sex of recipient	1960	1970	1975	1980	1982	1983	1984	1985	1986	1987	1988*
Medicine (MD):											
Institutions conferring degrees	79	86	104	112	119	118	119	120	120	122	120
Degrees conferred, total	7,032	8,314	12,447	14,902	15,814	15,484	15,813	16,041	15,938	15,620	15,091
Men	6,645	7,615	10,818	11,416	11,867	11,350	11,359	11,167	11,022	10,566	10,107
Women	387	699	1,629	3,486	3,947	4,134	4,454	4,874	4,916	5,054	4,964
Percent of total	5.5	8.4	13.1	23.4	25.0	26.7	28.2	30.4	30.8	32.4	33.0
Dentistry (DDS or DMD):											
Institutions conferring degrees	45	48	52	58	58	59	60	59	59	58	55
Degrees conferred, total	3,247	3,718	4,773	5,258	5,282	5,585	5,353	5,339	5,046	4,741	4,351
Men	3,221	3,684	4,627	4,558	4,467	4,631	4,302	4,233	3,907	3,603	3,216
Women	26	34	146	700	815	954	1,051	1,106	1,139	1,138	1,135
Percent of total	0.8	0.9	3.1	13.3	15.4	17.1	19.6	20.7	22.6	24.0	26.1

NA, Not available.
*Preliminary.
Data from: U.S. National Center for Education Statistics, *Digest of Education Statistics,* annual.

charges, whichever is less. Although malpractice rates may increase 50% in a given year, if the consumer price index increases only 5%, the increase cannot be passed along to the consumer. It must, in fact, be absorbed by the practitioner. In medicine, there is precedent for Medicare freezing fees for 2 consecutive years in 1984 and 1985. While other costs of practice and living continued to increase, reimbursement by Medicare remained fixed. In 1992 Medicare enforced a major restructuring of its reimbursement schedule, reducing payments to surgeons by as much as 30%. Medicare, a federally funded health insurance program for the elderly, does not cover any dental services, not even emergencies or prophylaxes.

MEDICALLY COMPROMISED PATIENTS

The responsibility of the dental professional in management of the medically compromised patient has clearly increased over the years. With medical advances in diagnosis and care of patients with systemic diseases, more patients being effectively treated for one or more medical conditions are currently being seen in dental offices. The discussion of medically compromised patients for the purpose of this chapter will be divided into two groups: those with systemic diseases and those with infectious diseases. The purpose of this section is to give the reader an overview of how management of these patients affects the practice of dentistry. For more information on specific disease entities, see references at the end of this chapter.

Table 2-7 Degrees conferred in selected professions: 1960 to 1988—cont'd

Type of degree and sex of recipient	1960	1970	1975	1980	1982	1983	1984	1985	1986	1987	1988*
Law (LLB or JD):											
Institutions conferring degrees	134	145	154	179	180	177	179	181	181	180	180
Degrees conferred, total	9,240	14,916	29,296	35,647	35,991	36,853	37,012	37,491	35,844	36,172	35,469
Men	9,010	14,115	24,881	24,893	23,965	23,550	23,382	23,070	21,874	21,643	21,124
Women	230	801	4,415	10,754	12,026	13,303	13,630	14,421	13,970	14,529	14,345
Percent of total	2.5	5.4	15.1	30.2	33.4	36.1	36.8	38.5	39.0	40.2	40.4
Theological (BD, MDiv, MHL):											
Institutions conferring degrees	(NA)	(NA)	(NA)	(NA)	(NA)	(NA)	(NA)	(NA)	(NA)	(NA)	(NA)
Degrees conferred, total	(NA)	5,298	5,095	7,115	6,901	6,494	6,878	7,221	7,283	7,181	6,474
Men	(NA)	5,175	4,748	6,133	5,817	5,395	5,673	5,886	5,865	5,794	5,088
Women	(NA)	123	347	982	1,064	1,099	1,205	1,335	1,418	1,387	1,386
Percent of total	(NA)	2.3	6.8	13.8	15.7	16.9	17.5	18.5	19.5	19.3	21.4

Systemic diseases

Among the systemic diseases frequently seen in dental practice are hypertension, bleeding disorders, diabetes mellitus, and patients with damaged hearts. The best way to identify patients at risk for these problems is by taking an accurate, thorough medical history. The information gathered through use of this tool, however, must be viewed with the understanding that the medical history is limited by the patient's knowledge and willingness to share that knowledge with the dental professional. A medical history form should be administered in an environment that implies and conveys a sense of confidentiality and privacy. The degree to which this environment is attained will enhance the reliability and validity of the medical history received. A thorough explanation of the implication of a medical history, as well as the nature of its intended use, will help to ensure an accurate medical history. Modifying the medical history form to include an explanatory statement addressing these issues may also be of assistance. Based on the current state of infection control practiced in dental offices, it is of limited value to include questions on the medical history form about sexual preference or history of intravenous drug usage. All patients should be treated with the same universal precautions (i.e., gloves, masks, and protective eyewear). A sample of the medical history form currently in use at the Boston University Goldman School of Graduate Dentistry is included as an example (Fig. 2-1). Positive response to one of the questions requires follow-up by the dentist for clarification. The dentist is *not expected* to diagnose a medical condition, but familiarity with signs and symptoms of systemic diseases is essential in knowing when to request consultation from the patient's physician in determining what mea-

Table 2-8 Active nonfederal physicians, and nurses, 1988, and dentists, 1989 by states*

Region, division, and state	Physicians, 1988† Total	Rate‡	Dentists, 1989 Total	Rate‡	Nurses, 1988 Total	Rate‡
U.S.	506,474	210	144,000	58	1,627,835	667
Northeast	135,543	270	36,280	71	424,876	842
NE	35,887	280	9,120	70	130,915	1,014
ME	2,036	173	570	47	9,639	805
NH	1,959	186	640	59	10,015	926
VT	1,334	244	320	57	4,490	805
MA	18,812	322	4,420	74	68,255	1,161
RI	2,393	244	560	56	9,149	927
CT	9,353	293	2,610	80	29,367	913
MA	99,656	267	27,160	71	293,961	783
NY	54,745	307	5,690	73	142,899	799
NJ	17,899	234	14,050	77	53,239	692
PA	27,012	227	7,420	61	97,823	816
Midwest	110,076	185	35,150	58	430,666	721
ENC	78,413	187	24,940	58	295,202	702
OH	20,598	191	6,050	55	80,095	738
IN	8,323	151	2,680	47	35,527	640
IL	24,194	210	7,230	61	84,779	732
MI	16,584	180	5,800	62	60,463	655
WI	8,714	181	3,180	65	34,338	711
DC	3,627	591	590	94	10,279	1,693
VA	11,701	204	3,180	54	33,500	573
WV	3,120	164	840	43	11,097	592
NC	11,276	179	2,700	42	37,568	588
SC	5,246	156	1,400	41	15,180	446
GA	10,294	167	2,920	46	33,860	540
FL	24,235	203	6,160	50	80,319	656
ESC	24,369	160	7,290	47	82,644	542
KY	5,953	161	2,000	53	19,495	528
TN	9,022	187	2,630	53	28,889	592
AL	6,137	151	1,680	40	22,113	542
MS	3,257	125	980	37	12,147	467
WSC	44,282	166	12,610	46	125,470	471
AR	3,414	144	960	39	11,292	473
LA	8,126	184	2,030	45	19,685	450
OK	4,691	145	1,560	47	15,036	469
TX	28,051	169	8,060	47	79,457	476
West	106,900	218	31,450	62	303,707	606
Mt	23,154	177	7,710	58	81,838	619
MT	1,207	150	510	62	5,275	659

WNC	31,663	180	10,210	57	135,464	766
MN	9,006	212	2,900	67	33,911	788
IA	4,096	145	1,590	55	22,770	805
MO	9,683	190	2,760	53	38,277	747
ND	1,101	167	320	47	6,239	950
SD	973	138	350	49	5,777	817
NE	2,655	168	1,020	63	11,627	731
KS	4,145	169	1,270	51	16,863	682
South	153,955	186	41,120	48	467,785	558
SA	85,304	207	21,220	50	258,671	620
DE	1,229	191	290	44	5,661	863
MD	14,576	325	3,140	66	32,207	704
ID	1,192	120	540	53	4,963	496
WY	648	134	260	52	2,697	567
CO	6,574	202	2,300	69	23,459	720
NM	2,554	173	690	45	7,489	501
AZ	6,422	191	1,770	51	23,191	671
UT	2,566	177	1,140	66	8,397	496
NV	1,571	158	500	49	6,367	609
Pac	83,746	232	23,740	64	221,869	801
WA	9,245	206	3,110	68	33,121	721
OR	5,325	196	1,950	70	20,446	740
CA	66,184	242	17,500	62	159,008	587
AK	588	138	340	66	3,351	670
HI	2,304	225	840	80	5,923	570

*As of December 31, except as noted. Excludes doctors of osteopathy, federally employed persons, and physicians with addresses unknown. Includes all physicians not classified according to activity status.

†As of January 1, 1988.

‡Per 100,000 civilian population. Based on U.S. Bureau of the Census estimates as of July 1, 1987 for physicians; July 1, 1988, nurses; and July 1, 1989, dentists.

Data from: Physicians: American Medical Association, Chicago, IL, *Physician Characteristics and Distribution in the U.S.*, annual (copyright); Dentists and nurses: U.S. Dept. of Health and Human Services, Health Resources and Services Administration, unpublished data. Dentists: Based on data supplied by American Dental Association, Bureau of Economic and Behavioral Research.

Table 2-9 Domestic services—establishments, employees, and payroll: 1987 and 1988*

1987 SIC code†	Kind of business	1987	Establishments (1,000) 1988					Employees, 1988 (1,000)
			Total	1-4 employees	5-19 employees	20-99 employees	100 or more employees	
(1)	**Services, TOTAL**	**1,990.1**	**1,937.5**	**1,150.1**	**596.2**	**155.2**	**36.0**	**25,143**
70	Hotels and other lodging places‡	51.4	49.0	23.9	13.5	8.7	2.8	1,385
701	Hotels and motels	(NA)	38.8	16.3	11.4	8.3	2.8	1,333
72	Personal services‡	184.4	177.3	112.4	57.2	6.9	0.8	1,101
721	Laundry, cleaning, and garment services‡	(NA)	48.1	28.2	16.0	3.5	0.4	406
7215	Coin-operated laundries and cleaning	(NA)	11.7	8.7	2.7	0.2	(Z)	45
7216	Drycleaning plants, except rug	(NA)	19.4	9.0	8.9	1.5	(Z)	158
723	Beauty shops	(NA)	75.3	48.4	25.2	1.7	(Z)	363
726	Funeral service and crematories	(NA)	15.1	8.8	5.8	0.4	(Z)	81
73	Business services‡	248.0	250.5	138.0	74.9	28.9	8.8	4,385
731	Advertising	(NA)	17.9	10.4	5.7	1.6	0.3	194
7311	Advertising agencies	(NA)	12.0	6.8	4.0	1.0	0.2	136
733	Mailing, reproduction, and stenographic services	(NA)	25.2	15.9	7.2	1.6	0.3	219
734	Services to buildings	(NA)	44.0	23.5	14.7	4.7	1.2	743
735	Miscellaneous equipment rental and leasing	(NA)	24.0	13.0	9.1	1.8	0.1	193
736	Personnel supply services‡	(NA)	24.4	9.3	5.7	5.8	3.6	1,247
7361	Employment agencies	(NA)	11.8	6.5	3.6	1.3	0.3	169
7363	Help supply services	(NA)	12.6	2.8	2.1	4.5	3.3	1,076
737	Computer and data processing services‡	(NA)	37.9	21.2	10.7	4.8	1.2	679
7371	Computer programming services	(NA)	13.2	7.9	3.4	1.4	0.4	203
7374	Data processing and preparation	(NA)	6.8	2.9	2.1	1.3	0.5	218
738	Miscellaneous business services	(NA)	60.5	33.0	18.2	7.3	1.9	1,001
7381	Detective and armored car services	(NA)	9.4	3.5	2.5	2.3	1.1	436
75	Automotive repair, services, and parking‡	149.8	145.5	94.1	45.9	5.1	0.4	813
751	Automotive rentals, no drivers	(NA)	11.4	5.5	4.4	1.2	0.3	150
753	Automotive repair shops‡	(NA)	106.2	72.6	33.5	2.0	(Z)	483

Table 2-9 Domestic services—establishments, employees, and payroll: 1987 and 1988*—cont'd

1987 SIC code†	Kind of business	1987	Establishments (1,000) 1988					Employees, 1988 (1,000)
			Total	1-4 employees	5-19 employees	20-99 employees	100 or more employees	
7532	Top and body repair and paint shops	(NA)	30.7	18.7	11.2	0.9	(Z)	162
7538	General automotive repair shops	(NA)	52.2	38.0	13.5	0.7	(Z)	202
754	Automotive services, except repair	(NA)	15.5	8.3	5.6	1.6	(Z)	128
76	Miscellaneous repair services	64.1	61.8	41.4	17.5	2.8	0.2	356
762	Electrical repair shops	(NA)	17.1	11.2	5.0	0.9	0.1	107
78	Motion pictures‡	34.9	33.5	18.4	12.1	2.8	0.2	370
781	Motion picture production and services	(NA)	9.0	6.5	1.8	0.6	0.1	159
784	Video tape rental	(NA)	15.5	8.8	6.3	0.5	(Z)	87
79	Amusement and recreation services‡	72.4	70.5	39.8	20.2	9.5	1.1	909
7997	Membership sports and recreation clubs	(NA)	13.5	6.8	3.4	3.0	0.3	223
80	Health services‡	424.2	417.2	244.1	136.6	25.3	11.2	7,222
801	Offices and clinics of medical doctors	(NA)	192.0	118.6	64.9	7.7	0.7	1,242
802	**Offices and clinics of dentists**	**(NA)**	**102.2**	**58.4**	**42.7**	**1.1**	**(Z)**	**499**
8041	Offices and clinics of chiropractors	(NA)	20.1	16.2	3.7	0.1	(Z)	61
8042	Offices and clinics of optometrists	(NA)	15.3	11.2	4.0	0.1	(Z)	58
805	Nursing and personal care facilities	(NA)	18.0	1.9	2.0	9.1	4.9	1,358
806	Hospitals	(NA)	5.2	0.2	0.1	0.8	4.2	3,213
807	Medical and dental laboratories	(NA)	14.3	8.7	4.4	1.0	0.2	139
808	Home health care services	(NA)	7.5	2.5	2.0	2.3	0.7	303
81	Legal services	139.8	135.7	98.8	30.1	6.0	0.8	849
82	Educational services‡	34.2	33.2	11.4	10.9	8.7	2.2	1,631
821	Elementary and secondary schools	(NA)	14.5	2.4	5.5	6.0	0.7	434
822	Colleges and universities	(NA)	3.0	0.4	0.5	0.8	1.3	1,013
83	Social services‡	104.2	104.8	43.7	44.2	14.6	2.3	1,532
832	Individual and family services	(NA)	25.9	12.3	9.8	3.3	0.5	355
833	Job training and related services	(NA)	6.7	1.9	2.3	1.8	0.7	271

Continued

Table 2-9 Domestic services—establishments, employees, and payroll: 1987 and 1988*—cont'd

1987 SIC code†	Kind of business	1987	Establishments (1,000)						Employees, 1988 (1,000)
				1988					
			Total	1-4 employees	5-19 employees	20-99 employees	100 or more employees		
835	Child day care services	(NA)	39.2	15.5	19.4	4.2	0.1		368
836	Residential care	(NA)	19.3	6.5	8.4	3.7	0.6		358
86	Membership organiza-tions‡	221.6	214.3	129.2	67.3	16.4	1.4		1,778
861	Business associations	(NA)	12.0	8.0	3.2	0.7	0.1		92
863	Labor organizations	(NA)	20.0	11.1	7.3	1.5	0.1		179
864	Civic and social associ-ations	(NA)	39.0	24.8	10.5	3.4	0.4		330
866	Religious organizations	(NA)	126.8	74.5	42.0	9.7	0.7		1,036
87	Engineering and manage-ment services‡	204.1	199.0	122.7	56.9	16.3	3.1		2,302
8711	Engineering services	(NA)	35.6	18.7	11.4	4.6	0.9		592
8712	Architectural services	(NA)	17.1	9.8	5.9	1.2	0.1		141
872	Accounting, auditing, and bookkeeping	(NA)	66.2	44.8	17.8	3.1	0.5		498
873	Research and testing services	(NA)	15.1	7.4	4.9	2.3	0.6		360
8731	Commercial physical research	(NA)	3.9	1.8	1.2	0.7	0.2		159
8741	Management services	(NA)	17.1	9.4	5.0	2.2	0.5		283
8742	Management consulting services	(NA)	26.0	18.3	5.8	1.6	0.3		218

*Covers establishments with payroll. Excludes government employees, railroad employees, self-employed persons, etc.
NA, Not available.
Z, Less than 50.
†Based on 1987 Standard Industrial Classifications.
‡Includes kinds of business not shown separately.
Data from: U.S. Bureau of the Census, *County Business Patterns,* 1988.

sures are necessary for optimum management of the patient in the dental setting. If it is determined that a medical clearance is appropriate, it should be requested in writing to include in the patient's chart for medicolegal reasons. An example of a medical clearance letter is included for reference (Fig. 2-2).

A medical clearance should be designed for clarity of response and ease of completion on the part of the physician. It is also important to provide space for the physician to print his or her name and phone number, should additional information

be required. It can be frustrating for the dentist and the patient to receive incomplete information and not to have the resources available to be able to follow up in a timely fashion. It is also important for the dentist to be as specific as possible in communicating to the physician about what dental procedures are expected in the patient's treatment and what medical information is needed in this regard. Finally, note that the patient must sign the medical consultation form authorizing the release of pertinent information to the dentist. It is considered a breach of the patient's right to privacy

HEALTH HISTORY   Record # _____

Patient Name: _____   Soc. Sec. No. _____

Age_____ Height _____ Weight_____   Birth Date _____

I. Circle Appropriate Answer (leave **blank** if you do not understand question): _____

1. Yes No Is your general health good?
2. Yes No Has there been a change in your health within the last year?
3. Yes No Have you been hospitalized or had a serious illness in the last three years?
    Why? _____
4. Yes No Are you being treated by a physician now? For what? _____
    Date of last Medical Exam? _____ Date of last Dental Appt.? _____
5. Yes No Have you had problems with prior dental treatment?
    Physician's name_____ Address_____
6. Yes No Are you in pain now?   Telephone # _____

II. Have you experienced?_____

7. Yes No Chest pain (angina)?	18. Yes No Dizziness?
8. Yes No Swollen ankles?	19. Yes No Ringing in ears?
9. Yes No Shortness of breath?	20. Yes No Headaches?
10. Yes No Recent weight loss, fever, night sweats?	21. Yes No Fainting spells?
11. Yes No Persistent cough, coughing up blood	22. Yes No Blurred vision?
12. Yes No Bleeding problems, bruising easily?	23. Yes No Seizures?
13. Yes No Sinus problems?	24. Yes No Excessive thirst?
14. Yes No Difficulty swallowing?	25. Yes No Frequent urination?
15. Yes No Diarrhea, constipation, blood in stools?	26. Yes No Dry mouth?
16. Yes No Frequent vomiting, nausea?	27. Yes No Jaundice?
17. Yes No Difficulty urinating, blood in urine?	28. Yes No Joint pain, stiffness?

III. Do you have or have you had?_____

29. Yes No Heart disease?	40. Yes No AIDS or ARC?
30. Yes No Heart attack, heart defects?	41. Yes No Tumors, cancer?
31. Yes No Heart murmurs?	42. Yes No Arthritis, rheumatism?
32. Yes No Rheumatic fever?	43. Yes No Eye diseases?
33. Yes No Stroke, hardening of arteries?	44. Yes No Skin diseases?
34. Yes No High blood pressure?	45. Yes No Anema, blood disease?
35. Yes No TB, emphysema, other lung diseases?	46. Yes No VD (syphilis, gonorrhea, chlamydia)?
36. Yes No Hepatitis, other liver disease, jaundice?	47. Yes No Herpes?
37. Yes No Stomach problems, ulcers?	48. Yes No Kidney, bladder disease?
38. Yes No ALLERGIES: to drugs, foods, medications?	49. Yes No Thyroid, adrenal disease?
39. Yes No Family history of diabetes, heart problems, tumors?	50. Yes No Diabetes?

IV. Do you have or have you had?_____

51. Yes No Psychiatric care?	56. Yes No Hospitalization?
52. Yes No Radiation treatments?	57. Yes No Blood transfusions?
53. Yes No Chemotherapy?	58. Yes No Surgeries?
54. Yes No Prosthetic heart valve?	59. Yes No Pacemaker?
55. Yes No Artificial joint?	60. Yes No Contact lenses?

V. Are you taking?_____

61. Yes No Recreational drugs?	63. Yes No Tobacco in any form?
62. Yes No Drugs, medicines, (incl. Aspirin)?	64. Yes No Alcohol?

Please list: _____

VI. Women only:_____

65. Yes No Are you or could you be pregnant or nursing?	66. Yes No Taking birth control pills?

VII. All Patients:_____

67. Yes No Do you have or have had any other diseases or medical problems NOT listed on this form?
    If so, please explain: _____

To the best of my knowledge, I have answered every question completely and accurately. I will inform my dentist of any change in my health and/or medication

Patients's signature _____ Date _____

Recall Review:_____

1. Patient's signature _____ Date _____
2. Patient's signature _____ Date _____
3. Patient's signature _____ Date _____

Faculty inspection _____ Date _____

Fig. 2-1 Sample health history form from the Boston University Medical Center, Henry M. Goldman School of Graduate Dentistry. (From Boston University Medical Center, Henry M. Goldman School of Graduate Dentistry.)

B O S T O N   U N I V E R S I T Y   M E D I C A L   C E N T E R

Boston University
Goldman School of
Graduate Dentistry

**Division of Oral Diagnosis
and Radiology**

100 East Newton Street
Boston, Massachusetts 02118-2392
617 638-5129

Dr. Fred G. Boustany, Chairman

Medical Consultation

Chart No. _____

To: _____   Date: _____

Reason for Consultation

_____ states that s/he:

_____ is currently under your care

_____ will seek a consultation at your office

Patients indicates a previous or current history of _____

_____

_____

This patient will require:

_____ routine dental care (fillings, prosthetics, etc.)

_____ periodontal treatment (possible surgery)

_____ oral surgery (extraction)

_____ use of local anesthesia with vasoconstrictor (epinephrine _____/ml)

_____ general anesthesia

Would you please provide:

_____ brief medical history

_____ list of current medications

_____ precautions which need to be taken

_____ prophylactic antibiotherapy/dose

_____ other(s) _____

Dr. _____   _____
       Division of Oral Diagnosis and Radiology   Patient signature: patient consent to release medical
                                                                        information to be sent directly to BUSGD

Report of Consultant:

Name of Responding Physician (please print): _____

Signature of Responding Physician: _____

Telephone number if we have further questions: _____

Thank You

Fig. 2-2 Sample medical consultation form from the Boston University Medical Center, Henry M. Goldman School of Graduate Dentistry. (From Boston University Medical Center, Henry M. Goldman School of Graduate Dentistry.)

(This side for Boston University School of Graduate Dentistry use only)

CLINICAL PROTOCOL TO BE FOLLOWED AT BUSGD

Date established _____

_____

_____

_____

_____

_____

_____
Dr. Fred G. Boustany

Note:
This Clinical Protocol should be approved and reviewed with Dr. F.G. Boustany (Rm G104, x5129) prior to the initiation of any treatment at BUSGD. It will also be discussed at the treatment planning session.

Fig. 2-2, cont'd. For legend see opposite page.

to divulge such information without the patient's consent, and most physicians will not do so.

Blood pressure should be routinely measured and recorded at the initial visit of all dental patients. Because hypertension is usually asymptomatic in its early stages, undiagnosed hypertensive patients may schedule office visits for routine dental care with no knowledge of their condition. Although "normal" blood pressure is generally defined as 120/80 mm Hg for adults over 18 years of age, attempts at defining "high blood pressure" have been less productive and are largely based on empirical evidence. A diastolic measurement of 90 and/or a systolic measurement of 140 are generally considered the upper limits of normal; however, a single high reading, especially in the potentially stressful dental office environment, is not diagnostic. Malamed recommends that blood pressure monitoring be done over several visits in an effort to determine whether elevations persist despite efforts to allay anxiety.

The implications of managing the hypertensive patient in the dental office include the following:

1. The patient's increased sensitivity to vasoconstrictors used in local anesthetics and some retraction cord and hemostatic pellets.
2. In patients who are being treated for hypertension with adrenergic inhibitors, xerostomia and postural hypotension are common side effects. Xerostomia can have ramifications in terms of burning mouth and tongue, root caries, and retention and comfort of prostheses. Postural hypotension must be considered when raising patients from a reclining position in the dental chair.
3. Minimizing pain or stress should be a primary concern in managing these patients. Length of appointment, amount and type of treatment rendered, and special efforts in making the patient comfortable should be considered by all office personnel.

Bleeding disorders may be caused by primary disease processes such as hemophilia, thrombocytopenia, or hematologic malignancies. They may also be the result of secondary processes, such as anticoagulant therapy or cirrhosis of the liver. In some cases, bleeding can be a manifestation of an oral infection related to human immunodeficiency virus (HIV) disease. Associating HIV disease with a bleeding disorder should not be the first differential diagnosis considered when confronted with a bleeding problem but should be a consideration when other etiologies have been ruled out. The important concept is not just to manage the bleeding problem but to recognize the etiology so that other treatment steps may be modified as appropriate. History taking is again of paramount importance. Anticipation of bleeding difficulties enables the

Table 2-10 Service industries—annual receipts of taxable firms: 1980 to 1989*

1972 SIC coded†	Kind of business	1980	1985	1986	1987	1988	1989
70	Hotels, camps, and other lodging places	(NA)	45,867	48,106	54,136	58,864	61,090
701	Hotels, motels, and tourist courts	26,952	43,472	45,779	51,633	56,065	58,138
72	Personal services‡	25,133	39,367	42,848	47,039	54,074	59,553
721	Laundry, cleaning, and garment services	9,213	12,841	13,279	14,160	15,796	16,732
723	Beauty shops	5,798	9,028	9,673	10,639	11,733	12,992
726	Funeral service and crematories	3,491	5,203	5,408	5,668	6,116	6,218
73	Business services‡	(NA)	207,311	226,923	247,841	289,144	318,234
731	Advertising	(NA)	14,941	15,804	16,803	18,340	19,023
7311	Advertising agencies	(NA)	11,100	11,748	12,019	13,154	13,627
733	Mailing, reproduction, and stenograhic services	(NA)	12,932	14,087	15,827	17,771	19,385
7333	Commercial photography, art, and graphics	(NA)	5,727	5,914	6,690	7,312	8,149
734	Services to dwellings and other buildings	(NA)	13,303	14,648	15,649	17,472	20,101
7349	Cleaning and maintenance services to dwellings, and other buildings, n.e.c.§	(NA)	10,467	11,725	12,313	13,811	16,197
736	Personnel supply services‡	(NA)	17,680	19,993	24,044	28,576	31,626
7361	Employment agencies	(NA)	3,414	3,705	3,940	4,801	5,598
7362	Temporary help supply services	(NA)	11,175	12,691	16,331	19,870	21,626
737	Computer and data processing services	(NA)	45,165	50,587	56,004	66,443	74,083
7372	Computer programming and other software services	(NA)	21,026	24,030	28,110	34,780	40,530

*In millions of dollars (estimated).
NA, Not available.
†Standard industrial classification.
‡Includes other kinds of businesses, not shown separately.
§N.e.c., not elsewhere classified.
‖Excludes nonemployers.

dentist to control the situation rather than having the situation control the dentist. With proper preparation, many dental procedures can be performed without untoward sequelae, even in patients with severe bleeding problems. For patients undergoing anticoagulant therapy, the dosage may have to be adjusted for several days before and after the dental visit. It is usually best to try to accomplish as much routine dental work as possible within a given appointment to minimize repeated disruption of the patient's anticoagulant regimen. All adaptations of anticoagulation regimens should be decided in conjunction with the patient's physician.

Implications for management of patients with bleeding disorders in the dental office include the following:

1. Tissues should be as healthy as possible before beginning operative or surgical procedures.
2. Maximize visualization of operative site to minimize tissue trauma.
3. Obtain primary closure of tissue whenever possible and stabilize with sutures.
4. Protect surgical site from trauma.
5. Establish a system for follow-up to ascertain patient status and mechanism for referral if professional support is needed if postoperative hemorrhage occurs.

Table 2-10 Service industries— annual receipts of taxable firms: 1980 to 1989*—cont'd

1972 SIC coded†	Kind of business	1980	1985	1986	1987	1988	1989
7374	Data processing services	(NA)	15,158	16,414	17,022	18,868	19,959
7379	Computer related services, n.e.c.§	(NA)	8,981	10,143	10,872	12,795	13,594
7391	Research and development laboratories	(NA)	7,661	8,824	9,198	11,236	12,941
7392	Management, consulting, and public relations services	(NA)	38,543	42,304	44,252	52,528	57,324
7393	Detective agencies and protective services	(NA)	7,327	8,161	9,303	10,881	11,416
7394	Equipment rental and leasing services	(NA)	15,702	16,294	16,893	20,043	21,326
75	Automotive repair, services, and garages‡	30,547	51,804	53,898	58,278	66,201	71,392
751	Automotive rental and leasing‡	8,759	14,620	15,497	16,679	18,733	19,364
7512	Passenger car rental and leasing	4,691	8,776	9,368	9,978	11,169	11,714
7513	Truck rental and leasing	3,988	5,485	5,793	6,451	7,283	7,358
753	Automotive repair shops	18,077	30,587	31,599	34,182	28,530	41,942
76	Miscellaneous repair services	15,424	20,726	22,445	24,599	27,351	29,374
78	Motion pictures	12,509	18,850	20,948	24,834	27,424	30,606
781,2	Motion picture production, distribution, allied services	(NA)	15,063	17,033	20,778	23,271	26,134
79	Amusement and recreation services‡	(NA)	29,756	32,170	34,476	37,820	39,969
792	Theatrical producers, bands orchestras, and entertainers	(NA)	6,381	7,623	7,725	8,183	7,636
794	Commercial sports	(NA)	5,029	5,054	5,966	6,691	7,315
80	Health services‡‖	(NA)	146,517	161,604	182,289	204,251	221,692
801	Offices of physicians	38,754	66,767	72,600	83,812	94,395	101,733
802	**Offices of dentists**	**12,639**	**20,377**	**21,691**	**23,787**	**25,733**	**27,592**
804	Offices of other health practitioners	(NA)	7,864	8,791	10,340	12,022	12,437
805	Nursing and personal care facilities	(NA)	17,462	19,040	20,063	21,246	23,104
806	Hospitals	(NA)	15,724	18,068	19,720	21,740	22,685
808	Outpatient care facilities	(NA)	7,118	8,814	10,654	12,596	15,484
81	Legal services‖	(NA)	52,842	58,897	66,998	75,953	83,066
891	Engineering and architectural services	(NA)	49,306	51,319	57,051	62,881	73,631
893	Accounting, auditing, and bookkeeping	(NA)	21,241	22,911	26,612	29,695	33,303
4722	Arrangement of passenger transportation	(NA)	6,078	6,424	7,053	7,819	8,654
653	Real estate agents and managers‖	(NA)	31,257	34,859	38,145	42,121	44,052

The dentist and dental hygienist are sometimes able to synthesize individual pieces of data obtained through the medical history to identify patients with undiagnosed diabetes mellitus. Even in the absence of a family history (but certainly in the presence of a hereditary pattern), positive responses to questions regarding frequent urination (polyuria) and having to get up in the middle of the night to urinate (nocturia), feeling thirsty or tired much of the time, and recent history of weight gain or loss should alert the diagnostician to the possibility of diabetes mellitus as an underlying process. Patients in whom diabetes mellitus is suspected should be referred for medical follow-up.

Treatment of a well-controlled diabetic for most routine dental procedures does not vary from treatment of a nondiabetic patient. However, one must be aware of the following implications for management of diabetic dental patients:

1. Appointments should be kept reasonably short and should not interfere with normal meals. Skipping breakfast or lunch can lead to a hypoglycemic state.

Table 2-11 Medical assistance (Medicaid)—recipients and payments, by basis of eligibility and type of service: 1980 to 1988*

Basis of eligibility and type of service	Recipients (1,000)					Payments (millions $)				
	1980	1985	1987	1988	1989	1980	1985	1987	1988	1989
TOTAL‡	**21,605**	**21,814**	**23,109**	**22,907**	**23,511**	**23,311**	**37,508**	**45,050**	**48,710**	**54,500**
Age 65 and over	3,440	3,061	3,224	3,159	3,132	8,739	14,096	16,037	17,135	18,558
Blindness	92	80	85	86	95	124	249	309	344	409
Disabled‡	2,819	2,937	3,296	3,401	3,496	7,497	13,203	16,507	18,250	20,476
AFDC§ program	14,210	15,275	15,767	15,541	16,036	6,354	9,160	11,100	11,731	13,788
Other and unknown	1,499	1,214	1,418	1,343	1,175	596	798	1,097	1,250	1,268
Inpatient services in										
General hospital	3,680	3,434	3,767	3,832	4,170	6,412	9,453	11,302	12,076	13,378
Mental hospital	66	60	57	60	90	775	1,192	1,409	1,375	1,470
Intermediate care facilities										
Mentally retarded	121	147	149	145	148	1,989	4,731	5,591	6,022	6,649
Other	789	828	849	866	888	4,202	6,516	7,280	7,923	8,871
Skilled nursing facility	609	547	572	579	564	3,685	5,071	5,976	6,354	6,660
Physicians	13,765	14,387	15,373	15,265	15,686	1,875	2,346	2,776	2,953	3,408
Dental	**4,652**	**4,672**	**5,131**	**5,072**	**4,214**	**462**	**458**	**541**	**577**	**498**
Other practitioner	3,234	3,357	3,542	3,480	3,555	198	251	263	284	317
Outpatient hospital	9,705	10,072	10,978	10,533	11,344	1,101	1,789	2,226	2,413	2,837
Clinic	1,531	2,121	2,183	2,256	2,391	320	714	963	1,105	1,249
Laboratory‖	3,212	6,354	7,596	7,579	7,759	121	337	475	543	590
Home health	392	535	609	569	609	332	1,120	1,690	2,015	2,572
Prescribed drugs	13,707	13,921	15,083	15,323	15,916	1,318	2,315	2,988	3,294	3,689
Family planning	1,129	1,636	1,652	1,525	1,564	81	195	228	206	227

*For fiscal year ending in year shown. Includes Puerto Rico and outlying areas. Excludes Arizona, which has no Title XIX (Medicaid) program. Medical vendor payments are those made directly to suppliers of medical care.
†Recipient data do not add due to small number of recipients that are reported in more than one category. Includes recipients of and payments for other care not shown separately.
‡Permanently and totally.
§Aid to families with dependent children.
‖Includes radiological services.
Data from: U.S. Health Care Financing Administration, *Health Care Financing Review*, quarterly.

2. A liquid containing sugar (juice, soda) should be available in the event hypoglycemia occurs.
3. Local anesthesia may be used in reasonable amounts without concern.
4. Diabetic patients have a greater likelihood of enhanced response to acute infections or of susceptibility to infections because of circulatory compromise. Routine prophylaxis with antibiotics is not indicated; however, active infections should be treated with antibiotics to prevent spread.
5. Diabetic patients may have a slower healing

process than nondiabetic patients, so they should be monitored closely following periodontal or oral surgery.

People with conditions such as congenital heart disease, rheumatic heart disease, and valve prostheses require special consideration in the dental office to prevent bacterial endocarditis. Most patients with these conditions are aware of their cardiac state. Because few dentists include auscultation of the heart as part of the initial dental workup, the medical history must be relied upon for the determination of the condition.

Antibiotic prophylaxis should be provided to all

Table 2-12 Employed civilians, by occupation, sex, race, and hispanic origin: 1983 and 1989*

Occupation	1983				1989			
	Total employed (1,000)	Percent of total			Total employed (1,000)	Percent of total		
		Female	Black	His-panic		Female	Black	His-panic
TOTAL	100,834	43.7	9.3	5.3	117,342	45.2	10.2	7.3
Managerial and professional specialty	23,592	40.9	5.6	2.6	30,396	45.2	6.1	3.7
Executive, administrative, and managerial	10,772	32.4	4.7	2.8	14,848	39.8	5.7	4.0
Officials and administrators, public	417	38.5	8.3	3.8	519	43.9	10.1	3.8
Financial managers	357	38.6	3.5	3.1	472	42.7	4.0	3.7
Personnel and labor relations managers	106	43.9	4.9	2.6	128	52.6	6.1	3.7
Purchasing managers	62	23.6	5.1	1.4	110	25.9	4.7	3.7
Managers, marketing, advertising and public relations	396	21.8	2.7	1.7	514	31.0	3.3	2.2
Administrators, education and related fields	415	41.4	11.3	2.4	585	53.4	9.9	4.0
Managers, medicine and health	91	57.0	5.0	2.0	188	67.6	6.7	3.1
Managers, properties and real estate	305	42.8	5.5	5.2	451	43.5	6.7	5.3
Management-related occupations	2,966	40.3	5.8	3.5	3,906	50.4	7.1	4.0
Accountants and auditors	1,105	38.7	5.5	3.3	1,416	48.6	7.5	3.2
Professional specialty	12,820	48.1	6.4	2.5	15,550	50.4	6.6	3.4
Architects	103	12.7	1.6	1.5	157	20.6	2.1	5.8
Engineers	1,572	5.8	2.7	2.2	1,823	7.6	3.6	2.3
Aerospace engineers	80	6.9	1.5	2.1	112	3.7	3.3	1.2
Chemical engineers	67	6.1	3.0	1.4	67	15.3	4.6	6.6
Civil engineers	211	4.0	1.9	3.2	249	5.4	4.2	3.6
Electrical and electronic	450	6.1	3.4	3.1	571	8.5	3.2	2.2
Industrial engineers	210	11.0	3.3	2.4	199	11.5	4.9	1.1
Mechanical	259	2.8	3.2	1.1	310	4.9	3.2	1.6
Mathematical and computer scientists	463	29.6	5.4	2.6	853	35.7	5.7	3.5
Computer systems analysts, scientists	276	27.8	6.2	2.7	566	32.4	5.7	3.0
Operations and systems researchers and analysts	142	31.3	4.9	2.2	239	41.1	5.8	4.9
Natural scientists	357	20.5	2.6	2.1	413	26.9	3.9	2.7
Chemists, except biochemists	98	23.3	4.3	1.2	122	27.8	5.9	5.2
Geologists and geodesists	65	18.0	1.1	2.6	52	15.4	2.9	0.5
Biological and life scientists	55	40.8	2.4	1.8	77	34.6	2.9	2.1
Health diagnosing occupations	735	13.3	2.7	3.3	854	16.5	3.2	4.4
Physicians	519	15.8	3.2	4.5	548	17.9	3.3	5.4
Dentists	**126**	**6.7**	**2.4**	**1.0**	**170**	**8.6**	**4.3**	**2.9**
Health assessment and treating occupations	1,900	85.8	7.1	2.2	2,242	84.8	7.3	3.1
Registered nurses	1,372	95.8	6.7	1.8	1,599	94.2	7.2	3.0

*For civilian noninstitutional population 16 years old and over. Annual average of monthly figures. Based on Current Population Survey. Persons of Hispanic origin may be of any race.

Continued.

Table 2-12 Employed civilians, by occupation, sex, race, and hispanic origin: 1983 and 1989*—cont'd

Occupation	1983				1989			
	Total employed (1,000)	Percent of total			Total employed (1,000)	Percent of total		
		Female	Black	His-panic		Female	Black	His-panic
Pharmacists	158	26.7	3.8	2.6	174	32.3	4.7	2.2
Dietitians	71	90.8	21.0	3.7	83	90.8	17.1	5.3
Therapists	247	76.3	7.6	2.7	324	76.3	6.4	3.0
Inhalation therapists	69	69.4	6.5	3.7	63	52.5	12.5	2.7
Physical therapists	55	77.0	9.7	1.5	90	77.3	4.8	6.1
Speech therapists	51	90.5	1.5	—	63	88.6	3.3	0.9
Physicians' assistants	51	36.3	7.7	4.4	62	26.6	6.9	6.2
Teachers, college and university	606	36.3	4.4	1.8	709	38.7	4.3	2.4
Teachers, except college and university	3,365	70.9	9.1	2.7	3,936	73.3	9.2	3.7
Prekindergarten and kindergarten	299	98.2	11.8	3.4	431	97.8	10.1	5.3
Elementary school	1,350	83.3	11.1	3.1	1,489	84.7	11.0	3.5
Secondary school	1,209	51.8	7.2	2.3	1,220	52.6	7.7	3.4
Special education	81	82.2	10.2	2.3	257	84.4	11.8	2.2
Counselors, education and vocational	184	53.1	13.9	3.2	214	60.4	12.0	6.2
Librarians, archivists, and curators	213	84.4	7.8	1.6	212	83.3	7.3	2.2
Librarians	193	87.3	7.9	1.8	188	87.3	7.6	2.3
Social scientists and urban planners	261	46.8	7.1	2.1	374	48.6	6.4	2.7
Economists	98	37.9	6.3	2.7	122	41.3	4.4	3.5
Psychologists	135	57.1	8.6	1.1	210	54.0	7.7	2.5
Social, recreation, and religious workers	831	43.1	12.1	3.8	1,043	48.8	12.4	3.6
Social workers	407	64.3	18.2	6.3	527	68.1	17.6	4.8
Recreation workers	65	71.9	15.7	2.0	101	74.4	9.8	3.3
Clergy	293	5.6	4.9	1.4	336	7.8	7.2	1.8
Lawyers and judges	651	15.8	2.7	1.0	774	22.3	3.2	3.3
Lawyers	612	15.3	2.6	0.9	741	22.2	3.0	3.4
Writers, artists, entertainers, and athletes	1,544	42.7	4.8	2.9	1,921	46.0	4.5	3.9
Authors	62	46.7	2.1	0.9	82	59.2	1.3	0.4
Technical writers	—	—	—	—	65	48.0	2.3	2.8
Designers	393	52.7	3.1	2.7	534	51.5	2.8	4.3
Musicians and composers	155	28.0	7.9	4.4	170	31.5	7.0	5.3
Actors and directors	60	30.8	6.6	3.4	96	34.6	7.2	3.8
Painters, sculptors, craft-artists, and artist printmakers	186	47.4	2.1	2.3	229	50.7	2.7	3.8
Photographers	113	20.7	4.0	3.4	112	30.3	4.8	7.6
Editors and reporters	204	48.4	2.9	2.1	253	49.2	5.6	1.6
Public relations specialists	157	50.1	6.2	1.9	159	57.1	5.5	1.3
Announcers	—	—	—	—	51	13.6	9.7	3.7
Athletes	58	17.6	9.4	1.7	74	19.4	8.7	6.3

patients who give a history of these conditions, consistent with the currently accepted regimen of the American Heart Association (see Tables 2-13 and 2-14).

The most frequent issue the practitioners face in treating patients with damaged hearts is when they require that patients take appropriate antibiotics prior to dental treatment and patients respond that they have had dental treatment performed before and never had to take antibiotics. In this situation patient education is of paramount importance. When the dentist explains that it is in the patient's best interest to protect the heart from any potential effects of dental treatment, most patients readily accept the recommendation. Although it may be tempting to think that if nothing happened to the patient before, nothing will probably happen now, the dentist should be cautioned that once a significant medical (cardiac) history has been elicited, it becomes the dentist's professional responsibility to follow all appropriate precautions. However, the patient cannot be forced to comply. A case study will illustrate the point:

A nurse sought dental care at a major Boston teaching hospital. She reported a history of heart murmur that was found to be of the type that required premedication (that is, not "functional" or benign). She refused to take the recommended antibiotics because she said that on previous occasions when she had done so, she got a severely irritating vaginal candidiasis that took weeks of Mycostatin therapy to clear up. It was felt that because of her profession and level of education, she was competent to make that decision. An entry was made in the chart indicating that the recommendation of antibiotic prophylaxis had been made, the possible adverse effects of lack of prophylaxis explained, and that the patient understood. The nurse signed the entry, it was cosigned by the dentist, and treatment was rendered.

Other prosthetic devices besides heart valves, including artificial knees, toes, hips, ureters, and surgically constructed systemic pulmonary shunts or conduits, are being placed with more frequency. It is thought that each of these may be the site of a bacterial cluster and resultant bacteremia. Therefore antibiotic prophylaxis is recommended in these instances as well. For those individuals known to be susceptible to endocarditis, the 1990 American Heart Association recommendation is that antibiotic prophylaxis be administered for all and any dental procedures known to induce gingival or mucosal bleeding, including professional cleaning.[9]

Infectious diseases

The oral cavity harbors microorganisms with potential to transmit a wide spectrum of infectious agents. Dental professionals are therefore at risk for any orally transmissible disease from the blood and/or saliva of the patients they treat.

The three infectious diseases that are currently of greatest concern to the dental professional are hepatitis B, AIDS, and herpes, although the list of transmissible diseases is more widely encompassing (see box below). Each of these three diseases will be discussed in terms of etiology, tests available for diagnosis, risk of transmission, and recommendations for prevention in the professional context.

Hepatitis B. The disease is produced by a virus known as the Dane particle. This intact virus consists of an inner core (HB_cAg) and an outer coat (HB_sAg) and is highly infective. As little as 0.00000001 ml of blood can transmit the disease. Initial symptoms may include the following: vague abdominal discomfort, myalgia, diarrhea, jaundice (30% of cases), lack of appetite, and low-grade fever. *However, approximately 80% of individuals*

TRANSMISSIBLE DISEASES OF CONCERN TO DENTAL PROVIDERS

Hepatitis (types B, A, non-A/non-B, C, E, Delta)
Acquired immunodeficiency syndrome
Syphilis
Gonorrhea
Influenzas
Acute pharyngitis (viral or streptococcal)
Pneumonias
Tuberculosis
Herpes
Chickenpox
Infectious mononucleosis
Rubella
Rubeola
Mumps

Table 2-13 Recommended standard prophylactic regimen for dental, oral, or upper respiratory tract procedures in patients who are at risk*

Drug	Dosing regimen†
Standard regimen	
Amoxicillin	3 g orally 1 hour before procedure; then 1.5 g 6 hours after initial dose
Amoxicillin/penicillin-allergic patients	
Erythromycin	Erythromycin ethylsuccinate, 800 mg, or erythromycin stearate, 1 g orally 2 hours before procedure; then half the dose 6 hours after initial dose
or	
Clindamycin	300 mg orally 1 hour before procedure and 150 mg 6 hours after initial dose

*Includes those with prosthetic heart valves and other high-risk patients.
†Initial pediatric doses are as follows: amoxicillin, 50 mg/kg; erythromycin ethylsuccinate or erythromycin stearate 20 mg/kg; and clindamycin, 10 mg/kg. Follow-up doses should be half the initial dose. *Total pediatric dose should not exceed total adult dose.* The following weight ranges may also be used for the initial pediatric dose of amoxicillin: <15 kg, 750 mg; 15 to 30 kg, 1,500 mg; and >30 kg, 3,000 mg (full adult dose).

infected with the virus are asymptomatic and unaware that they are infected. People who are infected with the virus can transmit hepatitis B whether they manifest clinical signs and symptoms or not.

A group of tests have been developed to determine the presence in the blood of hepatitis B antigens and antibodies to those antigens. The presence of hepatitis B core antigen (HB_cAg) is associated with active viral infection and infectivity. The hepatitis B surface antigen (HB_sAg) appears before acute illness and usually disappears quickly. Antihepatitis B core antibody (anti-HB_cAb) is not protective, appears early in the illness, and decreases in titer in those who become immune. Persistent high titer indicates ongoing infectivity. Hepatitis B surface antibody (HB_sAb) does not appear for several months and then rises to a high titer in those who become immune. The e-antigen (HB_eAg) is associated with lower risk of chronic liver disease and lower risk of infectivity. Table 2-15 summarizes the way to interpret results of blood tests for hepatitis B.

Fortunately for dental professionals, a vaccine has been developed to immunize recipients against hepatitis B. Three doses are given to confer immunity: an initial dose, followed by a second dose at 1 month, and then a third dose 6 months after the first. Given dental personnel's high risk of contracting hepatitis B, it is strongly recommended that all dental professionals be immunized. The risks of contracting hepatitis B include not only the morbidity of the acute phase of the disease but also the possible sequelae of chronic carrier state, cirrhosis of the liver, or primary hepatocellular carcinoma.

Acquired Immunodeficiency Syndrome (AIDS). No single factor has affected the practice of dentistry since the early 1980s more than AIDS. The impact of AIDS is poignantly expressed in the following: "Once upon a time, no one in the world had ever heard of the acquired immunodeficiency syndrome (AIDS). Neither was the human immunodeficiency virus (HIV) known. That state of innocence has ended forever."[6]

Dealing with the HIV epidemic and its consequences may prove to be the greatest challenge ever faced by the dental profession. The manner in which dentistry responds to this challenge may, to a large degree, shape dentistry's future. This RNA virus has forced dentistry to reassess its ethics, legal obligations, and ability to protect dentists, staff, and patients from transmissible disease. It has exposed innermost fears and prejudices and clouded the ability to distinguish fact from fiction.

HIV is an epidemic that must be understood within its historical perspective. In June 1981 the

Table 2-14 Alternate prophylactic regimens for dental, oral, or upper respiratory tract procedures in patients who are at risk

Drug	Dosing regimen*
Patients unable to take oral medications	
Ampicillin	Intravenous or intramuscular administration of ampicillin, 2 g 30 min before procedure; then intravenous or intramuscular administration of ampicillin, 1 g or oral administration of amoxicillin, 1.5 g 6 hours after initial dose
Ampicillin/amoxicillin/penicillin-allergic patients unable to take oral medications	
Clindamycin	Intravenous administration of 300 mg 30 min before procedure and an intravenous or oral administration of 150 mg 6 hours after initial dose
Patients considered high risk and not candidates for standard regimen	
Ampicillin, gentamicin, and amoxicillin	Intravenous or intramuscular administration of ampicillin, 2 g plus gentamicin, 1.5 mg/kg (not to exceed 80 mg), 30 min before procedure; followed by amoxicillin, 1.5 g, orally 6 hours after initial dose; alternatively, the parenteral regimen may be repeated 8 hours after initial dose
Ampicillin/amoxicillin/penicillin-allergic patients considered high risk	
Vancomycin	Intravenous administration of 1 g over 1 hour, starting 1 hour, before procedure; no repeated dose necessary

*Initial pediatric doses are as follows: ampicillin, 50 mg/kg; clindamycin, 10 mg/kg; gentamicin, 2 mg/kg; and vancomycin, 20 mg/kg. Follow-up doses should be half the initial dose. Total pediatric dose should not exceed total adult dose. No initial dose is recommended in this table for amoxicillin (25 mg/kg is the follow-up dose).

Centers for Disease Control (CDC) reported through their *Morbidity and Mortality Weekly Reports* (*MMWR,* the disease status and policy reports of the CDC) that five young homosexual men had required treatment for *Pneumocystis carinii* pneumonia, an opportunistic infection previously seen almost exclusively in immunodeficient patients, such as transplant recipients and those under treatment for cancer. Its occurrence in five previously healthy individuals without a clinically apparent underlying immunodeficiency was unprecedented. These men also had cytomegalovirus (CMV) infection and oral candidiasis, further indications that they suffered from a "cellular-immune dysfunction relative to a common exposure that predisposes individuals to opportunistic infections."[31] One month later the CDC reported the occurrence over a 30-month period of an uncommon malignancy, Kaposi's sarcoma, "among (26) previously healthy homosexual men."[21] The CDC noted that the clinical characteristics of these cases differed from that usually seen with Kapo-

si's sarcoma, which had generally been regarded as a disease of elderly men. Again, the situation suggested a common underlying factor—immune suppression.[16]

In 1984 evidence implicated a retrovirus as the etiologic agent of AIDS and two prototypes were isolated, LAV (lymphadenopathy-associated virus) in France and HTLV-III (human T-lymphotrophic virus type III) in the United States, which were later shown to represent the same virus.[39] In 1985 serologic tests became available to detect the presence of antibody to HTLV-III/LAV.[39] The availability of this test had many and varied consequences. First, it permitted investigation of the prevalence of the virus, and these studies demonstrated that infection with the virus itself was more common than the clinical illness (AIDS) in populations with an increased incidence of AIDS. Second, serologic testing gave an opportunity to study the progression of the disease within populations. Third, with the ability to detect antibodies, it became possible to screen blood

Table 2-15 Interpretation of results of serological tests for hepatitis B

			anti-HB$_c$			
HB$_s$Ag	HB$_e$Ag	anti-HB$_e$	IgM	IgG	anti-HB$_s$	Interpretation
+	+	−	−	−	−	Incubation period
+	+	−	+	+	−	Acute hepatitis B or persistent carrier state
+	+	−	−	+	−	Persistent carrier state
+	−	+	±	+	−	Persistent carrier state
−	−	+	±	+	+	Convalescence
−	−	−	−	+	+	Recovery
−	−	−	+	−	−	Infection with hepatitis B virus without detectable HB$_s$Ag
−	−	−	−	+	−	Recovery with loss of detectable anti-HB$_s$
−	−	−	−	−	+	Immunization without infection; repeated exposure to antigen without infection, or recovery from infection with loss of detectable anti-HB$_c$

From Dr. Richard Whitman, Boston University Medical Center, Goldman School of Graduate Dentistry.

and plasma donations for the virus. Surveillance of health care workers exposed to the virus also became possible.

Thus in June 1982 there was a hypothesis that a sexually transmitted infectious agent was causing disease in homosexually active men,[1] whereas in 1992 there is an identified agent, a case definition, and a realization that groups other than gay men are being affected. This realization was responsible for the focus on prevention to move from risk groups to risk behaviors, gay sex being one, as well as the behaviors of IV drug use and multiple sex partners. There are clinically defined signs and symptoms, some of which are oral. There are markers available for the disease, and there is some treatment, but no cure or vaccination.

The HIV antibody test was licensed in 1985.[11] The test detects the presence of antibodies to HIV, not the virus itself. The test indicates only that infection with HIV has occurred, not health status. A person who has antibodies to HIV is referred to as *seropositive,* and one without detectable antibodies is termed *seronegative.* Seroconversion is said to have occurred when an individual's test becomes positive following some time period previous to which test results had been negative. It is important to note that there is a window period in which one may be infected, but during which the body has not yet responded to the virus with detectable antibody response. This time period can

range from 3 to 12 weeks after infection, although reports of 6 months or more have been made. The screening test used is the ELISA, or enzyme-linked immunosorbent assay. If a specimen is positive, a repeat ELISA is generally performed. A persistent positive is confirmed by a Western Blot test. Although both the ELISA and the Western Blot test for antibody, the Western Blot is considered a more sensitive assay. Therefore persons testing negative on the ELISA are considered seronegative (at least for that point in time), and persons with a positive test confirmed by a Western Blot are considered seropositive. For those in whom the results are indeterminate, the tests are repeated.

As of 1992, more than 200,000 cases of AIDS have been reported to the CDC,[4] and the estimate of those infected with HIV—that is, seropositive but perhaps without signs and symptoms of AIDS—is about 1.5 million in the United States. It took 9 years for the first 100,000 cases to be reported, but less than 2 years for the second 100,000. By the end of 1990, 100,000 people had died of AIDS, and now there is an AIDS death every 15 minutes. Although the HIV epidemic still affects gay and bisexual men more than other groups, the spread of the disease into the heterosexual population is becoming more evident. Epidemiologic studies have shown an increase among IV drug users and disproportionate rates among minority groups. In *Living with AIDS*,[23] the National Commission on AIDS reported: "As of June 1991, women accounted for 10% of all AIDS cases . . . cases among women are growing faster than AIDS cases among men." Children are becoming infected as well: Nearly 70% of all pediatric AIDS cases are related to the mother's exposure to the disease.

What does this mean to dentistry? Several salient concepts emerge from the data provided by prevalence studies employing the HIV antibody tests: first, the concept of "risk groups" is of diminishing usefulness for evaluating who may be at risk; second, the vast majority of persons with serologic evidence of infection have no symptoms of infection; third, 9 of 10 infected persons are unaware that they are infected. Thus, while risk groups become less distinct, the asymptomatic population continues to grow and increasingly consists of individuals unaware of their status. It follows that dentists are treating many unknown HIV seropositive patients. With this knowledge, it becomes obligatory that all patients be treated as potentially infectious for HIV. There is simply no scientific rationale for selecting out certain patients or groups of patients to be subject to particular infection-control procedures. These arguments provide the basis for the use of universal rather than selective precautions in infection control.

Universal precautions have the added advantage of being effective against other viruses transmitted by blood and saliva during the course of oral health treatment. Infectious diseases are not a new threat in dentistry. Although HIV disease carries with it stigmas and fears that are a new phenomenon, hepatitis B (HBV) has always been an occupational hazard. State, federal, and local regulatory and advisory agencies have caused dental health care workers (DHCW) to change the way they practice and to alter the environment in which they place themselves, their staffs, and their patients.

In 1970 Congress passed the Occupational Safety and Health Act, creating, within the Department of Labor, the Occupational Safety and Health Administration (OSHA).[10] The charge to the OSHA was to protect workers and ensure healthful working conditions for every worker in the United States. This act required all employers to provide to all employees "a workplace that is free from recognized hazards that are causing or likely to cause death or serious physical harm." Prior to finalizing the bloodborne pathogen rule on December 6, 1991, the OSHA relied upon this general duty clause to enforce the use of recommended guidelines to control the spread of bloodborne disease among health care workers. Once the CDC published its first infection control guidelines in 1982,[2] standards of care evolved for the dental profession. The early guidelines did not specifically address dental care but outlined suggested precautions to be used when dealing with patients with AIDS, such as the use of gloves, refraining from bending or recapping needles, the use of gowns, and the use of extraordinary care to prevent injury. In general, early in the epidemic, the CDC recommended use of procedures known to be appropriate for persons infected with HBV. The first actual recommendations for dental care personnel in 1983 stated that

1. Personnel should wear gloves, masks, and protective eyewear when performing dental or oral surgical procedures.
2. Instruments used in the mouths of patients should be sterilized after use.[3]

State-of-the-art infection control guidelines did not emerge until April 18, 1986, when the CDC published "Recommended Infection Control Practices for Dentistry."[36] These recommendations were based on the use of a common set of infection-control strategies to be used routinely in the care of all patients in dental practices. This represented the shift to universal precautions from selective precautions. Of special interest is the editorial note that "All DHCWs (dental health care workers) must be made aware of sources and methods of transmission of infectious diseases."[36] It was emphasized that disease transmission in either direction (patient to DHCW or DHCW to patient) could be minimized by following the infection-control guidelines. In addition, vaccination for HBV was strongly recommended for dental personnel as a supplement to, not a replacement for, strict adherence to universal precautions.

The next major guidelines for infection control in dentistry came in 1987[35] and 1988[41] from the CDC and referred, in part, to all health care workers but also, in part, specifically to DHCWs.

The CDC now made note of the fact, cited previously, that the antibody status of most patients would not be known; therefore, these recommendations were to apply to all patients and all health care workers who performed or assisted in invasive procedures. The recommendations included the wearing of gloves and other personal protective barriers such as masks and eyewear, the handling of needles and other sharps in such a manner as to prevent injury, and the management of specific exposure incidents with a potential for disease transmission. In the recommendations specific to dentistry, it was emphasized that gloves were to be regarded as single-use items. Handwashing, the use of masks, protective eyewear, gowns where indicated, disinfection of environmental surfaces, and sterilization of instruments were more fully defined. The precautions recommended for dentistry began to recognize that blood, saliva, and gingival fluid should be considered infective. Handpiece sterilization and infection control procedures for dental lab cases emerged as important issues for dentistry. All these recommendations became the basis for the OSHA bloodborne standard.

It also became apparent during this period (1988 to 1990) that DHCWs were themselves susceptible to becoming infected.[22] Indeed, two dentists were reported to have most likely seroconverted as a result of occupational exposure. By December 1, 1990, 40 health care workers had been reported to the CDC as being occupationally infected with HIV through a special study set up to monitor health care workers. Among them, 27 reported needlesticks and 6 reported blood splashes to the eyes, nose, or mouth. Subsequently, three have developed AIDS. This report may not represent the total number of exposed and infected health care workers because it may not include those not reporting an occupational exposure or infection. No DHCWs have been reported through this surveillance system as occupationally infected. Of a total population of 213,357 professionally active dentists and dental hygienists, the current estimate of dentists and dental hygienists with AIDS is only 209.[4] There are possibly up to 2,090 dentists and dental hygienists with HIV. The best estimates of risk to HCWs is 0.3% for HIV transmission and 30% for HBV transmission after percutaneous injury from an infected patient.[14] From the data

available, it appears that the risk to DHCWs is extremely low.

DHCWs had already recognized the potential to transmit disease. HBV transmission had been well documented from dentists to patients, as well as herpes transmission from dental hygienists to patients. Indeed, health care workers (HCWs), primarily physicians and dentists, have a threefold to fivefold higher prevalence of HBV than the general population. However, transmission from HIV-infected health care workers to patients had not yet been reported. Since the early 1970s, when serologic testing became available for HBV, the CDC had reported on 20 clusters of HBV transmission to over 300 patients from infected HCWs. In 12 of the clusters, the HCW did not routinely use gloves, and some reported skin lesions that could have promoted the transmission. Nine of these clusters were linked to dentists or oral surgeons. Many of the transmissions could have been prevented by strict adherence to current universal precautions. Most of the reports were prior to the acceptance of universal precaution. The CDC[34] suggested: "The limited number of reports of HBV transmission from HCWs to patients in recent years may reflect the adoption of universal precautions and increased use of HBV vaccine."

Previous experience with HBV transmission suggested that the performance of invasive procedures was more likely to contribute to disease transmission,* that the use of universal precautions was likely to reduce the risk of transmission, and that this transmission would be expected to "occur only very rarely."[35] Therefore routine testing of HCWs was not recommended.

When the inevitable became the actual with the first report of transmission of HIV from an infected

---

*From the Centers for Disease Control: Recommendations for prevention of HIV transmission in health care settings, *MMWR* 36(2S):6S, 1987. An invasive procedure is defined as "surgical entry into tissues, cavities, or organs or repair of major traumatic injuries" associated with any of the following: "1. an operating or delivery room, emergency department, or outpatient setting, including both physicians' and dentists' offices; 2. cardiac catheterization and angiographic procedures; 3. a vaginal or cesarean delivery or other invasive obstetric procedure during which bleeding may occur; or 4. the manipulation, cutting or removal of any oral or perioral tissues including tooth structure, during which bleeding occurs or the potential for bleeding exists."

HCW to a patient during an invasive procedure,[18] it was indeed in dentistry. The first report of a "possible" transmission to "patient A" came in the July 1990 issue of *MMWR*.[32] By January 1991 the transmission was no longer considered merely "possible," and the report then read, "Update: transmission of HIV infection during an invasive dental procedure."[40] The concept of transmission from HCW to patient had progressed from highly improbable to possible to probable in less than a year, and the involvement had increased from one to five patients. These events, leading up to the death of patient A, Kimberly Bergalis, left an indelible imprint on dentistry.

The public outcry over the first real victim of AIDS was deafening. Conservative congressmen called for stiff measures, from jailing infected HCWs who continued to practice, to mandatory testing of all HCWs. One of the most serious consequences of this event for the health care field in general is that the professional future of infected HCWs may not be under professional control. At a minimum, proposals range from reviewing the health status of infected HCWs (HIV and/or HBV) by expert review panels to mandatory testing and patient notification. By an act of Congress in October 1991, states were given 1 year in which to adopt the CDC "recommendations for preventing transmission of human immunodeficiency virus and hepatitis B virus to patients during exposure-prone invasive procedures" or else to come up with their equivalent and have it approved by the CDC. In essence, the CDC recommendations cited by Congress are based on a series of assumptions as to the likelihood of transmitting disease from infected providers to patients.

- Infected HCWs who adhere to universal precautions and who do not perform invasive procedures pose no risk for transmitting HIV or HBV to patients.
- Infected HCWs who adhere to universal precautions and who perform certain exposure-prone procedures pose a small risk for transmitting HBV to patients.
- HIV is transmitted much less readily than HBV.

The key phrase is "exposure-prone procedures," and the problem is how to define them and how and when to restrict their practice by infected HCWs. The task may have seemed simple at first,

with the plan being to have the professions determine a list of exposure-prone procedures. It proved, however, to be far from a simple matter, and professional organizations either refused to produce a list, were unable to come up with lists, or felt that it was not in their best interest to list these procedures. Data from the CDC were challenged during public testimony by, for example, the ADA and the University of Texas Health Science Center at San Antonio, which presented testimony offering that the rates of injury were lower than those estimated by the CDC and that, therefore, their assumption that 13 to 128 patients were infected with HIV and 406 to 4,057 with HBV by surgeons and DHCWs during an invasive procedure were incorrect (*The Nations' Health,* April 1991). A more accurate measure of provider-to-patient transmission potential is not possible until a much larger sample of patients on whom exposure-prone invasive procedures were performed can be studied. With more than 9,000 patient lookbacks, no other case of transmission of HIV has been discovered. In 9 years, only one cluster of cases has been linked to provider transmission. The CDC cites the risk from an infected health care worker, more specifically, a dentist, to transmit HIV to a patient is between 1 in 263,100 to 1 in 2,631,000 dental procedures.

The recommendations are under revision, but the states must still comply with formalizing their plans to deal with the issue of infected health care workers. Whatever plan a state adopts, it must be in compliance with statutes and court actions on discrimination and disability such as Section 504 of the Rehabilitation Act of 1973, the Americans with Disabilities Act of 1990, and any pertinent state laws.

It is important to note that the recommendations of the CDC are not regulatory, only advisory. Although they may set professional standards, they do not have full legal force behind them. However, these recommendations became, for the OSHA, the basis for the final rule on occupational exposure to bloodborne pathogens, issued on December 6, 1991. As an OSHA administrator remarked, "We are providing full legal force to universal precautions—employers and employees must treat blood and certain body fluids as if infectious. Meeting these requirements is not optional. It's essential to prevent illness, chronic infection and even death."[29] The U.S. Department of Labor expects this standard to protect more than 5.6 million workers and prevent more than 200 deaths and 9,200 bloodborne infections each year.

The purpose of the OSHA standard is to minimize occupational exposure to blood or other potentially infectious body fluids or materials that pose a risk of transmission of bloodborne disease in a health care setting. It covers any employee exposed, or potentially exposed, during the performance of his or her duties, to blood, body fluids, or potentially infectious materials. Health and safety are recognized as one aspect of practice administration. Although the OSHA obligates the employer to provide for the employee, free of charge, a series of hazard abatement measures to diminish the risk of exposure, they are in the best interest of each DHCW and will pay for themselves by ensuring a safe dental practice. Some costs are one-time improvements (e.g., an eyewash station) and preventive measures (HBV vaccination), whereas others, such as gloves and masks, are recurring costs. The OSHA estimates that the annual cost per dental establishment, of which there are 100,174, to be about $873. The highest-cost area is personal protective equipment followed by vaccination and postexposure follow-up. Some costs may vary, dependent upon the length of employment, turnover, and actual office experience with injuries.

The hazard abatement measures include mandating the use of universal precautions, emphasizing engineering and work practice controls, providing and requiring employees to use personal protective equipment, making available the hepatitis B vaccination (and associated tests and boosters) at no cost to the employee, making available specific procedures for employees who sustain an occupational exposure (including confidential medical evaluation and follow-up), and the communication of hazards to employees by warning signs and labels. The OSHA further mandates that the training provided relate specifically to information about the standard itself, the particular office exposure control plan contemplated, and information about the transmission of bloodborne disease. There are requirements on identifying at-risk employees and their tasks within the context of a written exposure control plan. This plan must be specific as to how the office will comply with the standard. Employers have recordkeeping requirements including written schedules for housekeeping, plans for waste management, and exposure management.

Some states have their own occupational safety and health plans that may differ from the federal standard. DHCWs should become familiar with their state plan and/or the federal standard as appropriate. It will also be necessary to review individual state and local regulations on infectious and hazardous waste management and disposal because there is no federal standard on dental waste as yet. The Environmental Protection Agency did have a pilot medical waste tracking act and will consider whether to make it national in scope.

The OSHA bloodborne standard is not the only regulation from the Department of Labor of concern to dentistry. In 1987, the OSHA extended the hazard communication standard to the health care industry.[30] The standard became final for the health care industry in 1989. The intent of this standard is to protect HCWs from hazards associated with the use of chemical agents during the course of employment. The standard is based on the simple concept that employees have a need and a right to know the hazards and identities of the chemicals to which they are exposed. Employers are obligated to identify and list hazardous chemicals in their workplaces, obtain material data safety sheets (MSDSs) for these chemicals, develop and implement a written hazard communication program, and communicate hazard information to their employees through labels, MSDSs, and formal training programs. Employees must understand what personal protective equipment is necessary to prevent illness or injury and how to manage an exposure incident or an emergency. Unlike the bloodborne standard, training in hazard communication must occur prior to an initial assignment. Training in both bloodborne exposure and chemical hazard exposure must be renewed whenever the hazard changes. Training is required to be specific to the agents used by an employee.

AIDS and HIV disease have generated a new set of professional standards for infection control, a series of federal obligations to meet these standards, and other federal regulations to deal with the chemicals we use in controlling infection.

However, HIV disease has also presented dentistry with the insidious issue of discrimination. In their 1990 report on AIDS discrimination, the American Civil Liberties Union (ACLU) noted that the most frequent complaints were against dentists and nursing homes.[13] "Dentists turn AIDS patients away," noted Mitchell Karp, a supervising attorney for the New York City AIDS Discrimination Unit. There are many reasons given for refusal to treat: low reimbursement rates by Medicaid, a lack of understanding about the disease, fear of transmission, fear of becoming known as an "AIDS dentist," prejudice, and more.

Some examples of discrimination include the following:

- A dentist who refuses to treat a young woman who is unwilling to be tested for HIV as a precondition for treatment.
- A man who, while under treatment in a private office, informs the dentist that he has AIDS; his treatment is completed and payment accepted, but later that day the dentist sends him a letter with his check and radiographs explaining he does not treat people with AIDS.
- A dentist who charges a known HIV-infected person an additional $75 infection control fee.
- A man whose brother has AIDS is denied dental care.

The Americans with Disabilities Act of 1990 provides a national mandate for eliminating discrimination against persons with disabilities. Dental offices are considered places of public accommodation for the purposes of this act and, therefore, must be accessible to persons with disabilities. This access is not limited to physical accessibility but includes the denial of dental services or the treatment of someone in a different manner based on a disability or perceived disability, which includes HIV status. In some states the discrimination laws are more stringent than the Americans with Disabilities Act, and one would be bound to comply with the state laws. Whereas dentistry once dealt with the ethics of advertising dental services and painless dentistry, now the advertisement of negative HIV tests by dental offices is becoming an issue. More than one dental office has advertised in print, by letter, or on a wall of the office that the staff has been tested and is HIV-free. Not only is this offering the patient a false sense of security but also it violates the employees' right to confidentiality and detracts from the real issue of practicing safe dentistry as a means of controlling disease transmission, which is the rationale for the use of universal precautions.

The oral cavity harbors microorganisms that have a potential to transmit a variety of infectious diseases. In addition, the trauma of some dental procedures and the mixing of blood and saliva enhance the risk of bloodborne disease transmission. Any patient's blood or saliva is potentially infectious and puts the DHCW at risk.

The major infectious diseases that are of greatest concern to dentistry are hepatitis B, AIDS or HIV disease, and herpes. There are other diseases, however, that pose a risk to the HCW. Of emerging concern is tuberculosis (TB), which is making a comeback in direct proportion to AIDS cases.

"Tuberculosis is a recognized risk in health-care settings."[19] A 1990 report by the CDC was prompted by outbreaks of TB over recent years, including some multidrug-resistant strains. Transmission is most likely from patients without recognized disease, not from those on anti-TB therapy. Estimates are that for every active TB case there are 15 asymptomatic, yet infected, people. Basic approaches to minimize transmission include reducing aerosols, identifying and treating those with disease, and monitoring HCWs and settings for infection. TB is spread by airborne particles, such as those produced by a sneeze, a cough, or while speaking. The risk of disease progression after infection is heightened in persons with HIV disease. Environmental factors, such as inadequate ventilation and contact with patients in "small, enclosed areas," can play a part in transmission. A dental setting can be an ideal environment for transmission. The use of face masks is advised; however, their effectiveness is uncertain. Strict infection control and sterilization of critical items and instruments are necessary to assist in preventing transmission. Health care workers who have positive tuberculin skin tests should be evaluated for risk of HIV infection. Tuberculosis infection may indicate a need to restrict duties and patient contact until preventive treatment is in place.

Hepatitis viruses that were not A and not B became known as NANB, non-A, non-B. The diagnosis of these were by process of elimination, either serologic, as with HBV, or by transmission, as with A. Diagnosis was not based on identification of an agent. One NANB has been identified as hepatitis C, a single-stranded RNA virus that appears to have cytopathic activity and is transmitted in a fashion similar to HBV, primarily through intravenous drug use (IVDU), by blood and blood products, and by multiple sexual partner encounters. Studies indicate that hepatitis C virus may be responsible for 90% of the posttransfusion hepatitis.[15] The clinical course of the disease is similar to HBV. At least 50% will, however, develop chronic hepatitis, and 20% of these chronic carriers will develop cirrhosis or even hepatocellular carcinoma. A screening test for HCV antibody has been developed; however, the test fails to detect 100% of infections. A supplemental or confirmatory test as is available for hepatitis B is needed to eliminate false positives and identify true positives.

Also of concern is delta hepatitis, a single-stranded circular RNA virus. Often referred to as the "delta agent," this is a defective virus that relies on HBV for its pathogenicity. It is a piggyback virus that cannot infect on its own but depends on the presence of HBV for infectivity. The combination results in a "supervirus" and a more fulminant course of disease.

Because many diseases can go undetected for long periods of time, the focus must be on preventing disease transmission from providers to patients, from patients to providers, and between patients and families. Again, it is important to emphasize that one of the most important personnel barriers is the HBV vaccine, so much so that the CDC has recommended its inclusion in the childhood vaccination series.[20]

Herpes. Herpes is included in the discussion of infectious diseases because of its high prevalence (antibodies to herpes simplex virus are present in 95% of the population). The route of transmissions may occur both from dental professional to patient and from patient to dental professional by way of saliva. Herpetic lesions may occur periorally, on fingers (herpetic whitlow), and in the eye. All these potential sites of infection are high-risk areas for the dental professional as a result of direct contact with saliva (fingers) or splattering forma-

tion, erythema, edema, lymphadenopathy, and low-grade fever. The most frequent complication of a herpes simplex infection is recurrence.

Diagnostic testing for herpes simplex may be done with a Tzanck smear, tissue culture, or fluorescent antibody tests.

Treatment of herpes is largely symptomatic, although research on the efficacy of two antiviral agents, acyclovir and idoxuridine, may provide valuable information on their application in recurrent oral herpes simplex infections.

PREVENTION: INFECTION CONTROL

Because treatment of hepatitis B, AIDS, and herpes is symptomatic at best, prevention of the processes is the most important aspect of the discussion of these diseases. Even if a curve were available, protection from the untoward effects and discomfort of each disease would be desirable.

The following recommendations should be used routinely in the care of *all* patients in dental practice to control the spread of infection:

1. Always obtain a complete medical history. Include specific questions about lymphadenopathy, recent weight loss, and infections. Follow up on all positive responses. Remember that an individual may not be aware of an infective state, so diagnostic acumen may be required.

2. Use protective attire and barrier techniques. To protect yourself and patients, wear gloves, surgical masks, and protective eyewear. Change gloves between patients to minimize the transmission of disease from one patient to another. Cover all surfaces touched by instruments or that may be contaminated by blood or saliva with materials impervious to fluids (plastic, aluminum foil) and discard these after each patient.

3. For routine dental procedures, handwashing with ordinary soap before gloving and after degloving is adequate. Handwashing is important even after gloves have been used because there may be small tears or openings in the gloves that would allow microorganisms to enter.

4. Use disposable needles. Do not recap needles; this will minimize needlestick injuries. Do not purposely bend or break needles. Dis-

posc of them in a special puncture-resistant container after each patient.

5. Decontamination of surfaces should be accomplished through a solution of sodium hypochlorite (household bleach). Dilutions of 1:10 to 1:100 have been shown to be effective. Caution should be used because sodium hypochlorite is corrosive to metals, especially aluminum.

6. All instruments should be scrubbed to remove blood and saliva before sterilization. It is recommended that heavy rubber gloves (household gloves) be worn for this purpose to prevent inadvertent skin punctures.

7. Disinfection or sterilization of instruments should occur at the highest appropriate level for the material in question. Use the autoclave, dry heat, or chemical vapor for metal and heat-stable dental instruments and immersion in boiling water for 10 minutes or an EPA-registered disinfectant or sterilant chemical for the exposure time recommended by the chemical's manufacturer for instruments and materials that cannot be heat sterilized.

8. Dental handpieces must now be sterilized as well. Manufacturers have responded to the need for increased levels of infection control by producing handpieces that can be sterilized, not just disinfected. Washington was the first state to require dentists to autoclave handpieces after each treatment.[33] In addition, the following items will require sterilization: low-speed handpieces, contra angles, prophy angles and nosecone sleeves, high-speed handpieces, hand instruments, burrs, endodontic instruments, air-water syringe tips, high-volume evacuation tips, surgical instruments, sonic or ultrasonic periodontal scalers and tips, and surgical handpieces.[33]

There are four basic types of sterilization methods available for use in dentistry: steam autoclave, dry heat sterilizer, chemical vapor sterilizer, and ethylene oxide chamber. The ethylene oxide chamber method is the most costly to purchase and maintain, has the largest "footprints" (i.e., the amount of floor space occupied), and takes the longest time per load to achieve sterilization, and

its use is generally limited to hospital operating room support. It is important to use biologic indicators to verify that sterilization has been achieved.[7]

Table 2-16 provides the currently accepted parameters for achieving sterilization under different conditions.[8]

These guidelines are meant to provide the reader with an awareness of the precautions that should become a routine part of the daily practice of dentistry. Variations on these basic precepts may exist within certain school, clinic, or hospital settings. However, common sense and good judgment will help each professional determine the best preventive techniques for each environment.

ENVIRONMENTAL FACTORS

The environment in which dentistry is practiced has changed dramatically over the past decade. Some of the issues affecting that change have already been addressed: demographics, malpractice, educational process, and health status of patients. Other issues that have had a major impact on the professional environment have been prepaid dental care programs, advertising of dental services, emphasis on cosmetic dentistry, and development of alternative delivery systems for dentistry.

Alternative delivery system is a term that describes the new settings for dental care that have evolved since 1980. Prior to that, the dental office was most likely located over the corner drugstore, in a home-office combination, or perhaps in a professional building. Since 1980, dental offices have appeared in retail settings—in shopping malls (within chain stores like Sears or Zayres) and in major downtown business districts as independently standing offices, not part of a dental-medical complex.

The alternative delivery system of dental care has had an interesting history. When alternative delivery systems first developed, dental students were told that the era of the solo practitioner had come to an end, the private practice of dentistry as a cottage industry was a thing of the past, and that the future was "retail dentistry." All dental patients would be given beepers to carry to let them know when the dentist was ready or when their child's treatment had been completed. They could shop at leisure before and after their appointment

Table 2-16 Summary of sterilization conditions

Sterilizer	Temperature	Pressure	Time
Steam autoclave (unwrapped items)	121° C (250° F)	15 psi	15 min
	132° C (270° F)	30 psi	3 min
Steam autoclave (lightly wrapped items)	121° C (250° F)	15 psi	20 min
	132° C (270° F)	30 psi	8 min
Steam autoclave (heavily wrapped items)	121° C (250° F)	15 psi	20 min
	132° C (270° F)	30 psi	10 min
Dry heat	170° C (340° F)		60 min
	160° C (340° F)		120 min
	150° C (300° F)		150 min
	140° C (285° F)		180 min
	121° C (250° F)		12 hours
Dry heat (rapid flow, unwrapped items)	190° C (375° F)		6 min
Dry heat (rapid flow, packaged items)	190° C (375° F)		12 min
Chemical vapor	132° C (270° F)	20-40 psi	20 min
Ethylene oxide	Ambient		8-10 hours

From Council on Dental Materials, Instruments, and Equipment: Sterilization required for infection control, *J Am Dent Assoc* 122:80, 1991.

in the mall, and parking would never be a problem. Moreover, because these new dental settings all advertised, a price war would erupt, patients would flock to the least expensive dentist, and quality care would become an anachronism.

A few years later, we see that the retail dentistry paradigm has indeed contributed to the practice of dentistry, but seemingly not in the way initial predictions foretold. In 1984 Friedman and others conducted a study funded by the American Fund for Dental Health to investigate what effect advertising had on dental consumers. New patients ($N = 3,287$) in offices that advertised were surveyed for their demographic characteristics and their reasons for having chosen the practice.

Managing a retail practice is more complex than managing a traditional practice. In that these locations are frequently open up to 14 hours a day (7:00 A.M. to 9:00 P.M.) and up to 7 days per week, the issues involved in hiring, training, scheduling, and retention of personnel increase exponentially. Quality control is always a concern in multiperson organizations. Initial capitalization of the operation can exceed $250,000, and monthly overhead is proportionally large. The areas of personnel management, financial management, and organizational administration are ones in which the dentist has historically had minimum preparation and experience.

Another alternative delivery system that has been developing is one in which dentistry can be delivered to the patient at home through use of portable dental equipment. These systems have proven especially helpful in providing dental services to frail elderly in their homes, to nursing homes that do not have adequate space for a permanent dental facility, and in rural settings where access to centralized dental care would otherwise be difficult. The systems are flexible, relatively inexpensive, and provide a good alternative to equipping a mobile dental van (which can cost in excess of $80,000). The ADA has prepared information on manufacturers of portable dental equipment.

A chapter on factors affecting the practice of dentistry would not be complete without addressing two additional topic areas: biotechnology and dentally underserved populations.

Biotechnological advances are pushing the active practice of dentistry into directions previously considered to be areas of experimental research for basic scientists: new applications of pharmaceutical agents in addressing better techniques for managing periodontal disease; development of new and better types of composite resins; utilization of resins in areas such as root surfaces and large posterior restorations, which were previously thought unsuitable for nonmetal restorations; the engineering of appropriate shapes and biocompatible metals for dental implants; and the integration of interactive computer graphics, computer-aided design, and computer-aided manufacturing (CAD-CAM) in the dental practice to enable inlays, onlays, and crowns to be fabricated and seated with a single appointment. The scope of the biotechnology and the challenge of biotechnology transfer are beyond the scope of this chapter; for more information, the reader is encouraged to read current dental journals and participate in seminars and courses. However, a summary of several dental CAD-CAM systems is provided in Table 2-17 to give an introductory overview of what lies ahead in dental armamentarium.[37]

THE FUTURE

In the past 10 years, significant changes in the style of dental practice have occurred. Fluoridation of water supplies, the increase in number of dental professionals, and dental health education have all had an impact on the incidence of caries. New emphasis is placed on cosmetic dentistry in addition to treating dental disease. The biotechnology of dental implants has provided a new dimension to the practice of dentistry. The practice setting is more varied, and advertising is now accepted as a normal part of many dental practices. An increasing number of women are entering the profession and it will be interesting to observe how their presence affects the educational process and the practice of dentistry. Our population is aging, and the medical complexity of the patients we treat is increasing, as is the sophistication of the patients and their dental needs. In many ways the practice of dentistry is even more closely linked to the practice of medicine than before. We must be vigilant in our knowledge of medical conditions, pharmacologic agents, and infection-control procedures.

As the turn of the century approaches, dental professionals will be challenged by new events, new research, and new discoveries. The pace at which new information is affecting the practice of dentistry is so rapid that no dentist can accept the awarding of a diploma and the granting of a license

to practice dentistry as the termination of the educational process. Taking advantage of continuing education opportunities on a regular basis is absolutely necessary. Many of the current techniques, materials, and approaches to patient care did not exist even 5 years ago. Through courses offered by dental schools or proprietary groups, attending professional meetings, reading professional journals, and informal sessions with local study groups, the dentist can keep abreast of new research, new methods, and new skills. Many states require documentation of *at least* an established number of continuing education courses as a condition for license renewal. The growth of the profession within the last decade and the changing demographics both within and outside the profession foretell a stimulating, challenging practice environment for the future.

Dental public health serves communities on a group-by-group basis rather than individual patients on a one-to-one basis.[5] Activities of dental public health workers include studying the epidemiology of dental disease and changing disease patterns; developing programs for preventive dentistry, such as sealants and fluoridation; establishing policies at local, state, and federal levels to improve the dental health of the nation; and increasing access to dental services for all, especially those who have been historically underserved and remain so. Who are the dentally underserved populations? Among the many who do not receive adequate, regular dental services are the following groups: those on low and/or fixed incomes (including the working poor, many elderly, and often college students); those with infectious diseases; nursing home residents; frail, homebound elderly; the homeless; runaway teens; inner-city residents, especially children; those for whom language is a barrier; residents of our penal system (jails, prisons, penitentiaries); those who do not know they have dental needs or care, even if they do know; and those who believe that it is a normal part of the aging process to lose their teeth. In reviewing this sample list, it should be very clear that large numbers of individuals need dental services. One of the implicit responsibilities of dental health professionals is to contribute some of their time and abilities toward the betterment of those who could not otherwise obtain care. Dr. Abraham Kobren,

Table 2-17 Dental CAD-CAM system comparison

	Cerec	Duret	Dux	Celay	Procera	Denticad
System configuration						
Data acquisition	Optical	Optical	Mechanical—on impressions, milling	Mechanical—direct acrylic	Mechanical—on waxup	Mechanical—direct
Fabrication	Milling + hand finish	Milling		Milling	EDM	Milling
System capabilities						
Restoration type	Inlay, onlay	Crown, inlay, coping	Coping	Inlay	Crown	Crown, coping
Material	Dicor,* Vita†	Dicor, Aristee‡	Titanium	Ceramic	Titanium	Metal, ceramic, composite
Design automation	Moderate	Moderate	Low	Low	Low	High
Data acquisition	<5 min	<5 min	<15 min + model	15 min + model	20 min + model + waxup	<5 min

Restoration design	<10 min	50 min	<5 min	Waxup	Waxup	<3 min
Fabrication time	<15 min + grind in occlusion	30 min	30 min	5 min	90 min	<20 min
Total time: prep-seated in patient	90 min	50 min	50 min + model	20 min + waxup	110 min + waxup + model	<30 min
Learning curve— new technologies	Optical impressions, CAD, milling	Optical impressions, CAD, milling	Mechanical digitizer milling	Milling	EDM, milling, digitizer	Mechanical digitizer milling
System costs						
Initial§	Mid	High	Low	Low	High	Mid–high
Operator	Clinician	Clinician	Clinician or technician	Clinician	Clinician, technician	No special expertise

From Rekow DE: Dental CAD-CAM systems: what is the state of the art? *J Am Dent Assoc* 122:46, 1991.
*Machinable Glass Ceramic, Dentsply International, York, Pa.
†Vita Porcelain, Vita Zahnfabrik, Bad Sachingen, Germany.
‡Aristee, Spad Dijon, France.
§Initial costs: low, <$50,000-$100,000; high, >$100,000.

past president of the ADA, stated that the public health dentist serves as the dental conscience of the nation.[5] Should not all dental professionals serve in that capacity?

REFERENCES

1. A cluster of Kaposi's sarcoma and *pneumocystis carinii* pneumonia among homosexual male residents of Los Angeles and Orange Counties, California, *MMWR* 31:1982.
2. Acquired immunodeficiency syndrome (AIDS): precautions for clinical and laboratory staffs, *MMWR* 31:1982.
3. Acquired immunodeficiency syndrome (AIDS): precautions for health care workers and allied professionals, *MMWR* 32:1983.
4. AIDS information hotline, Personal Communications, *BBC,* March 13, 1992.
5. American Association of Public Health Dentistry and American Board of Dental Public Health: Dental public health: the past, present, and future, *J Am Dent Assoc* 117:171, 1988.
6. As AIDS epidemic approaches second decade, report examines what has been learned, *JAMA* 264:431, 1990.
7. Council on Dental Materials, Instruments and Equipment: Council on Dental Therapeutics: Biological indicators for verifying sterilization, *J Am Dent Assoc* 117:653, 1988.
8. Council on Dental Materials, Instruments and Equipment: Sterilization required for infection control, *J Am Dent Assoc* 122:80, 1991.
9. Dajani AS and others: Prevention of bacterial endocarditis: recommendations by the American Heart Association, *JAMA* 264:2920, 1991.
10. Department of Labor, 1970.
11. Diagnostic tests for evidence of HIV infection. Project Inform, Supplement on Testing, San Francisco, October 11, 1988.
12. Dolan TA: Gender trends in dental practice patterns, *J Am Coll Dent,* 58:12, 1991.
13. *Epidemic of fear.* Report from ACLU.
14. Estimates of the risk of endemic transmission of HBV and HIV to patients by the percutaneous route during invasive surgical and dental procedures. Draft, January 30, 1991, The CDC.
15. *FDA Drug Bulletin* 20:9, 1990.
16. Follow-up on Kaposi's sarcoma and pneumocystis pneumonia, *MMWR* 30:40, 1981.
17. Forbes RJ: Shattering myths about the mature market, *Destinations,* April 1985, p 28. Reprinted by permission of *Destinations* and the American Bus Association.
18. Gebert B and others: Possible health care professional to patient HIV transmission: dentists' reactions to a CDC report, *JAMA* 265:1845, 1991.
19. Guidelines for preventing the transmission of tuberculosis in health care settings with special focus on HIV related issues, *MMWR* 39:RR-17, 1990.
20. Hepatitis B virus: a comprehensive strategy for eliminating transmission in the United States through universal childhood vaccination, *MMWR* 40:RR-13, 1991.
21. Kaposi's sarcoma and pneumocystis pneumonia among homosexual men: New York City and California, *MMWR* 30:305, 1981.
22. Klein RS and others: Low occupational risk of human immunodeficiency virus infection among dental professionals, *N Engl J Med* 318:86, 1988.
23. Living with AIDS, report of the National Commission on Acquired Immune Deficiency Syndrome, Washington, DC, 1991. US Government Printing Office, Superintendent of Documents.
24. Meskin LH: Where the women are or where are the women? *J Am Dent Assoc* 122:8, 1991.
25. *Money,* February 1992, pp. 67-72.
26. Nash DA: The feminine mystique in dental education: a feminist's challenge, *J Am Coll Dent* 58:33, 1991.
27. Niessen LA: Women dentists: from here to the 21st century, *J Am Coll Dent* 58:37, 1991.
28. *1992 AADS House of Delegates Manual,* p 49.
29. Occupational exposure to bloodborne pathogens, final rule, Department of Labor, OSHA, Part II, 29 *CFR* Part 1910.1030.
30. OSHA Hazard Communications, final rule, standards only, Department of Labor, OSHA, 29 *CFR,* August 24, 1987.
31. Pneumocystis pneumonia—Los Angeles, *MMWR* 30:250, 1981.
32. Possible transmission of human immunodeficiency virus to a patient during an invasive dental procedure, *MMWR* 39:489, 1990.
33. Ramirez L: Mandatory sterilization, *Dentistry Today* 11:18, 1992.
34. Recommendations for preventing transmission of HIV and HBV to patients during exposure prone invasive procedures, *MMWR* 40:RR-8, 1991.
35. Recommendations for prevention of HIV transmission in health-care settings, *MMWR* 36:2S, 1987.
36. Recommended infection control practices for dentistry, *MMWR* 35:15, 1986.
37. Rekow DE: Dental CAD-CAM systems: what is the state of the art? *J Am Dent Assoc* 122:43, 1991.
38. Solomon E: Promotion and appointment to administrative positions of dental school faculty by gender, *J Dent Educ* 54:530, 1990.
39. The HIV/AIDS epidemic: the first 10 years, *MMWR* 40:22, 1991.
40. Update: transmission of HIV infection during an invasive dental procedure—Florida, *MMWR* 40:21, 1991.
41. Update: universal precautions for prevention of transmission of HIV, HBV, and other bloodborne pathogens in health care settings, *MMWR* 37:24, 1988.
42. US Bureau of the Census: *Statistical Abstract of the United States: 1991,* ed 111, Washington, DC, 1991, Bureau of the Census.

3   Role of Auxiliaries in Dental Care

Demand for dental care and consumer awareness in the area of health services have been steadily increasing. The public is no longer content to view health care as a luxury, available only to those people who can pay the rising costs, but rather sees it as a necessary service that should be accessible and affordable to all. Increased demand places a strain on the traditional methods of health care delivery. This is especially true of dentistry, which has largely existed as a private-practice, solo cottage industry. With new emphasis on cost effectiveness and more efficient means of delivery, dentistry has little choice but to respond to the pressure from the public and professional sectors.

Several alternatives to increasing and upgrading the delivery of services have been proposed in recent years. Other professions have delegated services to the various auxiliaries employed in that profession or created new paraprofessionals who can assume duties formerly performed by the highly trained and educated professionals. The federal government provided impetus to this movement in the medical field with the Health Professions Act of 1976. This stimulated the emergence of the physicians' assistant and the nurse practitioner, who were able to provide more extended care yet remained under the supervision of the physician. Furthermore, the Health Professions Educational Assistance Act made a team approach to the delivery of care more feasible through the training and use of new health personnel.

To help the dentist in the delivery of dental care, three types of supportive care providers have evolved: the dental assistant, the dental hygienist, and the dental laboratory technician. Dental assistants and hygienists comprise almost two thirds of the dental work force. In 1988 the active dental labor pool consisted of 142,200 dentists and 268,540 dental hygienists and assistants (Tables 3-1 and 3-2).

A subcategory of auxiliary is the expanded function dental auxiliary (EFDA), a hygienist or assistant who has completed advanced training beyond the basic professional education. Most EFDAs have been trained through federally funded programs and, once trained, must work under the supervision of a licensed dentist. Their skills vary according to the program in which they were trained, and they are able to use their skills according to the state law governing their place of employment.[7]

Dental technicians are generally not considered auxiliaries because their work, in most cases, is performed in a private commercial laboratory rather than in a dental office. They work according to a written prescription or work order from a licensed dentist. Laboratory technicians who are working toward establishing independent professional licensure allowing them to provide care directly to the public are called *denturists*.

The cost and length of training of health professionals are factors that substantiate efforts to concentrate on the development of the auxiliary to increase health care services to the public. The average total undergraduate cost (tuition and fees) for all years of dental school is approximately $39,468 for state residents and approximately $58,788 for nonresidents.[5] In comparison, a dental hygiene education costs roughly $5,945, and a dental assisting education costs roughly $2,468.* Educational programs for the dentist take 7 to 8 years as compared with 2 to 4 years of education for the dental hygienist and 2 years or less of education for the assistant.

Dentistry has looked at its resources, the trained auxiliaries, as a viable solution to the problem of

---

*Average of total costs, to students in district from American Dental Association, Council on Dental Education, Department of Educational Surveys: *Annual report on allied dental education,* 1990-91.

Table 3-1 Estimated number of active dental assistants and number per 100 active dentists: selected years, 1950 to 1988

Year	Number of active assistants	Number per 100 active dentists
1950	55,200	70.0
1960	74,000	82.0
1970	112,000	110.0
1980	155,500	123.0
1988	197,000	134.0

From U.S. Department of Health and Human Services, Public Health Service, Health Resources and Services Administration, Bureau of Health Professions: Fifth report to the President and Congress on the status of health personnel in the United States, *Dentistry,* March 1986, pp 5-31; Seventh report to the President and Congress on the status of health personnel in the United States, *Dentistry,* March 1990, pp VII-18.

Table 3-2 Estimated number of active dental hygienists and number per 100 active dentists: selected years, 1950 to 1988

Year	Number of active hygienists	Number per 100 active dentists
1950	3,190	4.0
1960	8,800	9.8
1970	15,100	14.8
1980	38,400	30.4
1988	71,540	50.3

From U.S. Department of Health and Human Services, Public Health Service, Health Resources and Services Administration, Bureau of Health Professions: Fifth report to the President and Congress on the status of health personnel in the United States, *Dentistry,* March 1986, pp 5-30; Seventh report to the President and Congress on the status of health personnel in the United States, *Dentistry,* March 1990, pp VII-17.

providing increased and more efficient delivery of services. How to use these auxiliaries effectively has generated considerable conflict and controversy within the dental profession itself and is still far from enjoying a consensus of opinion.

How can the dental auxiliary be used effectively and efficiently to meet the health care needs of the public? Both auxiliaries evolved in response to unmet need in the dental care system and have continued to develop in accordance with need. To understand the issues, it is important to review the development of each auxiliary.

DENTAL ASSISTANT

The first dental assistant was hired in 1885 by Dr. C. Edmund Kells of New Orleans. Kells hired a woman as a "lady in attendance" so that female patients could respectably come to his office unattended. It was found that these individuals could be enlisted to perform routine dental office chores in the operatory as well as in the business office. Dental assistants continued to serve as office helpers until World War II, when there was a crucial shortage of labor to meet the dental care demands of the military service. Thus use improved in the armed forces, where assistants were trained to work at chairside in an attempt to increase productivity. Dentists who had trained with assistants retained the concepts of auxiliary use on returning to civilian practice.[18]

Dental assisting has experienced a number of significant changes in more recent years. The first was during the 1960s, with the advent of four-handed, sit-down dentistry, which necessitated that a dental assistant be actively employed in the delivery of patient care. Operatory design and the use of work simplification principles made for a more efficient method of working. In 1961 the federal government supported a grant program that was designed to train dental students to work using the concept of four-handed dentistry. Since that time, other programs have been developed and supported in an attempt to increase the use of auxiliaries.

The first organization of dental assistants, the Education and Efficiency Society, was formed in 1921 by Juliette Southard in New York City. Others began to form, and in 1924 the societies met together for the first time on a national level.[18] This organization, the American Dental Assistants' Association (ADAA) remains the recognized professional association of dental assistants. The ADAA met for the first time in conjunction with the American Dental Association (ADA) in 1924. Since that time, the two organizations, as well as the American Dental Hygienists' Association, continue to meet simultaneously at annual sessions.

The ADAA took as its motto "education, efficiency, loyalty, and service." From its beginning the organization has worked arduously at developing dental assisting as a competent and acknowledged component of the dental profession and at advocating dental health care for the consumer.

The need for educational guidance was recognized in 1930, when the National Curriculum Committee of the ADAA was formed. This committee consolidated in 1937 with the National Education Committee to become the Education Committee, which initiated a program providing official recognition of educationally qualified dental assistants—a program of individual certification. As a result, the Certification Board was established in 1948 to examine individuals for knowledge and skills in dental assisting. The board was established as an independent corporation because its interests might conflict with those of the ADAA. The two continue to work closely with each other, although each remains autonomous.

Originally there were two routes to becoming certified. One was the *grandmother clause,* which meant that with 10 years of work experience, a dental assistant could become certified on request. The other was completion of a 104-hour course in addition to 2 years of verified work experience. This extension course was the first attempt to standardize the education of dental assistants. The program was developed in cooperation with the Council on Dental Education of the ADA. The courses were at that time the only means of getting a formal education that was approved by the ADAA.

In 1957 the ADA House of Delegates approved the standard for educational regulations of certification of the dental assistant. These regulations established a minimum length of 1 year for a training program that was to be offered in an academic institution. These requirements are now reviewed and established by the Commission on Dental Accreditation, which includes representation from the ADAA. Maintaining and improving the quality of dental auxiliary education are primary aims of the commission. Programs accredited by the commission must be at a postsecondary educational institution. There are presently about 244 accredited programs varying in length from 1 to 2 academic years. Graduates of these programs are eligible to sit for the Dental Assisting National Board Examination (DANBE). Programs offer either a certificate or, in the case of a 2-year institution, an associate's degree in dental assisting.

At one time it was possible to challenge a seven-course examination that was given as an accredited extension program through the University of North Carolina at Chapel Hill. By successfully challenging these, candidates were considered to have adequately exhibited the competencies necessary to take the certification examination. This route to certification was deleted from the 1982 certification examination application.

In 1978 the Certifying Board of the ADAA (currently DANB) opened the examination for a 3-year period, from 1979 to 1981, to allow anyone with dental experience to take it. The rationale in doing so was to provide a data base reflecting the examination results of students graduating from an accredited program and of those who were trained on the job. It was also stated by the Certifying Board that certification is a credential that indicates a level of knowledge, rather than how that knowledge was attained.

Basic eligibility pathways for the certification examination for Certified Dental Assistant are (1) graduation from a dental assisting or dental hygiene program accredited by the ADA Commission on Dental Accreditation or (2) high school graduation or equivalent and 2 years of full-time work experience (3,500 hours) as a dental assistant.

DANB reports that 125,000 dental assistants have been awarded the designation Certified Dental Assistant. Specialty certification examinations are also available. They include Certified Oral and Maxillofacial Surgery Assistant (COMSA), Certified Dental Practice Management Assistant (CDPMA), and Certified Orthodontic Assistant (COA).

The Dental Radiation Health and Safety Examination was developed by DANB to enable states to comply with requirements contained in the federal government's Consumer-Patient Radiation Health and Safety Act of 1981, which requires states to institute certification procedures for dental and medical personnel who operate radiographic equipment. This requirement can also be met by passing the basic Certified Dental Assistant examination.

Because of the escalating importance of infection control in the dental office, DANB has developed an Infection Control Examination (ICE) "for voluntary use by dental assistants and hygienists to discern knowledge in infection control including OSHA requirements and recommendations by the CDC and ADA. The ICE is also available for use by employers and state dental boards for regulatory purposes."[8]

There are no baccalaureate programs in dental assisting at this time, although degrees are offered in related areas such as dental auxiliary education, nutrition, management, and health science.

For an institution's program to be accredited, the institution must first submit a written document to the Commission on Dental Accreditation (CDA); if approved, it will then be subject to an on-site visit from a team of professionals (usually dental assisting educators). Full approval is given for a 7-year period, after which reevaluation is necessary. Although the CDA is not legally recognized in all states, the certificate is currently the only nationally recognized credential available to dental assistants.

The profession of dental assisting has continued to express its goals and objectives through the ADAA. The ultimate goal of the ADAA is to strengthen the association and to achieve recognition for the dental assisting profession. Member services and benefits have been revamped and made more responsive to member needs. Health and life insurance plans and a loan program are available.

In 1985 the organization began an intensive marketing program aimed at expanding its market base and making continuing education a viable revenue source. Long-range plans address the need for development, production, and marketing of continuing education products.[12] These activities indicate the Association's current emphasis on education to keep pace with the changing profession.

As the profession of dentistry has changed, so has the role of the dental assistant. Dental assistants are taking a stronger position concerning their rights and responsibilities, and with a workforce of 197,000, that position will not easily be overlooked.

DENTAL HYGIENIST

With the growing demand for increased capacity in the treatment of dental disease, the dental pro-fession in the early 1900s began to seek what Dr. Alfred Fones termed a *subspecialist*, whose primary function would be to serve in the prevention of dental disease. Fones conceptualized this subspecialty as one of training in health care education and oral prophylaxis, completely uninvolved with the treatment of disease. In 1906 he put these ideas into practice by training his assistant to provide these preventive services for his patients.

Subsequently, Fones developed a course for dental hygienists that stressed the value of oral health care. More specifically, he emphasized health care for children consisting of prophylaxis skills and dental health education programs in the public schools. At its very inception, then, the dental hygiene profession had a bearing on public health dentistry.

Although Fones is often credited with the development of the first course for dental hygienists and assistants in 1913, the Ohio College of Dental Surgery had developed a program for hygienists and assistants in 1910. However, as a result of strong pressure from local dentists, the Ohio program was dissolved.

After the third year of his hygiene program, Fones advocated that the training of dental hygienists be based within recognized education institutions, and in 1915 the Connecticut Dental Practice Act required licensure for dental hygiene. Thus the dental hygiene profession became securely established within the parameters of the dental profession's licensing and educational systems.

The number of dental hygiene programs began to increase slowly, and in the 1940s all programs were required to be 2 or 4 years in length and based within a college or university. Table 3-3 shows the marked increase in the number of programs from 1950 through 1981. The table also shows that the number of programs hovered around 200 during the 1980s and that the number of graduates began to decrease in 1982-83. The 1990-91 ADA Annual Report on Allied Dental Education states that there are 202 dental hygiene programs, indicating that two have opened since the 1984-85 report.

By February 1947 the ADA Council on Dental Education developed requirements for the accrediting of a school of dental hygiene, and since 1952 accreditation by the ADA Commission on Dental Accreditation Programs has been required for all schools offering programs in dental hygiene.[16]

Table 3-3 Dental hygiene programs and numbers of graduates: selected years, 1950 to 1990

Academic year	Number of programs	Number of graduates
1950-1951	26	632
1960-1961	37	1,023
1969-1970	100	2,465
1974-1975	160	4,568
1980-1981	200	5,088
1982-1983	202	4,652
1984-1985	200	4,024
1990	202	3,953

From American Dental Association, Department of Educational Surveys: Dental students' register for each selected academic year from 1950 to 1951 through 1961; Annual Report on allied dental education for all subsequent academic years.

Today, 202 accredited dental hygiene programs offer a curriculum leading to a 2-year associate's degree or a 4-year baccalaureate degree. In addition, there are opportunities for advanced education. Several institutions have programs especially designed to offer dental hygienists master's degrees with specialized training in public health, education, research, or administration. At the same time, the controversial concept of preceptorship training as an alternative to formal dental hygiene education is being explored. Clinical training would occur in private, for-profit dental offices, with practicing dentists as teachers. Advocates of preceptorship suggest that it is a solution to perceived personnel shortages and unmet needs. Opponents of preceptorship argue that there are legal risks and that it would offer many opportunities for charges of malpractice.[26]

Until 1969 dental hygiene was the only dental auxiliary acknowledged in the state dental practice acts. Dental hygiene licensure is required by the state after at least 2 years of training, and the profession is regulated by the state boards of dentistry through examination for licensure and regulation of the delivery of care. The functions that a registered dental hygienist is allowed to perform vary from state to state.

The ADHA has been the representative of the registered dental hygienist since 1923, when 46 hygienists met in Cleveland to discuss common professional issues. From this nucleus grew the association, which, as of February 1992, had approximately 30,000 members.

The ADHA has taken noteworthy steps toward equipping the hygienist to assume a role in dental public health. The association's Division of Professional Development serves as a resource to the dental hygiene community by providing current information to individuals, academic institutions, and government agencies. It also provides support for association efforts to achieve its goals of promoting education, research, and career development.

Employment patterns of hygienists have been fairly consistent over the years. They spend approximately 78% of the workday providing direct care to patients, primarily in private dental offices (95%). Of those in private offices, 73% are in solo practices and 27% are working in group practices. The remaining 5% are occupied in a diverse array of settings such as state and local governments, neighborhood health centers, hospitals, dental and allied dental education schools, research facilities, and business and industry. Although the percentage of hygienists working outside traditional private practice is small, a goal of the profession is to increase access to oral health care for special groups such as the homebound, individuals in nursing homes, and geriatric and day-care centers.[23]

The reasons that the majority work in private practice are essentially pragmatic. The employment setting has been primarily defined by the needs of the dental profession, and hygienists will shift from this practice setting when there is an increased demand for their skills elsewhere.

FACTORS INFLUENCING DENTAL AUXILIARIES

Both internal and external factors impinge on the dental auxiliary (Fig. 3-1). Internally, the professions of dentistry, dental hygiene, and dental assisting have repeatedly clashed over responsibilities and role delineations. Externally, federal and state governments, as well as consumers, have taken an active role in providing input into dental service delivery, thereby affecting the function of auxiliaries in the provision of dental care.

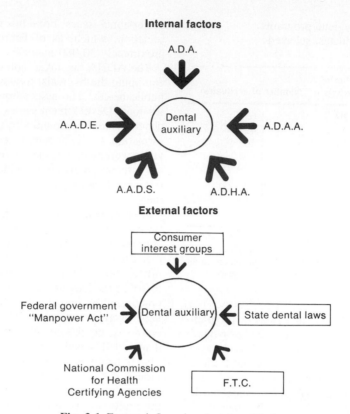

Fig. 3-1 Factors influencing dental auxiliaries.

Internal factors

Within the profession, the issue of auxiliary use remains who should provide what service.

A fundamental principle of auxiliary use is the realization that the dentist is ultimately responsible for the patient care provided and, furthermore, that there are aspects of a dentist's professional endeavor that should not be delegated to dental auxiliaries because these functions comprise the essence of the practice of dentistry.*

The dental auxiliary has been quick to assume that the dentist is anxious to delegate more repetitive functions to an auxiliary so that the dentist may be free to perform more advanced skills. In reality, many dentists may want to hold on to those

functions as their primary responsibility.[24] Many dentists perceive that the essence of the practice of dentistry is being taken from them by the specialist on one hand and claimed as a responsibility of the expanded-duty auxiliary on the other.

The dentist's attitude toward auxiliary use has vacillated. It can be reflected by the policies of the ADA between 1960 and 1980. The beginning of the 1960s was a time when professional policies, government support, and dental education focused on greater use of the dental auxiliary. The federal government's funding of dental auxiliary utilization (DAU) programs in 1961 met with such success in reducing the dentists' chair time that the ADA looked favorably toward research that would study additional methods of auxiliary use. In fact the 1961 House of Delegates of the ADA supported further research of dental auxiliary use and training.

As a result of this philosophy, various experi-

---

*Orientation remark by L. M. Kennedy, Chairman, Advisory Committee, Workshop on Dental Auxiliary Expanded Functions, sponsored by the American Dental Association, Council on Dental Education, Chicago, March 31 to April 2, 1976.

mental programs were conducted across the country at such institutions as the Forsyth Dental Center, U.S. Naval Training Center, University of Alabama, U.S. Division of Indian Health, University of Minnesota, University of North Carolina, University of Maryland, and University of Iowa. These research studies established that use of auxiliaries with expanded functions can increase productivity and quality of care and perhaps, contain the cost of dental care.

In 1969 the need to develop a model dental component for the impending national health insurance program was imminent and prompted the ADA to create the National Health Program Task Force. Its report supported a program that would experiment with the training and use of auxiliaries.

The following year, 1970, the Carnegie Commission Report reinforced the necessity to train auxiliaries by revealing the low level of health in the United States and by predicting a serious shortage of health care labor. The report proposed increasing the number of dentists and physicians being educated and providing funds for training programs that would expand the duties of auxiliaries. In light of these proposals, the ADA 1970 House of Delegates resolved that educational institutions should experiment with alternative methods of dental care delivery that use dental hygienists and assistants trained to provide additional functions.

To harness additional support for these programs, the ADA Council on Dental Education established the Inter-Agency Committee on Dental Auxiliaries. The committee was created to establish and support educational guidelines for the delegation of expanded functions to the dental auxiliary. This effort combined the leadership and resources of the various associations that are crucial to the education and regulation of dental auxiliaries: the American Association of Dental Examiners (AADE), the American Association of Dental Schools (AADS), the ADHA, and the Public Health Service, Division of Dentistry.

The Inter-Agency Committee concluded that more research was necessary to determine which auxiliary should perform what type of expanded function. Again, the necessity for research programs to evaluate efficient use of expanded-function dental auxiliaries was evident. The committee report concluded that the dental profession was more willing to delegate expanded functions for

auxiliaries than the individual state laws allowed.[2]

As the economy worsened in 1972, the attitude welcoming experimentation with expanded function auxiliaries changed. This gradual reduction of support was reflected in the ADA 1973 House of Delegates' resolution that the association stands in opposition to programs that permit a research program using auxiliaries to cut hard or soft tissues.

Finally, in 1975 a resolution passed by the House of Delegates[3] stressed "the termination of research in expanded functions and a return to traditional roles and responsibilities of dental auxiliaries." The dental profession's support for so many years in seeking alternative delivery systems by using expanded-function auxiliaries was ending, while at the same time the government, through the Federal Health Manpower Legislation (1974), was encouraging dental schools to develop new programs and to remodel present programs to train expanded-function auxiliaries. In agreement with the government legislation the 1975 House of Delegates of the AADS resolved that curriculum in dental hygiene schools should include instruction in all expanded functions, even though the legality of performing such functions varies from state to state. Such a curriculum would provide future graduates the flexibility to become licensed in any state and to perform the functions legalized within the state. More important, the AADS resolution highlights the professional dichotomy between dental educators and the ADA. By withdrawing support of programs that experiment with the delegation of functions to auxiliaries not legal within the state practice act, dental educators believe that the ADA is restricting academic freedom. During this period, while the ADA and the AADS were making these policy statements, the ADAA and the ADHA were vying with each other and with the ADA for recognition as the expanded-function dental auxiliary representative.

The authors of a 1979 ADA article reported that all study results showed that properly trained auxiliaries could provide the same quality of care for specific reversible and irreversible procedures as is provided by a dentist.[20] As the research programs proved that auxiliaries could perform expanded functions, the debate grew over *which* auxiliaries should have which expanded functions delegated to them. It was argued that dental assistants should be selected because (1) there are more of them,

(2) they are not restricted by licensing requirements, and (3) they command a lower salary than dental hygienists. The proponents for delegating expanded functions to dental hygienists argued that the hygienist (1) has a professional education, (2) is subject to licensure, and (3) is trained as a direct care provider.

The ADHA and the ADAA continue to represent their constituents in the battle over the right to perform various duties. Attempts to bring the dental auxiliaries together through their professional organizations to work on common issues was conceptualized in the form of an annual convention called Partners-in-Progress. However, after 3 years the meeting was curtailed because of a lack of cooperation between the associations.

While the auxiliaries discuss, debate, and dream about future roles, the dentist is no longer concerned about whether the auxiliary is capable of performing expanded functions, but whether these functions *should be* delegated at all.

The prediction of an increased demand for dental care faded during the 1970s with the postponement of a national health insurance program, a drastic drop in the birthrate, an increase in water fluoridation, and a sharp setback in the economy. While dentists became frustrated by their decreasing workload, the government was encouraging dental schools to increase the number of students or to develop remote sites for training by funding schools on a capitation basis. Traditionally in favor of these programs, the ADA and the AADE no longer supported the capitation program.[25]

When the number of dentists providing care exceeds the demand for care, the question of the delegation of duties becomes a moot point. As the economy worsens, dentists who find more free time in their work schedule start to perform the services that they used to hire hygienists to provide.

From 1960 through the 1980s there was a reversal in the policies of the ADA, moving from an invitation to experiment with expanded-duty dental auxiliaries to a moratorium on research and training in expanded functions and a watchful eye turned toward the number of dentists graduating from the dental schools. During these decades, the policies of the AADS, ADHA, and ADAA became more supportive toward examining alternative methods of providing dental care and increasing

available labor with the hope of ultimately providing optimal dental health for the public.

In the 1980s there was a decrease in caries prevalence, and the dentist-to-population ratio increased from 53.4 per 100,000 in 1980 to 58 per 100,000 in 1988.[22,23] The dental profession is grappling with the issues of an increased supply of dentists and a decrease in the rate of population growth, thereby taking the focus away from expanded use of auxiliaries. However, Table 3-4 indicates that a large percentage of dentists still rely on the use of auxiliaries. Dentists as well as hygienists and assistants are seeking alternatives to the narrow practice role of the auxiliary. The office job description may be expanding to include treatment coordinator,[11] human relations staffer,[13] cost containment advocate,[21] and manager of special patients, as well as general office manager.

From a public health perspective, it is difficult to discuss cutting back on the supply of dental labor—dentist or dental auxiliary—simply because the demand for care is not increasing. The need for greater access to dental care for people not previously receiving care or receiving insufficient care and the underuse of dental care systems are the real public health issues.

Table 3-4 Percent of independent dentists who employ auxiliaries: selected years 1955 to 1989

	Percent of dentists employing auxiliaries*		
Year	Dental hygienists	Dental assistants	Any type of auxiliaries†
1955	10.3	70.7	77.1
1961	15.0	76.7	82.6
1967	25.2	86.6	92.4
1972	36.9	90.2	93.6
1979	48.2	87.7	94.5
1981	50.7	87.2	95.5
1983	53.9	88.2	96.4
1988	57.6	91.4	97.1
1989	57.2	92.2	90.1

From American Dental Association, Bureau of Economic and Behavioral Research: *The 1990 survey of dental practice;* also prior reports of this series.
*Any of these employees may be either full-time or part-time.
†Includes dental laboratory technicians and secretary/receptionists, as well as dental hygienists and dental assistants.

External factors

The external factors that influence dental assisting and dental hygiene have continued to increase both in numbers and intensity. The dental profession has enjoyed relative autonomy until the past few years when various groups expressed interest in and a desire for input into all areas of health care. Dental auxiliaries have become a subject of controversy, caught between the conflicts of different interest groups. The factors that are involved in health care quality, labor, access, and cost are many. The ones that most directly affect the status of dental auxiliaries are federal government, state government, and consumers.

Federal government.

Program funding. The federal government has long played a role in the monitoring of health care delivery. One of its first efforts in dentistry was identification by Congress in 1950 of a dental labor shortage and the enactment of legislation dealing with that issue.[15] The major emphasis at that point involved the dental auxiliary in an attempt to increase dental care productivity through greater use of auxiliaries. The government began to support the development of programs that would promote the use of auxiliaries in expanding the dental work force capacity. The Dental Auxiliary Utilization (DAU) program was the first of its kind and was instituted in dental schools across the country. The program's primary purpose was to investigate the concept of four-handed dentistry and the feasibility of incorporating this type of delivery system into the practice of dentistry. When the program was proved to be sound and its goals of increasing productivity could in fact be realized, support for the program was gradually increased, until by the early 1970s, virtually every dental school had an operating DAU program.[3]

Two other programs sponsored by the federal government were training in expanded auxiliary management (TEAM) and expanded-function dental auxiliary (EFDA). Federal funding for these programs ended in the early 1980s, and most dental schools discontinued their efforts in this area of education.

Federal Trade Commission. The Federal Trade Commission (FTC) was originally established to monitor any violations of antitrust or fair trade laws. The Magnuson-Moss Act of 1965 gave the commission specific power to set minimum standards of conduct for an industry. This practice is the cause of much debate within the dental profession. The FTC has been conducting investigations into the provision of high-quality dental care at the lowest cost.

The independent practice of auxiliaries has been a major priority for the FTC. The FTC contends that to require dental hygienists to work under the supervision of a dentist unnecessarily limits the public's access to preventive care and may retard competition in the provision of dental services. If the FTC continues in its current path, auxiliaries may be more closely scrutinized to determine their role in providing competent, low-cost care.

National Commission for Health Certifying Agencies. This agency was formed in 1976 to establish criteria for professionals working in health areas. The ADAA and the ADHA are represented on the commission, which is involved in setting standards for certifying bodies that attest to the competency of individuals who participate in the health care system.[17] In April 1985, however, DANB relinquished its membership in the commission because it had not found membership of any direct value in promoting its examination programs and because of the high cost of membership.[9]

The issues of credentialing and educational requirements is an ongoing topic of debate. At a 1984 conference sponsored by the National Commission for Health Certifying Agencies, the ADAA president was informed of a move by the National Association of Health Career Schools to establish a new credentialing mechanism for their program graduates who cannot take the DANB certification examination unless they fulfill a 2-year work requirement. Rather than clarify the role of the dental assistant, a new credential could undermine the recognition of the CDA and legislative advances that have been established.[12]

State government. State governments have more direct control over the function and status of auxiliaries. Through the power vested in it, the state is responsible for the protection and safety of its citizens. Therefore the state hopes to ensure this protection by enacting laws that will prevent unnecessary harm to the public. Police power gives each state the right to enforce such laws. Thus state practice acts have evolved that would control the health professions, as well as other professions. These practice acts are intended to provide the general public with competent and standardized health care.

State dental practice acts establish minimum qualifications for and delineate the services performed by dental health care providers. In 1915 the state of Connecticut included a definition of dental hygiene in their state practice act. Since that time, every state in the country has written the practice of dental hygiene into its legislation with accompanying qualifications and licensing mechanisms. Despite the fact that dental hygiene statutes may vary from state to state, the educational and licensing requirements are relatively consistent. Dental assisting is not as universally defined, however, and state practice acts can be found that vary from a mere mention of a person labeled *dental assistant* to a person who is mandatorily registered, examined, and defined by statutes. The discrepancies in the boundaries imposed by state practice acts make the role of an assistant arbitrary, vague, and inconsistent.

The state board of dental examiners or board of registration is the appointed group responsible for enforcing a state's dental practice act. Members of state dental boards have traditionally been the gubernatorial appointments of nominees submitted by the state dental society. A board is theoretically representative of the state, not the profession. There has been increasing impetus to change the composition of boards in many states to include more representatives of the dental profession as well as lay appointees. It may very well be that the catalyst for more definitive and progressive state practice acts will be in the form of consumer board members rather than the dental profession itself.

State law also involves what is known as *sunset legislation,* which mandates periodic review of such regulating bodies as the professional licensing board. Therefore, even if the profession does not raise its own issues concerning the composition and function of state professional boards, they may be raised by the legislature itself. Depending on how states view the dental practice act, states may either give additional opportunities to dental hygienists or end licensing.

Dental hygienists have practiced under the supervision of dentists since the discipline was established many years ago. Legislation that would either modify supervision requirements or expand the scope of practice for hygienists has surfaced in Colorado and California. These state actions indicate a period of reassessment and change in the roles and responsibilities of dental hygienists.[23]

Consumers. As health care costs continue to spiral upward, efforts are directed toward finding a means of cost containment. In almost every area of health care it has been discovered that fuller use and delegation of additional functions to ancillary personnel is cost-effective and increases service provision. Naturally, the consumer is primarily concerned with having high-quality, low-cost care available to as high a percentage of the population as is feasible. One method that has been found to be appropriate in providing care on a local level has been the neighborhood health center. Some of these centers have operated successfully, free from professional control. Admittedly, there have been problems encountered when a center operates without adequately trained personnel, but many communities have found that their specific needs are best met when representatives of their own neighborhoods make the decisions through the actions of community boards.

Consumers have exercised more control in the delivery of dental care services through payment mechanisms. An increase in availability of care is a direct result of the growing variety of third-party payment plans.

Other external factors that have an impact on dental health care and its personnel include the increasing aged population and the acquired immunodeficiency syndrome (AIDS) epidemic (Chapter 2). The U.S. population is aging dramatically. By the year 2020, 18% of the population will be 65 years of age and older. Large increases in the demand for health services are expected.[23]

PLANNING THE FUTURE ROLE OF THE AUXILIARY

With an increase in third-party dental insurance and with the development of more alternatives to the traditional private solo practice setting, the dental auxiliary can be viewed in light of new roles and functions that may have a significant impact on the dental health of the public. In terms of function and capacity, these roles fall into three broad categories: community dental health advocate, educator, and dental care provider.

Community dental health advocate

Certainly the dental auxiliary can and should have a significant impact on and influence in the community in terms of promoting effective preventive dental care programs. The objectives of these programs include those aimed at achieving fluoridation, regular home-care procedures, periodic visits to the dentist, an awareness of nutrition as a factor in oral health, and screenings for oral cancer and hypertension.

The dental profession as a whole has made great progress since the time when simply sponsoring an annual National Children's Dental Health Week was deemed to be a sufficient contribution to the community's dental health. One of the indications of a more comprehensive approach toward improving the dental health of the community is the active role that the dental auxiliary takes in working with dental societies to secure political support for community fluoridation. Public acceptance of water fluoridation depends in large part on the dissemination of accurate information by committed dental health professionals and consumer groups.

With the signing into law of the National Health Information and Disease Prevention Act in 1977, which encourages the initiation and design of educational programs to help the consumer better understand qualitative health care, the auxiliary acquired another way to serve the community. Perhaps the most significant recent development in this area has occurred with the appointment of auxiliaries as members of the boards of registration in dentistry in several states. As board members, dental auxiliaries can help to establish rules and regulations that directly affect the delivery of dental care, as well as have a voice on such specific issues as licensure requirements and regulations of quality care (among others), which directly affect public dental health.

In addition to their service on boards of registration in dentistry, trained dental auxiliary personnel are needed to implement programs in public schools and to be administrators within the health components of programs such as Head Start, health maintenance organizations, health systems agencies, and professional standards review organizations. In the private sector, business concern about the rising cost of dental health care as an employee benefit is increasing, and the era of corporate-sponsored dental clinics and corporate dental health consultants cannot be far off. The dental profession's responsibilities to community needs and its increasing social awareness correspond to the expansion of the auxiliary's role as a community dental health activist.

Educator

The dental hygienist's or dental assistant's responsibility as an educator is well established. Traditionally, a young woman in a white uniform appeared in elementary school classrooms once or twice a year with a picture of Tommy Tooth and Old Mr. Tooth Decay. The presentation included toothbrush instruction, discussion of the process of tooth decay, and perhaps some reference to certain foods as recommended and certain others as not recommended. Today, with a command of modern educational methods and proven preventive measures, the corresponding presentation would include references to fluoride mouthrinse or tablet programs, home-care procedures, periodic dental visits, and more sophisticated nutritional counseling.

Perhaps the most significant trend is away from direct pupil contact and toward teaching and equipping the school nurse, the parent, the teacher of health courses, and even the classroom teacher and principal to convey the dental health message and to act as a dental hygiene model.

In the private practice setting, the auxiliary not only educates patients about their own dental health but also has the opportunity to inform the patient of the issues that are pertinent to the dental health of the community. The interaction between the patient and the auxiliary provides the best opportunity to answer questions and to present facts about such issues as water fluoridation, acceptance of expanded functions for auxiliaries, ionizing radiation, mercury toxicity, and the importance of screening programs for oral cancer and hypertension. When dental public health concerns such as water fluoridation become an issue in the community, the patient has already become an educated consumer and voter. By informing and educating each patient to facts about specific public health problems, the auxiliary can establish a powerful information network and thus effect changes within the community as well as within the individual.

Dental care provider

Rendering of direct dental care to patients falls into three broad categories: primary, secondary, and tertiary. Today the dental auxiliary is taking part in the provision of services that fall into the first two of these categories, with the possibility of providing care at the tertiary level in the near future. In addition to basic skills in prophylaxis, areas of primary care being provided by the dental hygienist or dental assistant include application of sealants, placement of interceptive orthodontic devices, administration of topical fluorides, and detection of oral cancer and hypertension.

From 1976 to the mid-1980s, the National Preventive Demonstration Program, administered by the American Fund for Dental Health and funded by the Robert Wood Johnson Foundation, was designed to provide preventive and restorative care to all children on a continuous basis. The program provided school-based preventive services for children, including systemic and topical fluorides, sealants, oral health education, diet regulation, and plaque control. With the advent of these types of programs, expanded-duty auxiliaries have been trained to provide these preventive services.

At the secondary level of care, the hygienist and the assistant may perform those expanded duties that are legal within the state where they practice. As consumer and professional acceptance of the delegation of additional expanded functions to the auxiliary increases, the public should benefit from an increase of available dental services.

Certainly, as the hygienist seeks alternative practice settings from those traditionally under the supervision of the dentist, the public will reap the benefits by receiving increased direct dental care. The concept was pioneered in California by Linda Krol (see case study on this page), who was the first dental hygienist to become an independent contractor. Krol established a separate office even though her work was under the supervision of a dentist. The alternative practice setting was de-

signed to solve the problems of patient load, insufficient work space, and insufficient dental hygiene personnel.[14]

In other areas the concept of the traditional private practice setting for the delivery of dental care is being modified to meet the needs of the public. Presently the law and regulations of some states allow hygienists to provide preventive services to patients in schools and institutions. Some of these patients would not normally receive care through the private practice system. This concept of the dental hygienist as a dental care extender is similar to the physician's assistant in medicine.

Case study: an alternative practice setting

A California dental hygienist, Linda Krol, was frustrated because new dental patients had to wait for 10 months until a hygiene appointment became available to see her. When office space adjoining her dentist's office became vacant, she discussed with her employer the possibility of her renting the office space and working for herself.

In California the state dental practice act requires that a dental hygienist perform services and practice only in a dental office or an equivalent facility approved by the state's Board of Dental Examiners. The two dentists by whom she had been employed for 13 years supported her desire to work independently on a professional level, and a contract was established between them. Because she planned to see patients of these dentists, the contract was an agreement by both parties stating the responsibilities of each party.

According to the Internal Revenue Service, this agreement designated Krol as an independent contractor. A copy of the contract was sent to the California Board of Dental Examiners for approval to remodel the adjoining office. The board approved the conditions outlined in the contract, contingent on the dentists' providing necessary supervision. Construction of three dental hygiene operatories, a laboratory, an office, and a reception room was completed, and the new office floor plan established the dental hygiene operatories closer to the supervising dentist than had previously been the case.

When Krol began providing services under the agreement, complaints came from members of the dental profession. Their concerns were that hygiene services were not being provided under the supervision and control of a licensed dentist. Finally, 13 months into her practice, Krol received a claim from the office of the state attorney general. Ultimately, this claim was set-

tled out of court on the conditions that Krol put on the door of her reception room the name of each dentist for whom she was contracting services; that 45 days before seeing a patient of a doctor other than the originally contracted dentists, the name of that dentist must be submitted to the board in writing; and that appropriate supervision and direction of services be maintained by the contracted dentist.[14]

In July 1986 an amendment to the Colorado Dental Practice Law that allows the independent practice of dental hygiene became effective. The ADA Commission on Dental Accreditation is challenging the amendment, and two patients with heart conditions are also plaintiffs in the case.

According to the amended statute, unsupervised dental hygiene practice includes scaling, smoothing, and polishing natural and restored tooth surfaces; gingival curettage; topical fluoride application; gathering patient history; oral inspection and dental and periodontal charting, and administering topical anesthesia. The law also allows the hygienist to own the hygiene office and to buy or lease equipment. Because dental hygiene education and accreditation are based on the fact that hygienists are supervised by dentists, the ADA is concerned that hygienists are not prepared to diagnose dental or periodontal disease or to monitor patients who need special care without the supervision of a licensed dentist.[19]

Although there are disputes over the establishment of the hygienist as an independent practitioner, each small advancement provides the consumer with another way of receiving dental care.

Alternative modes for delivering care may be modeled after examples in other professions. In medicine the Rural Health Clinic Services Act provides financial support for alternative practice settings. This bill sanctions payments by Medicare and Medicaid for care that physician extenders provide in remote health clinics and does not require the presence of a physician. If a similar policy is ever developed for dentistry, the dental auxiliary is well equipped to provide the labor.

Eventually, additional practice settings may be established in nursing homes, shopping centers, day-care centers, and other areas where previously the hygienist could not provide services without the dentist.

At the tertiary level the dental auxiliary is a likely provider of services with the expanded functions defined in the area of rehabilitation. The state

of Maine has passed a law in support of denturism, and as part of the educational guidelines the auxiliary must have completed a 2-year educational curriculum and be under the supervision of the dentist. The dental hygienist, who is already regulated in this manner, provides a ready resource for additional training as a denturist.

SUMMARY

Changes in the political, social, and professional climates affect auxiliaries and force more diversified roles. The political climate will play a major part in how involved the auxiliary will become in performing clinical tasks. For example, if Congress passed a national health insurance program including dental services, increased demand would dictate an increased need for service providers. The social trend would also promote expanded use of auxiliaries as the consumer insists on reasonably priced dental services. Societal trends have a great influence on where and how money is spent, and in the case of health care society is no longer taking a passive role. As a result auxiliaries may readily gain the support of consumer interest groups in promoting their cause.

The professional climate is the one most directly affecting the auxiliaries' role. As the number of dentists increases and the incidence of dental disease decreases, auxiliaries are looking outside the traditional practice setting for jobs. Two nontraditional areas opening up for auxiliaries are marketing and sales in the dental products industry and dental coverage review analysis in the insurance industry.

Underlying all these issues is, of course, the economic one. When the economy declines, everyone feels the pinch. Services that are not viewed as essential, such as dentistry, are historically the first ones sacrificed. Conversely, when the economy is strong, increased emphasis on dental care programs and services reflects prosperity. Dental research, education, and service provision are all dependent on the amount of public money available to support them.

There are interesting times ahead for dental auxiliaries—opportunities for greater involvement and growth at the same time as potential cutbacks in traditional practice opportunities. Auxiliaries will be best served by being articulate and outspoken advocates for themselves and their profession. Perhaps the real challenge and excitement will be in marketing their clinical and communication skills as a unique contribution to the dental profession.

REFERENCES

1. American Dental Association: Interagency committee report, *J Am Dent Assoc* 84:1027, 1972.
2. American Dental Association: *Report of the meeting of the House of Delegates, annual session,* Chicago, 1975.
3. American Dental Association, Commission on Dental Accreditation: *Memorandum,* Chicago, February 1980, The Association.
4. American Dental Association, Council on Dental Education, Division of Educational Measurements: *Annual report on dental auxiliary education 1985-1986,* Chicago, The Association.
5. American Dental Association, Department of Educational Surveys: *Annual report on dental education 1990-1991,* Chicago, The Association.
6. Boyer EM: *Dows Institute for Dental Research, College of Dentistry, University of Iowa, IA, Dent Hyg* 60:204, 1986.
7. Council of State Governments, National Task Force on State Dental Policies: Manpower utilization, *J Dent Educ* 43:85, 1979.
8. Dental Assisting National Board, *Certified Press,* 20:2, 1991.
9. Dental Assisting National Board: *Memorandum,* April 1985.
10. Dreyer R: RDHs in the dental industry, *RDH* 6:22, 1986.
11. Feinman RA: An auxiliary for the 1980s—the dental treatment coordinator, *Dent Econ* 75:70, 1985 (abstract).
12. Jespersen K: President's address, *Dent Assist* 55:37, 1986.
13. MacLeod AE: Independent management consultants, Halifax, Nova Scotia, Canada: dental assistants and productivity, *Oral Health* 74:71, 1984 (abstract).
14. Mayuga PW: Linda Krol: independent contractor, *J Am Dent Hygienists' Assoc* 53:169, 1979.
15. Meskin LH: Focusing on the future: the dental hygienist as an office manager, *J Am Dent Hygienists' Assoc* 5:9, 1979.
16. Motley W: *Ethics, jurisprudence, and history of the dental hygienist,* ed 2, Philadelphia, 1976, Lea & Febiger.
17. National Commission for Health Certifying Agencies: Bylaws, Article 2, Section 1, 1976.
18. Peterson S: *The dentist and the assistant,* ed 4, St. Louis, 1977, Mosby–Year Book.
19. Shanoff C: Colorado statute opposed by ADA commission, *Dent Today* 5:1, 1986.
20. Sisty NL, Henderson WG, Paule CL: Review of training and evaluation studies in expanded functions for dental auxiliaries, *J Am Dent Assoc* 98:2, 1979.
21. Smith HL: Cost containment in the dental office, *Dent Assist* 55:17, 1986.
22. U.S. Department of Health and Human Services, Public Health Service, Health Resources and Services Administration, Bureau of Health Professions: Fifth report to the President and Congress on the status of health personnel in the United States, *Dentistry,* March 1986.
23. U.S. Department of Health and Human Services, Public Health Service, Health Resources and Services Administration, Bureau of Health Professions: Seventh report to the President and Congress on the status of health personnel in the United States, *Dentistry* 11:17, 1990.
24. Waldman BH: Is dentistry's future threatened? *Dent Surv* 51:50, 1975.
25. Woodall IR: *Leadership, management, and role delineation: issues for the dental team,* ed 3, St. Louis, 1987, Mosby–Year Book.
26. Zarkowski P, Sheperd KR: Legal considerations and preceptorship: not to be ignored, *J Dent Hyg* 64:358, 1990.

SECTION TWO

Social and Financial Aspects of Dental Care

Although dental disease is prevalent and oral health a worthy goal, not all people avail themselves of dental services. There are many barriers to dental care; some relate to education, some to finances, some to cultural habits, and some to the dental care delivery system itself.

This section begins with an around-the-world view of dental health. Chapter 4 focuses on two international aspects of oral health: dental care delivery systems of countries with diverse socioeconomic and political conditions, and international health organizations involved in the promotion and improvement of oral health globally.

Chapter 5 concentrates on a specific population group, the elderly, and describes their particular dental needs. The elderly are the fastest-growing age group in this country and at present receive less dental care than younger adults. This chapter investigates some of the reasons for the elderly's lower use of services and public health programs that might better address their needs.

Chapter 6 discusses the financial aspects of dental care and dental health programs. It describes the methods of payment for dental care and the history of third party reimbursement in the United States. It provides detailed information on a variety of reimbursement mechanisms and a case study of how dental insurance premiums are determined.

4 International Dental Health

All of us, from whatever country, profession, and walk of life, share rather precariously this highly interdependent planet that revolves through space and time. . . . Now we must learn from each other in many ways, particularly in this century, when human activity has truly transformed the nature of life.[19]

Worldwide, dental care delivery systems vary greatly. The dental health care delivery systems of developed nations such as Japan, New Zealand, and the United Kingdom differ considerably from systems in developing nations such as China and Venezuela. How each system functions depends on the particular political, socioeconomic, and cultural factors. Dental care delivery systems are also affected by external forces, such as whether a country is at war. Consequently, improving and promoting oral health continue to be a major challenge. Dental health care professionals need to be aware of current and changing conditions that may affect dental care delivery systems throughout the world.

International oral health is of increasing interest to dental professionals. Many nongovernment organizations, professional associations, and government agencies are concerned about oral health. Each is a vehicle of opportunity for dental professionals to participate in the international arena of oral health. Frequently, professionals volunteer their time and talents to assist in the development, implementation, and evaluation of oral health care delivery systems and activities associated with the promotion and improvement of oral health worldwide. To be of help one must first develop an appreciation for and a general understanding of the different dental care delivery systems.

Oral health is not universally considered to be

an important aspect of total health. However, global measures of dental caries and periodontal disease indicate major dental health challenges.[50] To reach the goal of improving oral health worldwide, it is necessary to develop and maintain collaboration among professionals in all fields, not just in the field of dentistry. Planning, implementing, and evaluating any dental health care delivery system require a multidisciplinary approach including the behavioral, political, and social sciences, as well as the dental sciences.

The International Collaborative Study of Dental Manpower Systems in Relation to Oral Health Status Part I (ICS I) is a landmark cross-sectional study that focused on examining characteristics of dental care delivery systems and the effectiveness of particular characteristics in improving the oral health status of each participating country's sample population.[5,10]

This study, which took place between 1973 and 1980 under the sponsorship of the World Health Organization (WHO) and the United States Public Health Service, was a major undertaking involving nine countries: Australia, Canada, the German Democratic Republic, the Federal Republic of Germany, Ireland, New Zealand, Norway, Poland, and the United States.

The results, which were published in 1985,[5] provide information that can assist any country in the development, application, modification, and/or evaluation of its dental health services.

The International Collaborative Study Part II (ICS II) began in 1988. Although the study has not been completed, information pertaining to its nature was published in the June 1990 issue of the *International Dental Journal*. It is a continuation of ICS I, with the addition of three new aspects: (1) middle developing countries, (2) an elderly population, and (3) research into deeper and more refined sociologic relationships within prototypic dental care delivery systems.[28]

The accurate assessment of a population's oral health needs, promotion of oral health services, and consumer-oriented prevention activities have contributed to lower caries prevalence rates and more adequate dental treatment.[32]

In 1978 proceedings from the previous year's 2-day colloquium, International Dental Care Delivery Systems, were published.[23] More than 125 dental and dentally related professionals presented and discussed 15 dental care delivery systems from throughout the world. One important topic was the need for international collaborative efforts.[23]

A formal announcement of support from the International Association for Dental Research (IADR) for further collaboration between developed and developing countries occurred in 1980.[26] For progress to be made it is vital that major institutions not only recognize the importance of collaboration but also lend their support and mutual cooperation to a focused vision of promoting and improving dental health globally. International collaborative research is an area of growing importance. The WHO and the Fédération Dentaire Internationale (FDI) are leaders in this area.

In June 1990 important guidelines for oral health promotion programs for professional dental associations were published in *International Dental Journal*. The guidelines cover areas of "policy formation and dissemination; planning group; information gathering; goal setting; strategic planning; implementation; and evaluation." Common to all areas was the emphasis on adaptation rather than adherence. Although an individual association's needs may be different, all are similarly concerned that "oral health promotion can demonstrate the benefit of self-care and emphasize the consumer's responsibility for personal health."[11]

An oral disease prevention program needs a strategy specific to its population. Møller[33] stresses that this is necessary to the strategy's effectiveness, in that every situation is different.

This chapter focuses on two international aspects of oral health: (1) dental care delivery systems of countries with diverse socioeconomic and political conditions, and (2) international health organizations involved in the promotion and improvement of oral health globally.

FIVE COUNTRIES AND THEIR DENTAL CARE DELIVERY SYSTEMS
Terminology

Countries belonging to the first world are nations with developed, free-market economies such as Japan and the United States. All first world countries achieved significant industrialization levels prior to the start of World War I. Countries belonging to the second world are nations with centrally planned economies. All socialist countries are second world nations. Countries that do not fit first or second world characteristics include wealthy countries such as Kuwait, poor countries such as Bangladesh, complex economically structured countries such as Brazil, and extremely simple economically structured countries such as Paraguay.

The third world is comprised of nations with undeveloped or developing free-market economies. Third world nations have "economies which are neither fully industrialized nor centrally planned."[27] The roots of third world conditions are entwined and bound by the modern world's economic, political, and social requirements.

By the 1980s, the third world had been subdivided into four groups:

1. Organization of Petroleum Exporting Countries (OPEC), whose members include superrich nations with high per capita gross national product (GNP) such as Kuwait and Libya and nations with lower per capita GNP such as Indonesia and Nigeria.

2. Advanced developing countries (ADC), whose members (such as Brazil, Singapore, and South Korea) may show an exceptional average annual per capita GNP but demonstrate uncontrolled population growth.

3. Middle developing countries (MDC) show

adequate economic histories but cannot make a significant entry into the world's economic marketplace.

4. Less developed countries (LDC) include the poorest countries of the world. They represent 35% of the world's population, contribute 5% of the third world's exports, and have an average per capita annual income of $176 during the 1970s, with only a $4 per year increase thereafter.

In 1945 the United Nations counted 31 third world countries among its members. By 1980 the number had grown to 118. Some vital statistics of these countries include

- 49% of the world's land surface
- 51% of the world's population
- 3% of the gross global product
- 40 of these 118 countries are the poorest in the world
- 1.2 billion people live in chronic poverty
- 800 million people live in absolute poverty
- 460 million people are malnourished, half of whom are children
- 75% have no access to safe water
- 50% of urban households have minimally adequate housing

In 1980 developing countries represented

- 21% of gross global product (100% = $8.8 trillion)
- 25% of total world export earnings (100% = $1.3 trillion)
- 22% of world military expenditures (100% = $433.9 billion)
- 16% of world educational expenditures (100% = $365.5 billion)
- 9% of world public health expenditures (100% = $235.7 billion)

The Physical Quality of Life Index is a composite indicator of infant mortality, life expectancy, and literacy. In 1960 the third world had an index score of 39 years. Almost 20 years later, in the late 1970s, the index score increased to 57 years. During the 1980s the infant mortality rate in developing countries was 5 times higher than in developed countries. The average life expectancy in developing countries was 16 years less than in developed countries. Only 52% of the third world's population can read and write, compared

with 99% in developed countries. The average educational expenditure in developing countries during the 1980s was $18 per capita, compared with $286 per capita in the developed world. More than 850 million people in developing countries have no access to schools.

Population growth is the third world's greatest problem, and its control is its greatest challenge. From 1965 to 1974 the annual population growth rate peaked at 2.4%, compared with 0.7% in developed countries. From 1974 to 1984 the growth rate in developing countries was 2%, and it is anticipated that this rate will further decline. Between the years 1975 and 2000, 92% of the world's population growth will occur within developing countries, compared with 8% in developed countries. In 1984 the third world's population (*not* including China) totaled 2.354 billion people, representing more than 52% of the world's population. By the year 2000, developing countries are expected to represent nearly 80% of the world's population.

The third world has made some significant growth rate achievements for annual GNP (5.7% in 1980, 2.1% in 1986), agricultural production (3.2% in 1980), manufacturing production (6.9% in 1980), gross investment (8% in 1980), and national income reinvestment (25% in 1980). Unfortunately, however, these numeric achievements are only superficial indicators of growth for the third world. When per capita figures are calculated, these achievements seem less significant, and by the latter half of the 1980s development declined.

Nonetheless, the colonial history that is shared by all developing countries unites their pursuit of a new international economic order to include

. . . nondiscriminatory and preferential treatment for their manufactured goods in the markets of industrialized countries, more stable and higher prices for their commodities, renegotiation of their external public debt, codes of conduct for the activities of multinational corporations, more transfer of technology to less developed countries, and a greater voice in the management of the world's monetary system.[27]

Simultaneously, developing countries want to distance themselves from their colonial history. Independence from the "mother country" is a valuable accomplishment, but it does not ensure economic success. It is important for developing countries to unify their efforts in the struggle toward upward economic growth.

Political repression is another serious common denominator among many developing countries. Between the years 1975 and 1986, 25 countries endured violent changes in their governments. Most of these countries are small, economically depressed, and without traditional political structures. Nevertheless, 18 developing countries have undergone peaceful government changes, and 74 developing countries had no change in government.

Protectionism is another important issue in the third world. A country's ability to generate revenue from trade is directly linked to the country's ability to repay its debt. Third world countries owe a debt of $865 billion. Debt service payments alone amount to $100 billion. The world's banking system is tempered by the probability that these debts will be repaid and also by the amount of time it takes for repayment.

Professionals in various fields have their own solutions to the problems of the third world. Economists suggest ways to promote industrialization to improve a nation's income. Sociologists and political scientists believe that political and social reform must occur before economic conditions can change. There are many solutions to the problem, but with each it is important to keep the country and its integrity intact, including culture, religion, attitudes, and beliefs.[27]

Country profiles with an overview of dental care delivery systems

The dental care delivery systems of China, Japan, New Zealand, the United Kingdom, and Venezuela have been selected for detailed examination, based on a comprehensive literature review, the country's political affiliation and socioeconomic status, and the country's representation in the WHO's geographic regions. Information was also obtained from each country's consulate in Boston and/or the country's embassy in Washington.

Each country is described in terms of its geographic and demographic characteristics, government structure, and socioeconomic conditions. The dental care delivery system of each country is described by its population's dental health status, financing mechanism, use of dental auxiliaries, and structure of formal dental education. Although it is not my intention to neglect representation from some WHO regions, only half the regions are represented: the Americas, the European region, and the Western Pacific region. The African and the Southeast Asia regions contain primarily third world countries, and current, relevant information pertaining to many of the Eastern Mediterranean region countries could not be obtained as a result of recent warfare in the Middle East. Therefore countries from these regions were excluded from examination.

Table 4-1 Characteristics of selected countries

Country	Area (square miles)	Estimated population (1990)	Population per square mile	Form of government	Capital and dominant language
China	3,706,564	1,133,682,511	306	Socialist republic (communist)	Beijing Chinese dialects
Japan	143,750	122,739,706	858	Constitutional monarchy	Tokyo Japanese
New Zealand	103,736	3,295,866	32	Parliamentary state	Wellington English and Maori
United Kingdom	94,525	57,365,665	610	Constitutional monarchy	London English
Venezuela	352,143	19,698,104	56	Federal republic	Caracas Spanish

Tables 4-1 and 4-2 present introductory information. Refer also to Table 4-3 and Figs. 4-1 to 4-6.

China. China is a Communist Socialist Republic and a third world country. Beijing, the capital city, is located in the eastern coastal section of the country. China is bordered by the Yellow Sea and the East China Sea to the east; North Korea to the northeast; Russia and Mongolia to the north; Kazakhstan, Kirghizia, Tadzhikistan, Afghanistan, Pakistan, Nepal, India, and Bhutan to the west;

and Myanmar, Laos, Vietnam, and the South China Sea to the south. China is a member state in the Western Pacific region of the WHO.

China is similar in size, although not in population, to the United States. There are presently approximately 1.133 billion people in China. By the year 2000, an estimated 1.3 billion people will be living in China. No other single country has a larger population. Life expectancy for those born in the year 1990 is 69.66 years, and in the year 2000 it is estimated to be 72.41 years. The infant

Text continued on p. 88.

Table 4-2 Fluoridation status of selected countries (as of June 1, 1989)

Country	Population using fluoridated water (in thousands)	1988 population (in thousands)	Percent of population on fluoridated water	Source
China	Not available	1,888,169	Not available	
Japan	Not available	122,626	Not available	
New Zealand	18	3,343	0.54%	CDC 1986
United Kingdom	80	56,936	0.14%	BFS 1988
Venezuela	49	18,776	0.26%	PAHO 1988

CDC, Centers for Disease Control-fluoridation census; *BFS*, British Fluoridation Society; *PAHO*, Pan American Health Organization.

Table 4-3 Health statistics (data for 1988)

	China	Japan	New Zealand	United Kingdom	Venezuela
Male life expectancy (years)	68	75	71	72	66
Female life expectancy (years)	68	80	77	77	73
Crude birth rate	21/1,000	11.4/1,000	16.3/1,000	13.3/1,000	29/1,000
Crude death rate	7/1,000	6.2/1,000	8.3/1,000	11.6/1,000	4.6/1,000
Infant mortality	44.3/1,000	5.2/1,000	10.8/1,000	9.5/1,000	36/1,000
Hospitals	66,662	9,483	318	2,262	444
Population per hospital	16,324	13,041	18,513	25,171	42,288
Hospital beds	2,109,571	1,401,999	23,052	426,594	41,386
Population per hospital bed	516	87	145	133	454
Physicians	587,564	161,260	5,210	Not available	14,771
Population per physician	1,852	760	642	Not available	1,271
Dentists	Not available	55,600	1,160	8,522	4,342
Population per dentist	Not available	2,282	2,882	6,681	4,324
Pharmacists	33,541	99,326	2,300	13,598	3,187
Population per pharmacist	32,443	1,235	1,453	4,187	5,891
Nursing personnel	849,652	560,108	22,000	272,384	38,061
Population per nurse	1,281	219	152	209	493

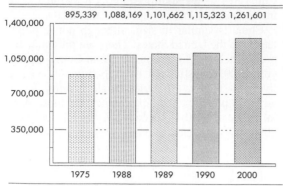

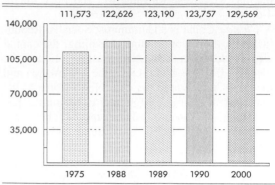

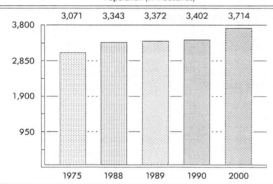

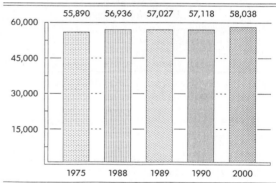

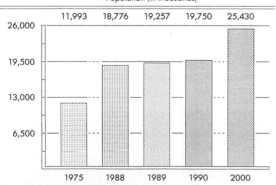

Fig. 4-1 A to **E,** Population statistics for 1975, 1988, 1989, and 2000. Data are from 1988 for annual population growth, population density, and population doubling time. (From PC Globe, Inc., Tempe, Arizona.)

CHINA
Age Distribution

Age	% of Pop'n	Male	Female	% of Pop'n	Age
70+	1.2%			1.6%	70+
60-69	2.4%			2.5%	60-69
50-59	3.9%			3.5%	50-59
40-49	5.1%			4.5%	40-49
30-39	6.6%			6.0%	30-39
20-29	8.5%			8.1%	20-29
10-19	13.1%			12.5%	10-19
0-9	10.6%			9.9%	0-9

160,000   80,000   0   80,000   160,000
(in thousands)

- Total population: 1,088,169,000
- Total male population: 559,319,000
- Total female population: 528,850,000
- Literacy rate: 75%
- Urbanization: 41.4%

JAPAN
Age Distribution

Age	% of Pop'n	Male	Female	% of Pop'n	Age
70+	2.7%			4.1%	70+
60-69	3.4%			4.5%	60-69
50-59	6.1%			6.3%	50-59
40-49	7.1%			7.2%	40-49
30-39	8.2%			8.1%	30-39
20-29	6.7%			6.5%	20-29
10-19	8.1%			7.7%	10-19
0-9	6.8%			6.5%	0-9

12,000   6,000   0   6,000   12,000
(in thousands)

- Total population: 122,626,000
- Total male population: 60,209,000
- Total female population: 62,417,000
- Literacy rate: 99%
- Urbanization: 76.7%

NEW ZEALAND
Age Distribution

Age	% of Pop'n	Male	Female	% of Pop'n	Age
70+	2.7%			4.1%	70+
60-69	3.6%			4.1%	60-69
50-59	4.5%			4.4%	50-59
40-49	5.4%			5.3%	40-49
30-39	7.4%			7.5%	30-39
20-29	8.6%			8.4%	20-29
10-19	9.4%			9.0%	10-19
0-9	8.0%			7.6%	0-9

320   160   0   160   320
(in thousands)

- Total population: 3,343,000
- Total male population: 1,658,000
- Total female population: 1,685,000
- Literacy rate: 99%
- Urbanization: 83.5%

UNITED KINGDOM
Age Distribution

Age	% of Pop'n	Male	Female	% of Pop'n	Age
70+	3.9%			6.7%	70+
60-69	4.7%			5.4%	60-69
50-59	5.3%			5.5%	50-59
40-49	5.9%			5.8%	40-49
30-39	7.0%			7.0%	30-39
20-29	7.9%			7.7%	20-29
10-19	7.6%			7.2%	10-19
0-9	6.4%			6.0%	0-9

4,600   2,300   0   2,300   4,600
(in thousands)

- Total population: 56,936,000
- Total male population: 27,728,000
- Total female population: 29,208,000
- Literacy rate: 99%
- Urbanization: 91.5%

VENEZUELA
Age Distribution

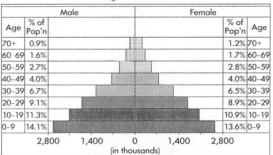

Age	% of Pop'n	Male	Female	% of Pop'n	Age
70+	0.9%			1.2%	70+
60-69	1.6%			1.7%	60-69
50-59	2.7%			2.8%	50-59
40-49	4.0%			4.0%	40-49
30-39	6.7%			6.5%	30-39
20-29	9.1%			8.9%	20-29
10-19	11.3%			10.9%	10-19
0-9	14.1%			13.6%	0-9

2,800   1,400   0   1,400   2,800
(in thousands)

- Total population: 18,776,000
- Total male population: 9,463,000
- Total female population: 9,313,000
- Literacy rate: 86%
- Urbanization: 82.3%

Fig. 4-2 A to **E,** Age distributions. Data are from 1988 for total population, total male population, total female population, literacy rate, and urbanization. (From PC Globe, Inc., Tempe, Arizona.)

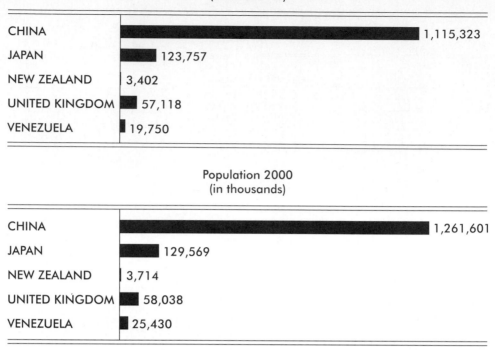

Fig. 4-3 **A** and **B,** Population comparisons: 1990 and 2000. (From PC Globe, Inc., Tempe, Arizona.)

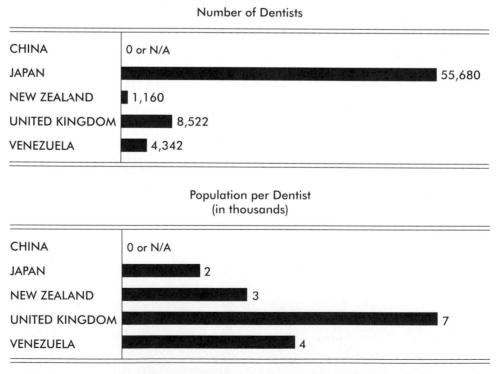

Fig. 4-4 **A** and **B,** Manpower statistics: dentists and provider-patient ratios (data for 1988). (From PC Globe, Inc., Tempe, Arizona.)

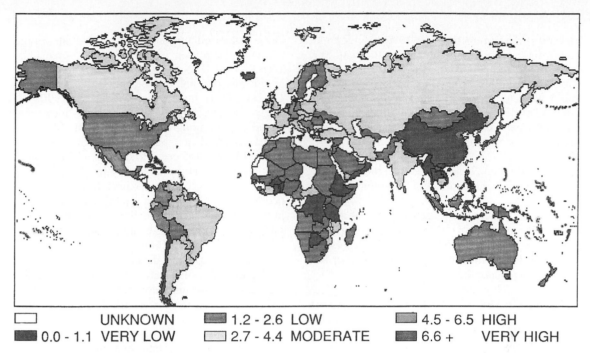

UNKNOWN   1.2 - 2.6 LOW   4.5 - 6.5 HIGH
0.0 - 1.1 VERY LOW   2.7 - 4.4 MODERATE   6.6 +   VERY HIGH

Fig. 4-5 Global map showing dental caries prevalence rates (DMFT) for children at age 12 years (data up to 1970). (From World Health Organization, Oral Health Unit.)

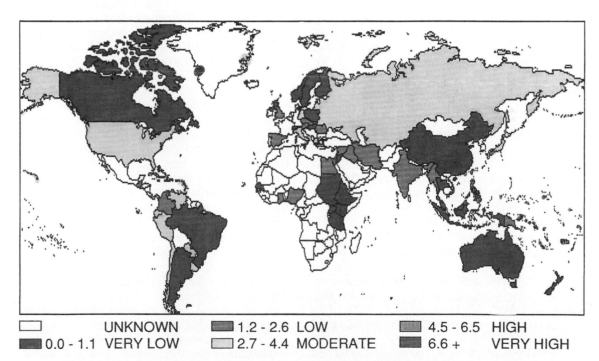

UNKNOWN   1.2 - 2.6 LOW   4.5 - 6.5 HIGH
0.0 - 1.1 VERY LOW   2.7 - 4.4 MODERATE   6.6 +   VERY HIGH

Fig. 4-6 Global map showing dental caries prevalence rates (DMFT) for children at age 12 years (data up to 1990). (From World Health Organization, Oral Health Unit.)

mortality rate during the year 1990 was approximately 34 (per thousand) and during the year 2000 it is expected to be almost 25. The median age of China's population for the year 1990 is 25.4 years and is expected to be 29.4 years in the year 2000. Because of the government policy of no more than one child per family, the fertility level is barely higher than replacement level, the death rates at all ages are low, and the Chinese people seem to enjoy healthier and longer lives than those in other countries with similar levels of economic development.[46]

As to be expected, a greater number of sophisticated medical resources are located in the larger cities. The rural communities have the fewest resources, whereas the municipal and provincial levels fare somewhere between.

China's health care system is a product of its history and its culture, and the Chinese assume an active role in their health care. The individual is treated like an equal by health care providers and encouraged to take part in treatment decisions.

The country and the people of China are very much controlled by the central government. The central government regulates fees, salaries, and even practice locations of health care providers. Education is also regulated by the central government. The exact number of dentists is unavailable, although estimates place it at 104,000 (1981) for a dentist-to-population ratio estimated at one dentist to every 100,000 people. This is due partially to the relatively low number of dentists educated in China. This ratio will continue to improve to the extent that China's educational capabilities improve.

Children are especially important in China as a result of the government's strict law permitting only one child per family. Education is taken very seriously as one of the ways China will progress and grow as a nation. A 1987 study of the oral health habits of 14- and 15-year-olds in Beijing showed that surveyed children visited the dentist mostly for relief from a toothache or to have fillings or extractions. Although all children surveyed brushed with toothpaste, only 23% used fluoridated toothpaste. Additionally, gingival bleeding was observed in more that 50% of the surveyed children.[1]

The Chinese people have a need and demand for dental care. Major dental decay has been observed in the primary dentition of schoolchildren, yet the permanent dentition is virtually caries-free. The WHO's Oral Data Bank indicates a very low decayed, missing, and filled teeth (DMFT) index (0-1.1 DMFT) for the 12-year-old child in 1990. Dietary changes, however, seem to be increasing dental decay among certain populations.[23]

Inadequate dental personnel appears to be the greatest barrier to access to dental care. In China, dentists trained at the university level are referred to as *stomatologists*. Approximately 296.5 million people, or 25% of China's total population, live in the urban, nonagricultural areas of China.[8] The majority of stomatologists are located in urban areas, whereas 75% of the population, including those with the greatest dental needs, are located in rural areas. The distribution of dental health practitioners is inadequate and presents an additional barrier to access of dental care for China's rural populations.

China's first formalized dental hygiene education program was established in 1983 by Dr. Chong Ren Huang, a practicing periodontist and Associate Dean of the Faculty of Stomatology at Shanghai Second Medical College. The program is located in the Shanghai People's Ninth Hospital. The first class of students contained 30 pupils, with an average age of 15. The equivalent of high school education in the United States, the completion of a difficult test of manual dexterity, and a difficult entry examination were required of these dental hygiene pupils.

The dental hygiene program requires 3 years of study. The comprehensive curriculum includes didactic and clinical courses. Prerequisite courses (English, mathematics, biology, and physics) are completed in the first year, dental sciences (basic and clinical) in the second year, and clinical extrinsic exposure (in hospitals and schools, 6 days a week) in the third year. Graduates receive a certificate in dental hygiene from the vocational school system in Shanghai.

The term *dental nurse* has been traditionally used to signify the trained dental auxiliary used in developing nations. This term comes from New Zealand's Dental Nurse Program. Huang's choice of the term *dental hygienist* indicates a positive and progressive view in the perception of the American-trained dental hygienist. As a periodontist, Huang is aware of the dental hygienist's significant contribution to the treatment of periodontal disease. He also promotes the teaching of basic restorative skills to dental hygiene students in China. In this way, dental hygienists are able to provide schoolchildren with needed basic restorative dental treatment.[22]

Considering the shortage of stomatologists in China and their disproportionate distribution, use of dental hygienists appears to be a logical choice to improve personnel ratios and to provide a more equitable distribution of dental services. One positive aspect of the health care system is the current incorporation of Western medicine with traditional Eastern medicine.

Japan. The highly industrialized first world country of Japan has a population of approximately 122.6 million people. Japan is a member state of the WHO Western Pacific Region. The four main and several smaller islands of Japan are situated east of Russia, North Korea, and South Korea, between the Sea of Japan and the Pacific Ocean. Most of the terrain is mountainous, with only 17% of the land suitable for cultivation and habitation. About 75% of Japan's population lives in urban areas, and 50% of the total population is centered in and around the major cities of Tokyo, Yokohama, and Osaka. The capital city of Tokyo, with 8.3 million inhabitants, has the largest population. In 1986 Japan was the sixth most populated nation in the world. Japan's population density of 844 persons per square kilometer ranks it among the most crowded in the world.[30] Total population is projected to be 126.6 million people in the year 2000.[46]

The government system, based on the idea of popular sovereignty, has been described in two ways: as a constitutional monarchy and as a parliamentary democracy. Japan's constitution sets forth the supreme law of the country. Constitutionally, the emperor is a powerless figurehead acting only in special matters of state. Since the end of World War II, Japan had adhered to pacifism; it "will not maintain any form of war potential." Freedoms and rights include "the right to life, liberty, and the pursuit of happiness; freedom of thought and conscience; economic freedom; social rights (the right to enjoy a minimum standard of living, the right to receive education, etc.); suffrage rights; and the right of petition (such as the Diet)."[16]

Japan's government has three main branches: legislative, executive, and judicial. The Diet, or legislature, holds the highest state power. The legislative branch contains a House of Representatives and a permanent House of Councillors. The cabinet, in the executive branch, controls and supervises the 13 ministry offices (including the Ministry of Education and the Ministry of Health and Welfare) and their subdivisions. The independent Supreme Court of Justice is the highest judicial authority.

Since 1922 Japan has maintained a social health insurance system, although most of the country's population was not covered by the system until the 1960s. Various health insurance plans are available, most of which require both the employee and the employer, or the government, to contribute to the cost of the plan. Dentists are paid by the plan based on a fee-for-service scale. Insurance covers the majority of officially authorized dental treatments; however, special procedures, such as orthodontic and advanced prosthodontic care and preventive services, are paid for by the patient. The social health system does provide free care to the elderly (age 70 and over), the indigent, and the handicapped.[5]

In 1980 there were 72 dental technician schools, each school accepting an average of 50 students each year. There were 102 oral hygiene schools, each school accepting an average of 45 students each year. High school graduation is a prerequisite for a 2-year paradental program.

In 1980 there were 29 dental schools in Japan; 11 schools are national, 15 schools are private, and 1 school (located in Kitakyushu) is supported by the prefectural government. The national dental schools accept up to 80 students; the private schools accept up to 160 students. Tuition varies also, with the national schools costing approximately the equivalent of $780 per year and private schools costing the equivalent of $6,800 or more per year. The dental program requires 4 years of education. Schools are in session for 8 months a year, with a 6-day week (half a day on Saturday). After graduation, each student must pass Japan's National Board Examination before receiving a dental license from the Ministry of Welfare. Approximately 3,500 dental students graduated in 1980.[26]

In 1986 Japan's Ministry of Health, Personnel

Bureau, reported that 66,797 dentists were practicing in the country. With a population of approximately 123 million, the average dentist-to-population ratio is one dentist for every 2,000 people. In 1986 the Personnel Bureau reported 31,139 practicing dental operating auxiliaries and 32,666 practicing oral-dental hygienists.[42] The typical general private dental office team, with three or four dental chairs, may consist of one dentist, one oral hygienist, and one dental technician.

All elementary and middle schools have a school dentist who examines each pupil once a year. Parents are notified if their child requires dental treatment. The Japanese Dental Association and the Association of School Dentists stress and support early detection and prevention of dental caries, dental health education, and nutrition and dietary counseling.[26]

As of 1980, community water fluoridation was not enforced. To compensate, topical application of 2% sodium fluoride or an 8% stannous fluoride solution, 4 times a year until age 13 or 14, was widely accepted as standard preventive treatment.[26] Data from the WHO Global Oral Data Bank indicate that the dental caries rate among children 12 years of age has increased from a moderate level (2.7 to 4.4 DMFT) in 1970 to a high level (4.5 to 6 DMFT) in 1990. This change seems to be related to the increase of refined sugars and carbohydrates in the diet.

Takada and associates[43] reported a decrease in the incidence of caries in first and second permanent molars of senior high school students (grade 12), from 7% to 9% in 1975 to 3% in 1986. The incidence of caries for the same group of teeth in freshman high school students (grade 9) was 8% in 1976 and 5% in 1986. Students in grades 11 and 12 had the greatest number of treated teeth.

New Zealand. Midway between the equator and the South Pole, in the Pacific Ocean, is the country of New Zealand. New Caledonia is 900 miles to the north across the Tropic of Capricorn, Australia is more than 1,000 miles to the west over the Tasman Sea, and South America is approximately 4,500 miles to the east across the Pacific Ocean. New Zealand is a member state of the WHO Western Pacific Region. Approximately 3.4 million people[46] live within the 103,883 square miles of three islands: the North Island, the South Island, and the smallest, Stewart Island. More than 80% of the population lives in urban settings, mostly in the lower hill areas around the perimeter of the islands, and 75% of the total population lives on the North Island, with a distribution of approximately 137,000 people in Wellington, the capital; 149,000 people in Auckland; and 168,000 in Christchurch. Much of the countryside is unpopulated, especially the mountain ranges and surrounding hills. The South Island has a more historic flavor and more of an agricultural economy, accompanied by a slower-paced life-style.

New Zealand is an independent member of the British Commonwealth. The governor-general, as Queen Elizabeth II's representative, holds the traditional parliamentary and legislative role in the government.[31] Most people are of British descent; however, New Zealand was originally settled by the Maori people, of Polynesian descent.

In 1921 the prototypical New Zealand Dental Nurse Program was established. For the first time a person other than a dentist was legally able to perform dental procedures. These dental nurses, allowed to perform simple dental restorations, visited every school in New Zealand with mobile dental units. Proper dental treatment and services were provided for the children, resulting in a decline in the dental caries prevalence rate.[41] In 1966, "1,118 [dental] nurses treated 480,000 children, inserted 2½ million fillings, and extracted only 558 carious permanent teeth."[47] School dental nurses currently are prepared during a 2-year intensive training period; they are then able to provide the following routine dental services to schoolchildren:[5]

• Oral examination
• Oral prophylaxis
• Topical fluoride application
• Primary and permanent teeth restoration with silver amalgam and synthetic fillings
• Pulp capping
• Extraction of deciduous teeth
• Individual patient counseling and classroom dental health education

In a nonfluoridated area a school dental nurse can treat 475 children per year, whereas in an area that had been fluoridated for 10 years, 690 children have been treated yearly by each dental nurse.[12] In 1968 Beck[6] reported that positive and permanent benefits from New Zealand's dental program were gained by most adolescents and young adults. More than two thirds of 20-year-olds continued with regular dental care after dental services were no longer paid for by their parents, indicating a high interest in oral health.

New Zealand's water fluoridation program originated in 1954, and according to the Center for Disease Control's (CDC) 1986 fluoridation census, 1.8 million New Zealanders (54% of the total population) live in fluoridated communities. Data from the WHO Global Oral Data Bank categorized New Zealand's 12-year-old population as having a very high dental caries prevalence rate (6.6+ DMFT) in 1970; in 1990, data for the same population indicated a low dental caries prevalence rate (1.2 to 2.6 DMFT). The 1975 results from ICS I indicate 36% of New Zealand's 35- to 44-year-olds are edentulous. The increased use of fluoridated water and fluoridated toothpaste, combined with the school dental service's preventive approach, has contributed significantly to the decline of dental caries over a period of 30 years.[7]

Children (age 2½ to 13½ years) receive free routine dental services from school dental nurses (orthodontic coverage is excluded). Adolescents (age 13½ to 18) receive dental health services from private-practice dentists, who are reimbursed by the state. Adults (over age 18) are provided dental health services based on a fee-for-service payment from the Ministry of Health, most likely at a private-practice dental office. In 1988 approximately 1,160 dentists were licensed to practice dentistry. With a total population of 3.3 million people, the dentist-to-population ratio is about 1:3,000. Almost 90% of the dentists in New Zealand are in a private practice setting, and nearly all participate in the government's dental service for children and adolescents.[31] Each of New Zealand's 14 dental districts has its own dental officer, who handles general public health matters and is responsible for the school-based dental program, along with the management of the dental program provided to adolescents. The minister of health is advised on dental health program matters by a Dental Benefits Advisory Committee.

Major changes within New Zealand's long-standing centralized organizational structure of health services may occur relatively soon. The situation as of 1985 was such that the minister of health was responsible for the three main components of the health care system: the public health services, the hospital boards, and the private and voluntary sector. Changing community needs, combined with an increasingly complex health care system, appear to have contributed to the current inappropriateness of this organizational structure for health care services. New Zealand's health care system seems to be having problems similar to those of other developed countries:[29]

- Inadequate control of costs
- Failure to guarantee value for money
- Lack of professional accountability
- Imbalances in care between and within services
- Gross overinstitutionalization of some services
- Disproportionate geographic distribution of services and resources
- Uncoordinated components of care, complicated by numerous voluntary and private agency services
- Lack of community involvement in the planning and provision of services.

Policymaking and planning has begun, but an "overall, explicit statement of national health policies and strategies" has yet to be seen.[29]

United Kingdom. "United Kingdom" and "Britain" both mean the United Kingdom of Great Britain and Northern Ireland. "Great Britain" comprises England, Wales, and Scotland. The United Kingdom is a member state in the European region of the WHO.

The United Kingdom is a constitutional monarchy, currently ruled by Queen Elizabeth II, who is the head of the executive legislature, head of the judiciary, the commander in chief of armed forces, and the supreme governor of the Church of England. Separate central government departments do exist for Wales and Scotland. The Parliament is the supreme legislative authority, consisting of three separate elements: the Queen, the House of Lords, and the elected members in the House of Commons. Basically, the political parties are the Conservative, the Labour, the Liberal, and the Social Democratic parties. There are other smaller parties as well, from Scotland, Wales, and Northern Ireland.[44]

The population of the United Kingdom in 1990

was just over 57 million people. The projected population estimate for the year 2000 is just over 58 million people. Social indicators such as infant mortality rate (per 1,000 births) and life expectancy at birth are 9.1 and 75.2, respectively, for the year 1987.[48]

The British social welfare system is made up of three components: National Health Service (NHS), personal social services, and social security. The NHS provides a comprehensive range of medical services that are available to all residents, regardless of socioeconomic status. Personal social services, provided at the local level and in conjunction with voluntary organizations, provide help and advice to the elderly, the disabled, and the children in need. The social security system provides a standard level of living by giving financial support to those who are unable to earn income and to those who are disabled.

Britain's government is directly responsible for the NHS, and it is administered to the people through a range of agent health authorities and boards throughout Britain.

The NHS is based upon the principle that there should be a comprehensive range of publicly provided services designed to help the individual stay healthy and to provide effective and appropriate treatment and care where necessary while making the best use of available resources. All taxpayers, employers and employees contribute to its cost so that those members of the community who do not require health care help to pay for those who do.[45]

General taxation pays for about 80% of the cost of health services in Great Britain. The remaining 20% is paid for by the NHS insurance contribution and from the charges toward the cost of certain items, such as prescription drugs and dental treatment. The NHS is able to provide dental care to many people at a low cost.

Some forms of treatment, such as hospital care, are provided free; others (forms of treatment) may be charged for. . . . The Health and Medicines Act 1988 introduced charges for dental examinations and a system of proportional charges for all types of dental treatment. However, women who are pregnant or who have had a baby in the last year, anyone under the age of 18 (or 19 if in full-time education), and people receiving income support or family support, continue to be exempt from charges.[45]

Dentists providing treatment in their own operatories are paid on a prescribed scale of fees.

On October 1, 1990, general dentists providing care through the NHS began working under a new contract. The original had been in effect since the establishment of the NHS in 1948. First, this new contract provides the dental patient with a 2-year commitment of continuing care from the dentist. This care includes the free replacement of restorations up to 12 months after initial placement and the provision that emergency dental treatment must be provided to the patient within 24 hours after it has been requested. In addition to the traditional fee for service, the dentist receives an additional payment for each patient registered with him or her under the new continuing care plan. Second, this new contract establishes a capitation plan for child patients. The dentist receives an initial "entry fee," which is applied toward the patient's fee for service. Hereafter, the dentist is paid annually, based on the number of children in particular age groups. Generally, British dentists have been proponents of this more preventive type of program for quite some time. The effects of this new plan on the participation of providers under the NHS system and the use of dental care are yet to be seen.[20]

Primary health care is offered by doctors, dentists, opticians, and pharmacists working within the NHS as independent practitioners. Family practitioner services are those given to patients by doctors, dentists, opticians, and pharmacists of their own choice. Family doctors provide the first diagnosis in the case of illness and either provide treatment or refer the patient to a specialist and/or hospital consultant.

There are approximately 8,500 dentists in the United Kingdom, with a ratio of one dentist to every 7,000 people. Private medical and dental treatment is encouraged by the government to meet a larger share of the nation's health needs. In this way the private sector adds to the total resources available and offers alternatives in the delivery of services. There are more than 2.5 million private-practice subscribers; including dependents of the subscriber, about 5.3 million people are covered by Britain's private medical insurance.

Four or more years of training at a dental school are required for full registration as a dentist in the NHS. The General Dental Council is the regulating body for dentists. The British Dental Association is the principal professional association for dentists, and the British Dental Hygienists' Association is the principal professional association for dental hygienists. "Dental therapists (who have undergone a two-year training course) and dental hygienists (who have undergone a training course of about a year) may carry out some simple dental work under the direction of a registered dentist."[45] As of 1978 there were two accepted dental auxiliaries: dental hygienists and "New Cross dental auxiliaries." The dental hygienist is able to work in a variety of settings, such as the Hospital Service, the School Service, or in the General Dental Service. New Cross dental auxiliaries are only able to work in the School Dental Service, where they provide basic restorative treatment to schoolchildren.[23] The government is no longer training New Cross dental auxiliaries.

Information from the British Fluoridation Society reports as of 1989 approximately 8 million people in the United Kingdom receive fluoridated water. An overview of DMFT scores in the United Kingdom among the adult population, age 16 years and older, reveals mean scores of 19 in 1978 and 17.2 in 1988. The highest DMFT scores were found in the group of people age 55 years and older: 23 in 1978 and 22.6 in 1988. The lowest DMFT scores were found among the age 16 to 24 group: 14.9 in 1978 and 10.8 in 1988.[13]

For the 12-year-old child in the United Kingdom, the WHO's Oral Data Bank indicates a high DMFT score (4.5 to 6.5 DMFT) in 1970 and a moderate DMFT score (2.7 to 4.4 DMFT) in 1990. A study by R.J. Anderson and associates[4] indicates that between the years of 1965 and 1980 dental caries prevalence rates among 5- and 12-year-old children throughout England decreased significantly. Anderson's findings are surprising when juxtaposed with results of a study carried out in the mid-1980s, which indicated that children between the ages of 11 and 16 in England consume high amounts of sweets and soft drinks.[21]

Venezuela. Venezuela is located in northeastern South America. With a total area of 352,143 square miles, Venezuela's northern border runs 2,175 miles along the shores of the Caribbean Sea. Columbia lies to the west, Brazil lies to the south, the southern tip of Venezuela nearly reaches the

equator, and Guyana lies to the east. The Republic of Venezuela also includes 72 islands in the Antilles. The capital city of Venezuela is Caracas, situated in a valley on the Caribbean Sea, with a 1982 population of approximately 3 million. The country's 1990 population estimate is 19,750,000 with a projected estimate for the year 2000 of 24.5 million. Prior to the 1950s, most of the country's population lived in rural sections of the country. During the 30 years from the 1950s to the 1980s, the population shifted to predominantly urban locations in the northern part of the country; pockets of small villages remain in isolated areas in the south.[46] Venezuela is both a member state of the WHO region of the Americas and of the Pan American Health Organization (PAHO).

Although the government may be considered a democracy, one political party is repeatedly elected. Like most South American countries, the economy is based on capitalism and the people are divided unequally into the very rich and the very poor.[27]

In 1987 a national health system was put into effect, making the Ministry of Health and Social Welfare the new coordinator and manager of all separate groups (72 in total) involved in providing health care services, including related activities of government agencies (except the National Armed Forces) and self-controlling institutions.[37] Specialty dental education programs are now available in the Venezuelan dental schools; however, training in the United States remains a far more valuable asset for assuring an economically successful dental practice. Foreign education credentials are highly advertised and helpful in attracting clients. The dentist is the primary provider of dental care. Dental assistants do not receive any formal training, and dental hygienists, as such, are not used in Venezuela. The typical dental office is predominantly a solo private practice setting. There are few private group practices, exclusively located in the higher income areas of the major cities. Those able to afford dental care prefer a private practice setting to a community dental clinic. Financing mechanisms do not involve the concept of dental insurance as it is known in the United States. Instead, a fee-for-service structure is used in both the private and public sectors.[9,25]

Approximately 4.9 million people receive fluoridated water, based on 1988 PAHO data. For both 1970 and 1990, data from the WHO Global Oral Data Bank indicated moderate levels of caries prevalence (2.7 to 4.4 DMFT) at age 12 years.

With approximately 4,342 dentists and a population of nearly 20 million, the overall dentist-to-population ratio is 1:4,000. This ratio assumes that an equal distribution of and access to dental services exists. In Venezuela, equal distribution and access is not the case. Dental personnel are primarily situated in the urban areas, and rural populations are at a distinct disadvantage in accessing care. Complicating the already economically depressed situation, a doubling inflation rate during 1988 negatively altered the course of many planned health care activities. However, the universities with dental education programs are using their resources, including dental students, to train dental auxiliary personnel at the local community level. With the community leaders' cooperation, these auxiliaries are able to provide the dental treatment so desperately needed by populations in the country's rural communities. Care among the poor consists primarily of emergency treatments and extractions requested by the patient. Dental health needs are greatest among populations in low socioeconomic positions, where preventive care is not widely available.[23]

INTERNATIONAL HEALTH ORGANIZATIONS
World Health Organization

The WHO, with a staff of approximately 5,500 people, is the largest, most prominent, and most influential international health organization. "In addition to providing direct cooperation to every country that requests it, WHO promotes, coordinates and carries out a series of 'global' functions that no individual country could undertake."[53] At present, approximately 160 nongovernment organizations maintain official relations with the WHO. Established on April 7 (now World Health Day), 1948, as a self-governing, specialized, multilateral agency within the United Nations, The WHO is responsible for public health and international health matters. With 166 member countries, the WHO contributes in two main ways: by carrying out specific member country government-requested projects and by promoting coordination

of community health programs within and among these countries. Thus the WHO's actions make many projects logistically and politically possible.[41]

The WHO's primary objective is the attainment of health for all by the year 2000. The organization is dedicated to the belief that every person has a fundamental right to primary health care services to attain complete physical, mental, and social well-being, thereby allowing the opportunity of a socially and economically productive life.

The WHO activities invest in member countries and their people by using the WHO's resources to assist and educate people and to develop community health policies and strategies. The overall goal is to establish self-sufficiency among member countries in successfully carrying out health programs.

The WHO has various responsibilities:

- To act as the directing and coordinating authority on international health work
- To promote technical cooperation
- To assist governments, upon request, in strengthening health services
- To furnish appropriate technical assistance and, in emergencies, necessary aid, upon the request or acceptance of governments
- To stimulate the eradication of epidemic, endemic, and other diseases
- To promote, in cooperation with other specialized agencies where necessary, the improvement of nutrition, housing, sanitation, recreation, economic or working conditions, and other aspects of environmental hygiene
- To promote and coordinate biomedical and health services research
- To establish and stimulate the establishment of international standards for biological, pharmaceutical, and similar products and to standardize diagnostic procedures
- To foster activities in the field of mental health
- To develop international standards for food, biological, and pharmaceutical products
- To propose international conventions and foster cooperation among scientific and professional groups that contribute to the advancement of health.[54]

The structure of the WHO has three levels. The World Health Assembly, a delegation of representatives from all WHO member countries, meets once a year in Geneva, Switzerland. The agenda focuses on major policy matters and the biennial budget. The executive board, which meets twice a year, is comprised of 31 member country representatives, elected with staggered 3-year terms, with the function to advise and carry out the decisions of the assembly. The secretariat, headed by a director-general, represents all WHO staff, related professionals, and general personnel at headquarters (30%), regional offices (30%), and in individual member countries (40%). The director-general candidate, who is nominated by the executive board and then formally appointed to the position by the assembly, is assisted by one deputy director-general and five assistant directors-general.[55]

In addition to maintaining headquarters in Geneva, the WHO decentralizes itself into six regions, each having a regional director, a regional committee, and a regional office.

The regional offices include:
• Africa, Brazzaville, Congo
• Americas, Washington, D.C.
• Eastern Mediterranean, Alexandria, Egypt
• Europe, Copenhagen, Denmark
• Southeast Asia, New Delhi, India
• Western Pacific, Manila, Philippines

The Oral Health Unit within the WHO maintains the computerized Global Oral Data Bank as a means of accumulating initial and future standardized statistics on the oral health status of the world's population. Initial statistics are needed as a baseline for the evaluation and monitoring of oral health status globally over a period of time. Ever-improving computer technology and information services have, in theory, made the world smaller and remote areas more accessible. Data are directly entered into a standardized data entry program (MS-DOS), which is supplied to interested governments or dental professionals by the WHO Oral Health Unit. The data are transferred via computer disk to WHO Headquarters, where statistical analysis is performed. The Oral Health Unit stores the data in the Global Oral Data Bank and shares the results of the statistical analysis with the primary and subsequent investigators. Acquisition of standardized data is necessary to estimate global trends of dental caries and periodontal disease and to evaluate oral health programs.[49,52] Statistics from 173 countries, territories, or principalities are available through the data bank.

The following summarizes important dates in the history of the WHO and oral health:

1946	International Health Conference approves the WHO Constitution
1948	Birth of WHO (constitution ratified)
	First World Health Assembly is held in Geneva, Switzerland
1961	WHO publishes the first *World Directory of Dental Schools* (second edition published in 1967)
1969	Twenty-second World Health Assembly adopts a resolution supporting water fluoridation for dental caries prevention
	Initiation of the Global Oral Data Bank
1977	Thirtieth World Health Assembly targets health for all by the year 2000
1978	Joint WHO/UNICEF International Conference (Alma-Ata, USSR) adopts a declaration on primary health care as the key to attaining health for all by the year 2000
	Thirty-first World Health Assembly reinforces dental caries prevention
1979	The global goal for dental caries is established at no more than 3 DMFT at the age of 12 years
1981	WHO unanimously adopts the global strategy for health for all by the year 2000
	The United Nations General Assembly endorses the global strategy and urges collaboration with the WHO by other concerned international organizations
1987	International Development Program launched to help developing countries create a national oral health plan

Pan American Health Organization

The PAHO is the oldest international public health agency in the world. "The fundamental purposes of the Pan American Health Organization are to promote and coordinate the efforts of the countries of the Region of the Americas to combat disease, lengthen life, and promote the physical and mental health of the people."[37]

The PAHO concerns itself with basic public health matters such as provision of safe drinking water and adequate sanitation; nutrition, immunization, oral rehydration therapy, and acute respiratory infection treatment among children; and control of tropical diseases. Other health problems are addressed, such as cardiovascular diseases, cancer, accidents, and drug addiction. The seven project priority areas are health services, water and sanitation, child survival, human resources, tropical diseases, essential drugs, and food and nutrition.

Joint projects are pursued with local ministries of health, nongovernment organizations, universities, and local community groups to improve health systems and consequently to improve the health of the people. Collaboration among countries themselves is additionally important for the attainment of the common goals of primary health care. Target populations of the PAHO are mothers and children, the poor, the elderly, refugees, and displaced persons, all of whom represent our most vulnerable citizens. Health for all in the Americas by the year 2000 is the PAHO's regional overall goal, affiliated with the WHO's global goal of health for all by the year 2000.

The PAHO, an agency within the United Nations system, is located in Washington, D.C., and is the WHO's regional office for the Americas. The Pan American Sanitary Bureau (PASB) is responsible for executive matters of the PAHO.

The region for the Americas encompasses member states from the following nations:

Antigua and	Dominica	Panama
Barbuda	Dominican	Paraguay
Argentina	Republic	Peru
Bahamas	Ecuador	St. Kitts and Nevis
Barbados	El Salvador	Saint Lucia
Belize	Grenada	Saint Vincent and the
Bolivia	Guatemala	Grenadines
Brazil	Guyana	Suriname
Canada	Haiti	Trinidad and Tobago
Chile	Honduras	United States of America
Columbia	Jamaica	Uruguay
Costa Rica	Mexico	Venezuela
Cuba	Nicaragua	

In addition, there are three "participating governments"—France, the Netherlands, and the United Kingdom—and two "observing governments," Portugal and Spain.

The PAHO works closely with each member state, assisting in the planning, implementation, and evaluation of activities via 29 PAHO offices, including the PAHO headquarters in Washington, D.C.; the Caribbean Program Coordination Office, in Bridgetown, Barbados; and the United States–Mexico Border Field Office in El Paso, Texas. There are also 10 PAHO/WHO regional and subregional scientific and technical centers, institutes, and programs located in Latin America and the Caribbean.

The PAHO is a nonprofit organization whose budget is derived from three main sources. The PAHO member states contribute 34% and WHO member countries contribute 17% (contributions are based on the particular country's population and national income); 49% of the budget is derived from extrabudgetary sources, such as international development agencies, financial institutions, foundations, and corporations. The 1990-1991 PAHO budget ($145,599,550) is distributed into four operational areas: 64% for direct cooperation with member states, 19% for regional health programs (hemispherewide), 12% for program support, and 5% for policy and program direction.

Basically, the PAHO has two main technical and scientific program areas:

1. *Health Systems Infrastructure Area.* Programs in this area are concerned with developing and managing basic resources necessary for the implementation of national health policies.
2. *Health Program Development Area.* Programs in this area deal with high-risk populations with priority health problems.

The Oral Health Unit of the PAHO is included in the Health Systems Infrastructure Area, under the Organization of Health Services Based on Primary Health Care. The PAHO recognizes oral health as an essential component in total health of the individual. The two principal objectives of the Oral Health Unit are (1) "to promote oral health as an integral part of health," and (2) "to introduce oral health as a basic component of general health services for the prevention and treatment of the most common oral diseases, such as dental caries and periodontal diseases."[38]

Oral health program activities focus on prevention, education, service delivery, and research. Prevention programs include such projects as the production of fluoridated table salt in Jamaica to make fluoridated table salt available to the entire Caribbean community. In this region, fluoridated table salt is more cost-effective than fluoridated water as an efficient vehicle for administering fluoride. Very often water sources are inadequate and too numerous to treat with fluoride. Another concern would be that the fluoridated water source would not reach the country's rural population; therefore the population with the greatest need would remain unserved by the benefits of the fluoridated water.

Salt fluoridation is a much more effective means to disperse fluoride throughout an entire population. It is easily distributed and financially feasible to produce. The salt industry cooperates and participates favorably in the fluoridated table salt program. The accepted fluoride dose rate is 200 mg of sodium fluoride ion per kilogram of refined table salt. An antihumectant must be added to stabilize the fluoride. This ingredient makes the salt dryer, which dramatically improves the texture and appearance of the salt, thereby producing a much more attractive product for the consumer. Both the salt industry and the consumer benefit. By raising the cost of salt $0.01 per pound, the salt fluoridation program is able to pay for itself in a reasonable period of time. By shifting costs from the government (Ministry of Health) into the public and community sector, the costs are easier to absorb. The salt fluoridation program cost is approximately $0.01 per capita per year. The program is well accepted by both the population and the government, and the program fosters cooperation between the two parties. Jamaica, Costa Rica, and Brazil currently have salt fluoridation programs. Columbia, Mexico, and Peru have initiated programs.

Another prevention program has resulted in the successful reduction in the incidence of dental caries in schoolchildren in Bermuda. A multiple fluoride treatment program occurred over a period of 11 years and resulted in an 80% reduction in the incidence of dental caries. The type of fluoride provided with age and corresponding dosage is as follows:

Fluoride *drops*
  6–18 months: 1 drop per day
  18–36 months: 2 drops per day
    1 drop = 0.25 mg of sodium fluoride USP
    0.25 mg of sodium fluoride USP = 0.125 mg sodium fluoride ion
Fluoride *tablets*
  3–5 years: 1 tablet of 0.75 mg sodium fluoride per day
  5–11 years: 1 tablet of 1.00 mg sodium fluoride per day
Fluoride *mouth rinse*
  12–14 years: 10 ml 0.2% sodium fluoride twice monthly

Dental educational programs for children in the countries of Guyana and Suriname were initiated. Expanded-duty auxiliary schools in Jamaica, Suriname, and Trinidad provide personnel resources. More than 100 auxiliaries have been trained to provide basic dental treatment for children, and an auxiliary association has been formed. The first English language–based dental school has been opened in Trinidad. Service delivery programs carried out in Chile, Mexico, and Venezuela show that comprehensive primary oral health care is economically feasible, especially in communities with limited resources. Local dental schools can assist in the provision of dental treatment to underserved populations by modifying dental school curricula to combine formal training and community service.[18]

With the selection of Quito, Ecuador, as the site for the WHO's Collaborating Center in Oral Health, dental research in Latin America is expected to expand. Informational materials and courses on human immunodeficiency virus (HIV) infection and related oral manifestations were created through the collaboration of the PAHO's Oral Health Unit with the PAHO-WHO Acquired Immunodeficiency Syndrome Program, the U.S. National Institutes of Health, the Centers for Disease Control, and the WHO Collaborating Center on Oral Manifestations of HIV Infection.

From 1986 through 1989 the PAHO's Oral Health Program focused on the overall goal to "promote the integration of oral health services with other health services and the extension of dental care coverage and dental disease prevention efforts."[37]

Priorities of the PAHO's Oral Health Unit are as follows:[38]

- Developing national resources and collaborating centers within the WHO network
- Analyzing factors that affect the provision and coverage of dental care services in the developing countries of the region
- Establishing mechanisms for collection and transfer of information
- Incorporating oral health within the concepts and programs of local health systems
- Continuing studies on new teaching methodologies
- Promoting intercountry and subregional collaboration in the region

Fédération Dentaire Internationale

The FDI was founded in 1900 in Paris; it is the second oldest international health organization, after the International Committee of the Red Cross. The FDI "aims to advance the science and art of dentistry and the status of the dental profession in the interest of improved oral health for all peoples."[15] The WHO and the International Organization for Standardization collaborate with the FDI. Major developments resulting from such collaboration include the Community Periodontal Index of Treatment Needs (CPITN) screening method, the WHO-FDI AIDS initiative, and the International Oral Health Development Program (IDP) to promote oral health care in developing countries.

Headquartered in London, the FDI, a nongovernment organization, is the umbrella organization for national professional dental associations and individual supporting members. A total of 92 national member associations, representing 84 countries, have been voted into the FDI membership at annual congresses. The following five national associations became member associations during the 78th Annual Dental Congress in Singapore (1990): the Chinese Taipei Association for Dental Sciences, the Mauritius Association of Dental Surgeons, the Sri Lanka Dental Association, the Namibia Dental Association, and the Yemen Dental Association. Individual membership is open only to current members of national dental associations, such as the American Dental Association.

Delegates from the national member associations make up the General Assembly of the FDI, which meets annually at the World Dental Congress to make decisions on the FDI policies, the yearly program, and the budget. The FDI Council is responsible for administrative aspects. Each year, the FDI annual World Dental Congress convenes in a different country, providing an excellent opportunity to gain a greater understanding of the international aspects of the dental profession.

There are four scientific commissions within the FDI. The Commission on Oral Health, Research, and Epidemiology (CORE) maintains close collaboration with the WHO while attending to the functional issues of its title. The Commission on Dental Education and Practice (CDEP) concerns itself with issues such as "continuing education, supervision of dental auxiliaries, group practice, and dental health education for patients and the public." The Commission of Dental Products (CDP) has contributed significantly to the standardization of dental materials, instruments, and equipment. The Commission on Defense Forces Dental Services (CDFDS) "dedicates its efforts to the needs of military personnel of all nations."[14]

Working groups within one of these specific scientific commissions study specific research topics. Three working groups and their topics of study, added at the annual congress in Singapore (1990), follow:

- The working group (CORE) studying principal requirements for controlled trials of agents and procedures to prevent caries and prevent periodontal diseases
- The working group (CDEP) conducting a study of a preregistration and postgraduate training period for dentists
- The working group (CDP) investigating multicountry clinical trials on (dental) materials performance

Other new working groups include the following:

- The working group (CORE) studying aspects of nutrition and oral health

- The working group (CDEP) investigating quality assurance
- The working group (CDEP) researching computer-aided diagnostic instruments in dental practice
- The joint working group on international collaboration for oral health research (ICOHR) and standing activity on forensic odontology (CDFDS).[14]

The FDI and the WHO collaborated and formed the FDI-WHO Joint Working Group 10 (JWG 10). JWG 10 was established in 1986 with the following purposes:

- "To monitor existing or proposed programmes in different countries concerned with the prevention and treatment of periodontal diseases and evaluate the outcome of those programmes"
- "To review research into the identification of individuals or groups running a high risk of experiencing the destructive phases of periodontal diseases"[39]

The *International Dental Journal* is the official scientific bimonthly publication of the FDI. Contents of this publication include timely dental papers with significant global importance, including many papers presented at the FDI World Dental Congress, as well as reports from the commissions and working groups. The *FDI News,* published in four languages, is also a bimonthly publication; it contains articles about "the activities at the Congresses, the work of the commissions, current research of practical application, news about the profession worldwide, and a calendar of dental meetings."[15] The FDI also publishes technical reports prepared by the commissions, which, along with *FDI News,* are available free of charge to supporting members of the FDI.

An individual unable to become a supporting member of the FDI, yet desiring a subscription to the *International Dental Journal* can purchase the subscription directly from the publisher (Butterworth, 80 Montvale Avenue, Stoneham, MA 02180; telephone 617-438-8464) at an annual subscription rate of approximately $165.

International Association for Dental Research

Founded in 1920, the IADR has grown to include more than 8,000 members representing more than 60 countries. Members are primarily dental scientists in all disciplines and specialties in the dental research fields. The IADR's goal is to "promote research and the communication of results within the scientific community, to the dental professional, and to the public."[24]

Membership is open to any person who is interested in dental science and dental research, who conforms to the recognized standards of professional ethics, and who meets all divisional requirements. Joint membership in the IADR and the AADR (American Association for Dental Research) requires sponsorship from two current members of IADR and AADR. Members may enroll in a maximum of 3 of 17 IADR groups representing specialized research fields, such as behavioral science, geriatric dental research, mineralized tissue, and salivary research. Dues paid by American and Canadian members automatically include a subscription to the *Journal of Dental Research,* published monthly. Included in all memberships is a subscription to the newsletter, *IADReports,* which contains articles on current IADR activities, annual meeting details, other professional organizations' meeting information, division news, announcements, and a calendar of events.

The American members make up approximately 50% of the entire IADR membership, and subsequently the AADR has become a division of the IADR in its own right.[2]

International Federation of Dental Hygienists

The International Dental Hygienists' Federation (IDHF) was officially founded June 28, 1986, during the 10th International Symposium on Dental Hygiene, in Oslo, Norway. The American Dental Hygienists' Association (ADHA) is a cornerstone in the history of IDHF, extending back to the First International Symposium on Dental Hygiene in 1970. National dental hygiene associations and individual members make up IDHF active membership.

An individual member shall be from countries where there is a national organization or where the national organization is a Federation (IDHF) member. The applicant must be a member of a national organization to qualify for IDHF membership. The legally recognized title of the profession need not be "dental hygienist" but must meet the IDHF definition of dental hygienist.[17]

The seven founding national member associations are Norway, the United Kingdom, the Netherlands, Japan, Sweden, Canada, and the United States. Three additional national member associations from Australia, Denmark, and Switzerland joined at the IDHF chartering. South Korea has since become a member, and applications have been requested from Italy, Nigeria, and Portugal.

The aim of IDHF is not to impose one country's solutions upon another country, but to achieve the following five objectives (adopted June 27, 1986):

1. To promote access to high-quality preventive oral health services to all peoples
2. To represent and advance the profession of dental hygiene on a nongovernmental, worldwide basis
3. To promote and coordinate the exchange of knowledge and information about the profession and its education and practice
4. To educate the public that oral disease can be prevented through proven regimens
5. To foster the exchange of dental hygiene human resources

The official IDHF newsletter, *Contact International,* is published quarterly and contains sections on continuing education opportunities, topical dental issues, events of the International Symposium on Dental Hygiene, and contributions from individual members and national member associations.

The IDHF supports the United Nations' Human Rights statement of the International Bill of Rights and preventive oral health services for all people as a part of total health.

The Federation is beginning to establish an international professional profile preparatory to assuming a strong leadership position in the international professional world and is completing the collection and tabulation of data on world-wide dental hygiene education, licensure, practice and major issues of concern so that it will be recognized as the international dental hygiene information clearinghouse. There is every indication that the Federation will continue to grow and will serve not only its members but other segments of the world's population by promoting access to quality preventive oral health services and raise the level of awareness of the public that oral diseases can be prevented.[34]

A professional milestone for dental hygienists was reached when the FDI invited the IDHF to participate in the 78th Annual World Dental Congress in Singapore (1990). Ms. Ruth Nowjack-Raymer, represented IDHF at the annual congress. The overall assessment of the role dental hygienists may play in future contributions to oral health globally is very positive, especially in conjunction with the FDI–IDP, designed to aid developing nations[3]. "The Federation (IDHF) has established liaison with both the FDI and the WHO in hopes that members can become involved in oral health projects on a worldwide basis."[17]

National Institute of Dental Research

The National Institute of Dental Research (NIDR), as part of the National Institutes of Health in Bethesda, Maryland, is a governmental organization within the U.S. Department of Health and Human Services, Public Health Service. This institution has an annual budget of more than $135 million and employs approximately 340 full-time staff members. The NIDR currently supports more than 100 projects at its own laboratories at the National Institutes of Health campus and more than 1,000 research projects and training programs at over 200 institutions throughout the world.[36]

There are three main components of the NIDR: the Extramural Program, the Intramural Research Program, and the Epidemiology and Oral Disease Prevention Program. Extramural oral health research and training of research personnel are funded by the Extramural Program through grants, awards, and research contracts, representing almost 73% of the total NIDR annual budget. Scientific investigations range from basic laboratory studies to clinical trials. The program supports more than 190 research organizations, as well as university dental research centers.

The Intramural Research Program focuses on activities that increase basic knowledge of oral diseases and oral disorders. Current areas of research include molecular and cellular biology, neurobiology, microbiology, immunology, and biotechnology. Eight laboratories, a dental clinic, and a pain research unit are used for intramural research.

By conducting descriptive and analytical studies on the distribution, etiology, and prevalence of oral diseases, the Epidemiology and Oral Disease Prevention Program strives to expand and improve present information about the distribution, frequency, and prevention of oral diseases and oral disorders. Another aspect of this program is that of health promotion and application through field trials and demonstration activities.

The NIDR supported the landmark ICS I and the ongoing ICS II. Through participation with the WHO, the NIDR has formulated its research agenda for the 1990s, central to which is collaboration. The agenda includes topic areas such as "epidemiology, fluoride research, nutrition, and studies of oral cancer and other oral conditions that are more prevalent in parts of the world outside the United States." All parties involved have only to benefit by such an arrangement.[35]

In the research area of dental use and treatment outcomes, recommendations for international collaborative research include the following:

Analyze in relation to oral health status the variations in treatments by providers in different organizational settings, with different training, and practicing in different cultural contexts. Opportunities exist for cross-national and cross-cultural oral health studies to validate measures of health outcomes and underlying determinants of oral health status and to understand the processes and outcomes of oral health systems and programs not generally available in the United States.[35]

The NIDR also collaborates with many international entities, including the FDI, the PAHO, and the WHO.

Project HOPE

Project HOPE (Health Opportunity for People Everywhere), founded in 1958 as a nonprofit health organization by William B. Walsh, was designed to provide medical care via the world's first peacetime hospital ship, the S.S. Hope, to populations in coastal areas that asked for assistance.

Through the continued activities of Project HOPE, health personnel in developing areas learn current techniques in pediatric and adult intensive care, cardiovascular surgery, preventive dentistry, nursing, maternal-child health, biomedical engineering, community health improvement, medical relief, and health care administration. Operating programs in approximately 20 countries, Project HOPE activities include support for training workshops and organization of conferences for government health personnel and technical assistance in

methodology, evaluation, and project design of training programs, education that can then be passed on to others. The desired end result is for the newly trained personnel to assume complete responsibility for the country's health improvement programs. A school-based preventive dentistry program in Shanghai, China, and a stomatology and oral oncology training program in Cheng Du, China, have been established through the efforts of Project HOPE volunteers.

Project HOPE also contributes to building libraries and learning resource centers. Its International Textbook Program has distributed more than 720,000 health sciences textbooks and journals to more than 45 countries. Material is also disseminated via computer information resources, such as the conference network of the University of the West Indies Distance Teaching Experiment (UWIDITE). In addition, Project HOPE's international electronic mail system links the HOPE Center to Africa, Central and South America, the Caribbean, Europe, and the Pacific.

The People-to-People Health Foundation, Inc., is an independent international corporation that provides funding for Project HOPE activities. Additional funding is received from the U.S. Agency for International Development and from private contributions. More than $40 million each year is needed to maintain Project HOPE activities globally. Project HOPE and People-to-People Health Foundation headquarters is now at the HOPE Center in Millwood, Virginia, located 60 miles west of Washington, D.C. In 1981 the Center for Health Affairs was established as a division of Project HOPE to provide objective research and analysis of global health issues. The Center for Health Affairs is located in Washington, D.C.[40]

CONCLUSIONS

This chapter presents many, but certainly not all, aspects of oral health on a global level. It was not feasible to include all organizations involved with the promotion and improvement of oral health globally. Many individuals, groups, and organizations have made significant contributions in the arena of international oral health. Many international organizations provide opportunities for one to become involved intimately with the promotion and improvement of oral health globally. The FDI, the PAHO, and the WHO are among the most influential international health organizations. Local and national levels of participation and cooperation also deserve recognition.

Dental health is an important part of an individual's total health. Dental health programs are a necessary and important part of community health programs. Successful community health programs require commitment and broad-based support from private, government, education, and research sectors. In many countries, dental health programs must compete with other desperately needed health programs for limited resources.

George M. Gillespie, Chief of the Oral Health Unit at the PAHO, suggests that one way the dental personnel shortage issue, especially critical in underdeveloped countries, can be addressed is by the creation of a dental auxiliary university. This university would be an institution in which dental assistants, dental hygienists, and expanded-duty auxiliaries could become educated and trained to provide desperately needed dental services to populations worldwide. Dental hygiene professionals worldwide can best contribute to overall oral health by vigorously promoting the importance of effective plaque removal.

Countries such as Grenada, Saint Lucia, and Jamaica are interested in accessing assistance from dental hygienists. Most countries would benefit by program activities in (1) nutrition education to lower caries activity; (2) water or salt fluoridation, school-based fluoride programs, and home use of fluoridated toothpaste; (3) education of children and adults to increase and maintain effective oral hygiene practices, along with education about the proper use of dental services; and (4) school dental programs providing education and treatment.

Expanded-duty auxiliary programs are already in place in Jamaica, Trinidad, and Suriname. Aux-

iliaries are able to perform basic dental restorations and treatment for children. More than 100 auxiliaries have been trained, and have already established their own association.

Dental hygienists are largely an untapped resource, capable of significantly reducing dental personnel shortages in many countries. However, a new role for the dental hygienist must evolve into a broader, less traditional type of dental care provider. Many people in developing and undeveloped countries do not understand the necessity for or the concept of the role and function of the traditional dental hygienist. This lack of understanding can be explained in two ways. First, dental disease is historically caries oriented, with the dentist providing treatment. Second, in many places periodontal disease and oral hygiene have not been recognized as health issues. A clear goal is to increase interest, motivation, and participation in improving oral health.[18]

This chapter presents some representative examples of underdeveloped and developing nations, such as China and Venezuela; of developed nations, such as New Zealand; and of highly industrialized nations, such as Japan and the United Kingdom. The dental health status of these nations is not solely governed by socioeconomic conditions. For example, during the past 20 years, Japan's DMFT level for the 12-year-old population negatively progressed from what was a moderate DMFT level (2.7 to 4.4) in 1970 to a high DMFT level (4.5 to 6.5) in 1990, surpassing the WHO global indicator of oral health (3 DMFT per 12-year-old child). During the same time frame, New Zealand's DMFT level for the 12-year-old population has impressively improved from a very high level (6.6+) to a low level (1.2 to 2.6), thereby attaining a level lower than the global indicator.

Table 4-4 A 20-year comparison of dental caries prevalence rates (DMFT) at age 12

Country	1970 DMFT level	1990 DMFT level
Japan	Moderate, 2.7 to 4.4	High, 4.5 to 6.5
Venezuela	Moderate, 2.7 to 4.4	Moderate, 2.7 to 4.4
United Kingdom	High, 4.5 to 6.5	Moderate, 2.7 to 4.4
New Zealand	Very high, 6.6+	Low, 1.2 to 2.6
China	Unknown	Very low, 0 to 1.1

According to the data available from the WHO Global Oral Data Bank, the United Kingdom and Venezuela DMFT levels for the 12-year-old populations are within range of the global indicator. New Zealand and China are below the indicator.

These particular data are not indications of dental personnel availability or periodontal status. A developing country such as China may appear to have a low prevalence of dental caries; however, the periodontal needs in older populations may be high and the dental personnel resources may be low. At the other end of the spectrum, a wealthy country such as Japan, which has financial resources for preventive programs such as education and fluoridation, does not seem to be able to control the dental caries prevalence rate of its youth (Table 4-4; Figs. 4-5 and 4-6).

A global mean for DMFT of the 12-year-old population has been calculated from the data contained in the Global Oral Data Bank. Separate means for developing countries and highly industrialized countries have also been calculated. In 1980 the global mean was 2.43 DMFT, the developing countries' mean was 1.63 DMFT, and the highly industrialized countries' mean was 4.53 DMFT. Five years later, in 1985, the means were 2.78, 2.43, and 3.82, respectively. It is important to note that not all member countries have contributed equally current data to the data bank. Therefore existing oral data bank statistics may indicate trends in oral health status rather than an accurate reflection of the oral health status of all member countries at the present time. Oral health surveys may not have been conducted recently in some countries.[51]

Modern technological advances in communication, information, and transportation systems provide greater access to the people of the world and assist in the identification and quantification of their health needs. The Global Oral Data Bank is still in need of data from populations in many countries. Using standardized data collection methods set forth by the WHO, initial oral health assessment surveys to establish baseline data are needed, as well as subsequent surveys at established intervals. Additionally, more complete and accurate data on the fluoridation status of countries are desirable. Modern technology provides the capability to help countries develop productive and cost-effective dental care delivery systems. By furnishing these countries with needed technical support, learning by trial and error can be eliminated.

REFERENCES

1. Ainamoj J and others: "Oral health habits among teenagers in Helsinki, Beijing, Hanoi, and Hochiminh City," *J Public Health Dent* 50:214, 1990 (abstract).
2. American Association for Dental Research: Membership services information, July, 1990.
3. American Dental Hygienists' Association: UPDATE: dental hygiene representative participates in FDI-World Dental Congress, *J Dent Hyg,* November-December 1990, p 404.
4. Anderson RJ and others: The reduction of dental caries prevalence in English schoolchildren, *J Dent Res* 61:1311, 1982.
5. Arnljot HA and others, editors: *Oral health care systems: an international collaborative study,* London, 1985, Quintessence, on behalf of the World Health Organization.
6. Beck DJ: *Dental health status of the New Zealand population in late adolescence and young adulthood,* Department of Health Special Report No 29, Wellington, 1968, Government Printer.
7. Brown RH: Evidence of decrease in the prevalence of dental caries in New Zealand, *J Dent Res* 61:1327, 1982.
8. Census of 1990: *The 1990 census,* Communiqué No 1, *Beijing Review* 33:17, 1990.
9. Clancy SA, Project Stretch: Personal communication, March 20, 1991.
10. Cohen LK: *Dental care delivery in seven nations: the international collaborative study of dental manpower systems in relation to oral health status.* In Ingle JI, Blair P, editors: *International dental care delivery systems: issues in dental health policies,* Cambridge, Mass, 1978, Ballinger on behalf of the WK Kellogg Foundation.
11. Cohen LK: Promoting oral health guidlines for dental associations, *Int Dent J* 40:79, 1990.
12. Denby GC, Hollis MJ: The effect of fluoridation on a dental public health programme, *N Z Dent J* 62:32, 1966.
13. Downer MC: The improving dental health of United Kingdom adults and prospects for the future, *Br Dent J* 170:154, 1991.
14. Fédération Dentaire Internationale: *FDI News,* November/December 1990.
15. Fédération Dentaire Internationale: *FDI: the world organization for dentistry. What does it do? How is it organized?* Leaflet E2/4/89, 1989.
16. Foreign Press Center: *Facts and figures of Japan,* Tokyo, 1989, Foreign Press Center.
17. Gardner J, International Dental Hygienists' Federation: Personal communication, March 3, 1991.
18. Gillespie GM, Oral Health Unit, Pan American Health Organization and World Health Organization: Personal communication, March 22, 1991.
19. Hamburg DA: *Greetings from the Institute of Medicine.* In Ingle JI, Blair P, editors: *International dental care delivery systems: issue in dental health policies,* Cambridge,

Mass, 1978, Ballinger on behalf of the WK Kellogg Foundation.

20. Hancocks S: New contract for U.K. dentists, *FDI News,* November/December 1990.

21. Honkala E and others: Dental health habits in Austria, England, Finland and Norway, *Int Dent J* 38:131, 1988.

22. Huntley DE: A scientific exchange with the People's Republic of China, *Dent Hyg* 58:156, 1984.

23. Ingle JI, Blair P, editors: *International dental care delivery systems: issues in dental health policies,* Cambridge, Mass, 1978, Ballinger on behalf of the WK Kellogg Foundation.

24. International Association for Dental Research: Membership services information, July 1990.

25. Kane JF, Project Stretch: Personal communication, March 20, 1991.

26. Kawamura Y, editor: *Chronicle of the 58th IADR general session,* Osaka, 1980.

27. Kurian GT: *The encyclopedia of the third world,* vol 3, New York, 1987, Facts on File.

28. Leclercq MH, Barmes DE: International collaborative studies in oral health: a practical illustration of WHO research policy, *Int Dent J* 40:167, 1990.

29. Malcolm LA: *Decentralization of health service management: a review of the New Zealand experience,* In Mills A and others, editors: *Health system decentralization: concepts, issues and country experience,* Geneva, 1990, World Health Organization.

30. Management and Coordination Agency: *Kokusai tokei yoran (International statistics manual),* 1988.

31. Ministry of Foreign Affairs: *About New Zealand,* Wellington, 1987, Ministry of Foreign Affairs.

32. Møller IJ: Impact of oral diseases across cultures, *Int Dent J* 28:376, 1978.

33. Møller IJ: Preventive responses to various national problems, *Int Dent J* 29:208, 1979.

34. Motley WE: *Brief history: international liaison committee/International Dental Hygienists' Federation,* Unpublished manuscript, 1989.

35. National Institute of Dental Research: *Broadening the scope: long-range research plan for the nineties,* Bethesda, Md, NIH Pub No 90-1188, 1990.

36. National Institute of Dental Research: *Dental science–dental health: NIDR at 40,* Bethesda, Md, NIH Pub No 88-1868, 1988.

37. Pan American Health Organization: *Report of the director: quadrennial 1986-1989, annual 1989,* Washington, DC, Official Document No 234, 1990, Pan American Health Organization.

38. Pan American Health Organization: *Pan American Health Organization: oral health program,* Washington, DC.

39. Pilot T: Reaching out to the community: the activities of the FDI-WHO joint working group 10 on periodontal health services, *Int Dent J* 39:52, 1989.

40. Project HOPE Development Office, Carolyn Heisey and Nicki Peterson: Personal communication, February, 1991.

41. Siegel MP, World Health Organization: Personal communication, February and June 1991.

42. Southeast Asian Medical Information Center, International Medical Foundation of Japan: *SEAMIC health statistics, 1987,* Pub No 52, Tokyo, 1988, SEAMIC/IMFJ.

43. Takada K and others: Use of students' oral health information data base at high school, *J Public Health Dent* 50:215, 1990 (abstract).

44. United Kingdom, Central Office of Information: *Britain's system of government,* Reference Pub No 21/88, London, 1988, Her Majesty's Stationery Office.

45. United Kingdom, Central Office of Information: *Social welfare in Britain,* Reference Pub No 70/89, London, 1989, Her Majesty's Stationery Office.

46. United States Department of Commerce, Bureau of the Census, International Demographic Data Center, China Branch Office: *Summary tables,* Washington, DC, 1991, China Branch Office.

47. Walsh J: International patterns of oral health care: the example of New Zealand, *N Z Dent J* 66:143, 1970.

48. World Bank: *World tables,* Baltimore, 1990, The John Hopkins University Press.

49. World Health Organization: *A guide to oral health epidemiological investigations,* Geneva, 1979, World Health Organization.

50. World Health Organization: *Fluorine and fluorides,* Geneva, 1984, World Health Organization.

51. World Health Organization: *Evaluation of the strategy for health for all by the year 2000: seventh report on the world health situation, vol 1, Global review,* Geneva, 1987, World Health Organization.

52. World Health Organization: *Oral health surveys,* ed 3, Geneva, 1987, World Health Organization.

53. World Health Organization: *Four decades of achievement (1948-1988): highlights of the work of WHO,* Geneva, 1988, World Health Organization.

54. World Health Organization: *WHO: what it is, what it does,* Geneva, 1988, World Health Organization.

55. World Health Organization: *Facts about WHO,* Geneva, 1990, World Health Organization.

5 Geriatric Dental Health

Interest in the provision of care for the elderly began in the 1960s, when the two federally sponsored health programs, Medicaid and Medicare, underscored the enormous and disproportionate cost of health care services to this group. Since then, both the dental and the medical professions have attempted to develop rational systems for training personnel and establishing delivery systems that meet the needs of the elderly.[42] This chapter considers some of the social and economic issues affecting the elderly, as well as the medical and psychological considerations that affect the practice of dentistry. The elderly are not simply another version of younger individuals who happen to have a greater incidence of disease. They are human beings who have attained a stage of life characterized by unique social and biological conditions.

In part, the high cost of care to the elderly is a result of their increase in numbers during the twentieth century. In the early 1900s the ratio of individuals older than age 55 to the rest of the population was 1 to 10, and for the over-65 age group it was 1 to 25. By 1984 the population older than 55 accounted for one in five Americans, and the over-65 age group accounted for one in nine.[47]

Table 5-1 shows the country's age distribution in 1984 and provides some basis for assessing the future. The increase in the number of elderly is a result not only of increased longevity but also of population spurts caused by periods of increased numbers of births. The data reflects the baby boom generation or those individuals born between 1946 and 1962, who in 1984 constituted the 20- to 39-year-age group. This group will be eligible for Social Security during the early part of the twenty-first century.

In 1984 21% of the U.S. population was older than age 55 and approximately 12% was older than age 65 because of increased longevity, an increase in births after World War I, and a decline in births during the 1960s. All these factors have contributed to a steep rise in the median age of the U.S. population. In 1970 the median age of the U.S. population was 28; in 1984 this number jumped to 31. This last number represented a singularly large increase in U.S. demographic history.[47]

In 1989 the Bureau of the Census[44] projected that over the next 20 years the elderly population would grow more slowly than it has in many decades and that the "percentage of the population that is elderly would change from 12.4% in 1988 to 13.9 in 2010. Between 1995 and 2005, the proportion of the population that is elderly would remain virtually unchanged, rising from 13.1 to 13.2 percent."

"From 2010 to 2030, the number of people 65 and over is projected to increase substantially—from 39.4 million in 2010 to 65.6 million in 2030. Nearly 22 percent of the population would be 65 or older in 2030."[44]

The aging of the U.S. population is changing in other respects as well. Not only is the over-65 population growing but also among the over-65 groups the over-75 group is growing the fastest. For example, in 1980 the "young" old group (65-74) outnumbered the older group (75 plus) by a 3 to 2 ratio. In the year 2000 the number of individuals over age 75 will equal the number of individuals between 65 and 74.

As the population ages the distribution by sex also changes. The elderly population is comprised of many more women than men. According to the 1980 census, at age 65 there were 79.4 men for every 100 women. By age 85 there were only 48.5 men for every 100 women. Of the women over age 65, the majority (66%) were widowed and living alone. Men are more likely to live with a spouse, and about 30% continue to work.[30]

Approximately 20% of those older than age 65 spend some time in a nursing home or extended care facility. At any point in time, about 5% are

105

Table 5-1 Distribution of the population by older age groups, 1984

Age group	Number	Percent
All ages	236,416	100
0-54	186,220	79
55-64	22,210	9
65-74	16,596	7
75-84	8,793	4
85 plus	2,596	1
55 plus	50,195	21
65 plus	27,985	12

From U.S. Senate Special Committee on Aging: *America in transition: an aging society*, 1984-85 edition, Washington, DC, 1985, US Government Printing Office.

institutionalized.[30] Most dependent elderly are cared for by relatives, and home health care services provide support for those who live alone and require assistance.

Many of the elderly suffer from chronic disease. About 90% have one chronic disease or more. Although a majority of the elderly remain active, almost 17% are unable to carry on major activities. Chronic ailments and associated limitations contribute to the dependence of the elderly and also have major impacts on treatment modalities, treatment plans, and preventive therapy.[30]

LEVELS OF DEPENDENCE

Most individuals older than 65 function without assistance. Many, however, although not institutionalized, have major activity limitations as a result of chronic conditions.[40] Elderly people living in the community are categorized according to degrees of dependence. *Dependence* is defined as the "need for assistance in bathing, dressing, eating or transferring from bed to chair."[36] The functionally dependent are those who are seriously impaired and unable to maintain themselves. They are either homebound or institutionalized. The frail elderly are those who have chronic debilitating physical, medical, and emotional problems and a loss of their social support systems. They are unable to maintain their independence without help from others. Most of these individuals reside in the community; a small percentage are institutionalized.[12]

The elderly who are admitted to extended-care

facilities usually suffer from one or more of the following conditions: failing intellectual capacity and inability to make life-choice decisions, physical instability leading to falling episodes, immobility as a result of crippling conditions, and incontinence. These individuals have dental treatment needs somewhat different from those of the general elderly population.

A survey of nursing home patients disclosed the following regarding their dental health and treatment needs: 70.3% had no natural teeth, and 30% had some or all their natural teeth, most of whom believed that their teeth were in good or fair condition. About half these patients had been transported to a private office for care, and the other half had been treated at home. Approximately 40% of those with teeth had visited the dentist, whereas only about 19% of the edentulous patients had gone. This discrepancy in use between dentate and edentulous patients mimics the pattern of use among noninstitutionalized dentate and edentulous individuals.[9]

There is a vast gap between the institutionalized patients' perception of their treatment needs and professionals' perception of their needs. Of those who did not visit a dentist during the past year, examining dentists determined that 82.5% were in need of some type of dental treatment. Of those needing care, 71% could be treated in a dental chair, and 18.1% required bedside care. Four percent could not be treated because of a mental or physical condition.

As the elderly population increases, the number of institutionalized patients requiring care will also grow. This group is currently underserved, and there is a need for dentists and dental hygienists to be trained in the delivery of services to this group.[1]

USE OF DENTAL SERVICES

The increase in numbers of elderly and the shifts in social factors have been accompanied by changes in the numbers of individuals over age 65 who visit the dentist. In 1964 about 21% of the individuals over age 65 had visited the dentist during the previous year.[3,11] In 1979 this figure had increased to approximately 33%. A 1985-86 National Institute for Dental Research (NIDR) sponsored survey discovered that, among 5,000 well elderly, approximately 55% of the dentate elderly had visited a dentist within the past 12 months. Only 13% of the edentate elderly had seen a dentist over the same period. The well, dentate elderly used the services of a dentist at about the same rate as working adults and the population as a whole.[45] The increased use has generally been attributed to changes in the social, educational, and economic backgrounds of the newer generations of elderly rather than to any changes in the delivery system.[11]

Investigators describe use behavior as a function of socioeconomic factors such as income, age, race, and gender.[2,9,11,20] Other findings relate user behavior to use patterns that occur during earlier periods of the individual's life.[49] Although this is not surprising, it is helpful in forecasting behavior in future generations of elderly.

The assessment of treatment needs is a difficult and problematic task. Treatment needs are generally described in terms of professionally established criteria. The elderly, however, have less stringent standards in evaluating their oral health status. Perception of treatment needs affects use. In part, the perception of need may be influenced by education, but it is likely that there will always be a considerable gap between professional judgment and perceptions of the potential patient. This phenomenon, therefore, is an explanation of why there is often a difference between the behavior predicted by the professional and the actual behavior of the potential patient. The elderly also tend to have lower expectations for the outcomes of therapy than do the dental professionals, particularly with respect to periodontal and preventive services and especially among men.[49] This factor of decreased expectations may also account for the significantly lower use rates among edentulous and denture-wearing groups.

According to the elderly, the key impediment to seeking service is cost. Most elderly have fixed incomes and need to apportion this income among various options. Dental services, according to most polls, do not appear at the top of the priority list. However, the interpretation of cost as a factor in receiving dental care is confounded by the observation that in countries with publicly funded programs there is not a significant difference in the amount of use by the elderly. Use behavior, therefore, is determined by a combination of attitudinal and socioeconomic factors. Factors that contribute to low use by the elderly are fear of treatment, lack of transportation, lack of mobility by the individual, lack of a regular dentist, illnesses, and some concerns about bothering a busy dentist.

The use of dental services by the elderly is also partly determined by the education and attitudes of the dental professionals. Surveys of dental professionals indicate that many have little or no training in geriatrics and most accept popularly held aging myths.[13,21] Surveys on dental education reveal efforts at both the predoctoral and postdoctoral levels to remediate this situation. The lack of geriatric sophistication by dental professionals often results in dental offices that are poorly located or poorly designed for the purpose of accommodating the needs of the elderly. Adequate nearby parking is often missing. Ramps to assist those who are handicapped or hallways of sufficient width for the passage of wheelchairs may not be provided.[10,14] Many professionals feel that the elderly or the chronically ill cause discomfort for other patients. Treatment of the elderly is perceived as being more difficult and more time-consuming than treatment of other groups.

TREATMENT OF THE ELDERLY PATIENT

The aging adult must cope with an increasing number of physical and psychological problems. The average older adult living in the community suffers from 3.5 major disabilities; the average institutionalized elderly individual manifests six pathologic conditions.[36]

Aging also implies the modification or loss of cells of various organs of the body. The kidney, for example, over the course of a life span, loses nephrons. Most organ systems, however, function well with only 15% of their cells intact. The loss of cells does limit the reserve capacity of the involved organ and thereby compromises the ability of the individual to cope with stress. The dental practitioner, therefore, must consider this factor as a component of the office visit.

Symptoms of cognitive impairment occur more frequently in older individuals. These individuals may appear to be suffering from fluctuating levels of awareness, mild confusion, stupor, or delirium. Most of the time these symptoms are caused by malnutrition and anemia, congestive heart failure, infection, drugs, head trauma, alcohol, a cerebrovascular accident, dehydration, responses to surgery, and a host of other conditions. Often the health care practitioner may assume that these symptoms are manifestations of a chronic brain syndrome such as Alzheimer's disease. It is important to distinguish among the various causes of brain-related symptoms for the patient to receive the appropriate care.

Aging changes and disease

The interplay of aging changes and disease is of particular importance to the practitioner because the distinction between these phenomena permits accurate diagnosis and appropriate treatment. Physiologic changes related to aging influence the presentation of disease and the response to treatment and are associated with the complications that ensue. Generally, three related categories describe the impact of physiologic change on disease: (1) physiologic variables that remain constant throughout life; (2) physiologic changes that increase the likelihood of disease; and (3) physiologic changes that have a direct clinical relationship to the appearance of disease. An example of an incorrectly anticipated aging change is the diagnosis of senile anemia. In normal aging adults, blood sera factors such as hematocrit, fasting blood glucose, serum electrolyte concentrations, and blood gas values remain the same. A drop in the hemoglobin value should be evaluated for causative agents and not attributed to the aging process.

The changes that increase the likelihood of disease are generally those that deprive the various organ systems of their physiologic reserve because of the loss of cells. The systems affected in this manner include the renal, the pulmonary, the immune functions, and the homeostatic mechanisms. This reduction in reserve contributes to the increased vulnerability of the elderly to disease during acute illness, trauma as a result of burns, major surgery, and administration of medications. Visits to the dentist or dental hygienist, of course, are potential sessions of increased stress, and the practitioner must modify the management of the patient accordingly.

The purpose of the discussion on aging in terms

of physiologic change is to clarify the relationship of the aging process to disease. The aging process may have relatively no impact on the body's physiologic functions or, as in the case of the kidney, the process may compromise some organ systems so as to render them and the individual more vulnerable to stress and disease. In some cases physiologic changes may result in adverse symptoms. Examples of these types of changes include age-related menopause, arteriosclerotic changes, and modifications of the lens of the eye. The modifications of the lens have important implications for dentistry. Dentists and dental hygienists have observed the tendency of elderly patients to select denture teeth that are several shades too white. This occurs because of the increased opacity and amber tint of the lens of the eye. The patient sees the recommended denture teeth as being too yellow and therefore aesthetically unacceptable. This is but one example of how the understanding of aging changes are important to appropriate patient management.[23]

The relationship of physiologic change as a result of aging and disease, as previously discussed, does not account for all disease-related phenomena in the elderly. The complexity of the process is underscored by the following occurrences: (1) Several diseases occur less frequently in older adults, and (2) some diseases or conditions in the elderly initially have symptoms that are different from those found in younger individuals. The immune-mediated diseases such as myasthenia gravis or lupus erythematosus are found infrequently or not at all in older adults. Certain antibody titers are higher in the elderly, which suggests that older adults have increased resistance to some diseases.

With respect to the altered state of disease presentation, there are two interesting examples. The first is hyperthyroidism, found in younger individuals as an elevator of mood and various functions. In the older adult most functions are depressed by the condition. Patients with acute myocardial infarctions also show different symptoms. The elderly are less likely to manifest chest pain, although they are more likely to experience syncope. Findings such as these suggest that pain in the elderly needs to be evaluated differently than in younger individuals.

Dental disease in the elderly

Dental caries is thought of as a disease of youth that stabilizes in the middle twenties. Current information indicates a decrease in caries among 5- to 17-year-olds. These findings suggest that future generations of middle-aged and elderly individuals will have more teeth and more vulnerable tooth surfaces.

During 1985-86 it was discovered that there had been a dramatic decrease in the proportion of edentulous persons (when compared with studies done in the 1960s) and that there was an increase in the mean number of decayed and filled teeth among dentulous older adults. This latter finding was thought to be the result of the increased retention of teeth and use of dental services and not the result of increased caries activity.[39,45] Root caries has been studied for several years, but only recently has the root caries index (RCI) afforded the dental profession a realistic picture of root caries prevalence and location.[25-27] The RCI calculates the presence of root caries in relation to susceptible surfaces, that is, where gingival recession has taken place. The occurrence of root caries is age related (Fig. 5-1); its occurrence is related to the number of exposed root surfaces (at times caused by periodontal

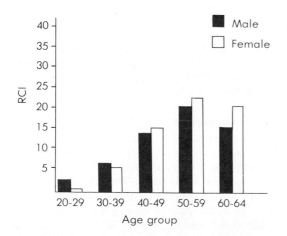

Fig. 5-1 RCI prevalence rates for males and females by age group. (From Katz RV: Root caries: clinical implications of the current epidemiologic data, *Northwest Dent* 60:308, 1981.)

surgery). Mandibular molars are the teeth most often attacked by root caries.

Strategies that are effective in the prevention of coronal caries are presumably effective in the prevention of root caries. There is evidence that both systemic and topical fluoride have the appropriate effect.[18] Antimicrobials are under investigation as caries-preventive agents.

Secondary decay is a considerable problem, and some researchers have suggested that restorations with overhanging margins are at increased risk of disease in the elderly. Prevention of these conditions should include the application of fluoride to the potential sites and the elimination of aberrant margins.[30] Periodontal disease occurs with more frequency and more severity with advancing age.[19,31,39,45] However, the rates and the degrees of severity, according to the national survey, were less than anticipated.[45] The prevalence of gingivitis (periodontal disease without pocket formation) has decreased.[39] The occurrence of periodontal disease is related to the increased rate of plaque accumulation that is observed in the elderly during periods of oral hygiene abstinence. There is also evidence that the appearance of gingivitis is more rapid and that bone loss and rate of gingival attachment loss are accelerated. Preventive therapy for the elderly needs to be more frequent and more vigorous.

The design of self-administered plaque-control programs must include consideration of the inability of many elderly to manipulate conventional self-cleaning devices. This is especially true among victims of stroke, arthritis, or palsylike conditions. In some instances, especially among institutionalized elderly, it is necessary for auxiliary personnel to attend to dental hygiene needs. Oral hygiene implements may be modified to facilitate use. Modifications or substitutes for the toothbrush include the following: an electric toothbrush; something placed over the handle such as a styrofoam ball, a bicycle handgrip, or a soft rubber ball; plastic tubing attached to the handle of the toothbrush to lengthen the handle; an Ace bandage or aluminum foil wrapped around the toothbrush handle; a bend in the toothbrush handle; and the creation of a cuff to fit around the handle. A floss holder may also be valuable (Fig. 5-2).

Oral examinations of older adults should include

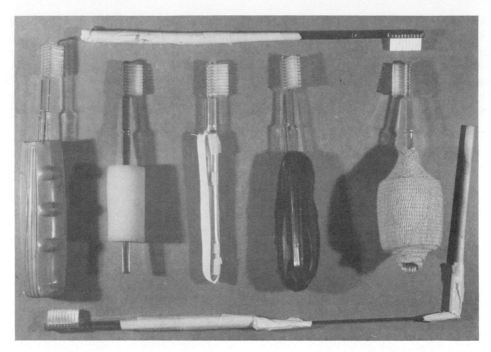

Fig. 5-2 Toothbrush modifications: *top,* plastic tubing extension; *left to right,* bicycle handle, Styrofoam ball, elastic cuff, Velcro cuff, Ace bandage; *bottom,* bent wire extension.

a thorough examination of anatomic sites that are potential tumor sites. Oral cancer accounts for 5% of cancer in men and 2% of all cancers in women. These lesions are more frequent in older adults. To minimize the effect of this disease, the patient should be informed of the hazards of tobacco and alcohol, the need for regular dental checkups, and the need to eliminate tissue irritants.

Discussion of dental treatment

Treatment of institutionalized patients is marked by a dramatic need for oral prophylaxis. Epidemiologists who have attempted to quantify dental disease in this group have commented on the difficulty of clinical examination because of the presence of plaque and debris.[26-28] In addition to preventive services, of those elderly who require services, about 24% need treatment of lesions that arc potential sources of pain or infection. Approximately 5% need relief from pain or infection, and 84% need treatment of pulpally involved teeth.[9] Nursing home patients, who are on the average older than the elderly who remain in the commu-

nity, generally are less able to practice personal hygiene and less able to manipulate dental appliances. Because of this, partial dentures for the handicapped elderly are reconstructed with wrought wire clasps to facilitate denture removal.

The types of dental services provided to well elderly are described in a program conducted in Minnesota in 1982.[48] The goal of this program was to establish a statewide dental program for the purpose of determining the dental needs of the elderly. In addition to testing the administrative feasibility of a statewide program, the project determined the frequency distribution of types of services. The program was offered to those who were 62 years of age or older and retired. These individuals also needed to pass a means test, and all services were paid for by the state of Minnesota. Of the 15,000 applications mailed, about 30% were returned (somewhat below the use rate determined by the NIDR survey of 1985-86), and about 40% of these were eligible for services. The mean age of the eligible population was 73.8 years. The services offered were routine examinations, emergency treatment, restorative services, oral surgery, surgical and nonsurgical periodontal treatment, endodontic treatment, and prosthodontic services. A summary of the dental treatment delivered to first-year users appears in Table 5-2.

An analysis of the services delivered reveals the following: men were the recipients of more removable prosthodontic and oral surgical services; women received more diagnostic, preventive, and restorative services; provision of diagnostic, preventive, restorative, endodontic, and fixed prosthodontic services declined with the advancing age of the participants; and provision of removable prosthodontic services increased as the average age of recipients increased. Although use among the participants declined during the second year, the service distribution profile remained about the same.

In 1990 Meskin and associates[33] described the results of a five-state survey of dental services provided to older adults in private practice. They discovered that the elderly required more removable and fixed prosthodontics and that there was more interest in implants. They also confirmed the increase in root caries among the elderly. More than 50% of the income in restorative dentistry was derived from the placement of re-restorations in patients 40 years of age or older.

The findings of the Minnesota project and the Meskin survey, as well as the shifts in the distribution of dental disease among the U.S. population, indicate that future generations of elderly will have significant needs for preventive and restorative services. The decrease in the number of the edentulous indicates that fewer elderly will require full dentures, and more elderly will be in need of partial denture construction. Moreover, with the increasing penchant of dentate elderly to use the services of dentists, it is probable that an increased proportion of the elderly will seek dental care.

Evaluation of the elderly patient

What is apparent in the provision of care to the elderly is that they are a heterogeneous group, both biologically and socially. The over-70 population demonstrates greater variation anatomically, physiologically, and biochemically than any other age category.[37] These differences may be functions of race, sex, geographic location, or socioeconomic factors. The multifarious nature of this segment of the population poses a management challenge to the dental practitioner.

The identification of patient diversity is further complicated by factors that impact on the ability of the patient to communicate with the practitioner. Of the population older than age 65, approximately 10% suffer from dementia, 22% suffer from impaired hearing, and about 15% have visual handicaps.[32] History-taking or interviewing of the elderly often requires increased interview time and dependence on other professionals (the dentist, for example, depends on the patient's physician as well as the dental hygienist). Thus one might conclude not only that there is more information to glean from an interview with an older adult but also that accessing the information is more complex.

Delivery of services to the elderly, more than any other aspect of dental care, requires that the practitioner consider several dimensions of the patient's life. The "dynamics of rational dental care" depicts the relationship of various factors that need to be considered in the development of a treatment plan (Fig. 5-3). Appropriate dental services for the elderly require a comprehensive evaluation of the patient's status.

Medical considerations. The international classification of disease published by the World Health

Table 5-2 Frequency distribution of use by category service

Service	Total claimants %
Diagnostic	80.7
Prophylaxis	56.3
Restorative	55.7
Endodontics (nonsurgical)	6.3
Periodontics (nonsurgical)	8.5
Oral surgery	27.5
Removable prosthodontics	62.2
Fixed prosthodontics	5.1

From Yellowitz JA and others: The Minnesota Dental Insurance Program for Senior Citizens: two year results for the utilization of services, *J Am Dent Assoc* 104:455, 1982. (Copyright by the American Dental Association. Reprinted by permission.)

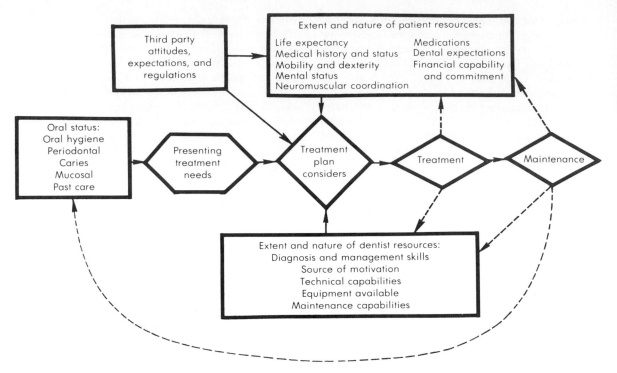

Fig. 5-3 Dynamics of rational dental care. (From Ettinger RL, Beck JD: Geriatric dental curriculum and the needs of the elderly, *Spec Care Dentist* 4:209, 1984. (Copyright by the American Dental Association. Reprinted by permission.)

Organization lists 120 diseases with oral manifestations.[31] The dental practitioner needs to be aware of these diseases, and medical and dental histories should reflect efforts to identify these conditions.

The most frequent causes of death in the elderly are cardiovascular disease, cancer, and stroke. Recently Alzheimer's disease has been implicated in the mortality rates of older adults. Other diseases or conditions that occur frequently in the elderly are thyroid cancer, breast cancer, cervical cancer, occult bleeding, hypertension, postural hypotension, oral disease and its relationship to malnutrition, wax impaction in the ears, auditory or ophthalmic disorders, bowel malfunctions, degrees of urinary incontinence, sleep disturbances, and postural instability that causes falling.[35]

Concurrent with the presence of disease is treatment with pharmacologic preparations. The elderly, because of altered metabolic rates, need to have their dosages modified. Patient compliance with drug regimens is an important issue, and many dental practitioners insist that their patients bring their medicines to the office so that a careful drug assessment can be made. The following is a list of drug-related phenomena that are of interest to the dentist or dental hygienist. Table 5-3 cites drug-induced changes in the tissues of the mouth. Following are other factors to keep in mind:

1. Antimicrobials are well tolerated, but reduced dosages are required.
2. Aspirin and Coumadin may contribute to hemorrhaging.
3. Stomatitis may be related to the administration of dentifrices, mouthwash, denture adhesives, toothache drops, ascorbic acid, intramuscular gold therapy, antineoplastic agents, and folic acid antagonists.
4. Pacemakers may be affected by equipment such as pulp testers and motorized chairs.

Table 5-3 Drug-induced changes in tissues of the mouth

Drug	Effect	Drug	Effect
Adrenal hormones		Cyclophosphamide (Cytoxan)	Stomatitis
Corticosteroids (general)	Oral candidiasis (thrush) Hairy tongue	Folic acid antagonists (e.g., methotrexate, fluorouracil, asparaginase)	Stomatitis Stomatitis
Beclomethasone dipropionate (Vanceril)	Oral, laryngeal, and pharyngeal candidiasis		
Analgesics		Mercaptopurine (Purinethol)	Stomatitis
Aspirin	Burns and ulceration of oral mucosa	Plicamycin (Mithracin)	Stomatitis
Phenylbutazone (Butazolidin)	Parotitis	Vinblastine (Velban)	Stomatitis
Antibiotics		*Gold therapy*	
Antibiotics (general)	Oral candidiasis Hairy tongue	Gold sodium thiomalate (Myochrysine)	Stomatitis, glossitis
Tetracycline	Oral candidiasis Hairy tongue Tooth pigmentation	Aurothioglucose (Solganal)	
		Heavy metal antagonist	
Erythromycin	Enamel hypoplasia	Penicillamine (Cuprimine)	Taste disturbances
Anticonvulsant		*Heavy metals*	
Phenytoin	Gingival hyperplasia	Lead, bismuth, mercury	Pigmentation of oral soft tissues
Antidepressants		*Hypotensives*	
Amitriptyline (Elavil, Endep)	Xerostomia	Clonidine hydrochloride (Catapres)	Xerostomia, parotitis
Imipramine (Tofranil)	Xerostomia	Reserpine (Serpasil)	Xerostomia
Desipramine (Norpramin)	Xerostomia	*Mouthwashes and gargles*	
Antifungal antibiotic		Hydrogen peroxide	Hairy tongue
Griseofulvin (Fulvicin U/F, Grisactin, Grifulvin V)	Hairy tongue	*Agents*	
		Lithium carbonate (Eskalith, Lithane)	Taste disturbances
Antineoplastics			
Doxorubicin (Adriamycin)	Stomatitis		
Bleomycin sulfate (Blenoxane)	Stomatitis		

5. Long-term administration of phenothiazines may lead to tardive dyskinesia, which is characterized by spastic, uncontrolled movements of the lips and tongue.
6. Several artificial salivas are available. These preparations alleviate some of the symptoms of xerostomia and serve as oral cavity moisteners.

Conditions requiring consultation with a physician. The elderly, more than other age groups, are at risk for infective endocarditis, late prosthetic joint infection, excessive bleeding as a result of anticoagulants, and complications from ischemic heart disease. All these conditions require consultation with the physician.

More than half of all endocarditis patients are elderly. Patients who have had synthetic arterial repairs or bypasses or who are immunosuppressed as the result of steroid treatment, poorly controlled diabetes, cancer chemotherapy, or transplant immunosuppression are also vulnerable and, after consultation with the physician, require prophylactic antibiotic therapy.[40]

Poor dental health and poor oral hygiene are factors in determining whether the patient requires antimicrobials. Dental or periodontal infections and the presence of debris as the result of poor oral hygiene increases the risks of bacteremias.[40] Frequent and intense dental hygiene therapy and physician advocacy of good oral hygiene are components of good treatment.

More than 100,000 joint replacements are performed in the United States each year, and a significant proportion are placed in elderly patients. Infection of joint prosthesis has been demonstrated experimentally, but the clinical evidence is spotty. There have been case reports of late joint infection, that is, 3 months after surgery. These infections have been staphylococcal and not from organisms found in the oral cavity. One survey reported that 93% of physicians felt that antibiotic therapy with cephalosporin was necessary. Prophylactic antibiotic therapy is, at this point, controversial, and therapy should be coordinated with the physician.[40]

Many elderly patients require anticoagulant therapy. Dental procedures that produce bleeding, such as extractions, periodontal therapy, routine dental cleaning, and some routine restorative dental procedures, need to be evaluated for their impact on these patients. Routine withdrawal from anticoagulants is not necessary for all dental treatment.

Mulligan and Weitzel[34] have designated the following categories in connection with risks of hemorrhage:

Low-risk dental procedures include supragingival prophylaxis, simple restorations without subgingival extensions, and local anesthetic injection in well-defined areas over bone.

Moderate-risk procedures include subgingival cleaning, complex restorative procedures with subgingival extensions, simple extractions where primary wound closure is achievable, and regional local anesthetic injections.

High-risk dental procedures include extensive oral surgical procedures.

Using the Mulligan and Weitzel scheme, low-risk category procedures should not require anticoagulant modification. Patients undergoing moderate-risk procedures must have their prothrombin times checked. Prothrombin times within the common therapeutic range (1.5 to 2.0 times normal) should permit treatment without modification as long as the operator has access to conventional antihemorrhage measures. Patients with prothrombin times more than twice normal require removal of anticoagulant 2 days prior to surgery. Anticoagulant may be restored after surgery.[40]

Patients on aspirin, dipyridamole (Persantine) therapy or, other drugs to inhibit platelet aggregation generally do not require special consideration. Patients undergoing extensive surgery generally should discontinue their medications. In all cases a physician should be consulted.

Elderly patients who have suffered ischemic heart disease pose a significant challenge to the dental hygienist or dentist. Dental treatment may provoke anxiety and psychological stress. Complex and lengthy procedures may produce stress in patients who are able to tolerate routine care. The physician must be contacted to determine the patient's stability and to gain a recommendation for minimizing patient stress.

Mental status. Because of the multiplicity of factors that relate to the treatment of the elderly, it is important to evaluate the ability of the patient to communicate and to comply with personal care behavior. The practitioner must determine, either through a psychological evaluation or through an interview, the capacity of the individual to respond to treatment. Although instances of senile dementia are rare, they do increase in frequency as the individual ages: 2% in those between 60 and 65 years of age, 5% in those over age 65, and between 20% and 30% in those over the age of 85.[15]

The most common type of dementia in the elderly is senile dementia of the Alzheimer type. This disease is characterized by a gradual deterioration of almost every function of the brain.[7] The patient progresses through a series of behavioral changes and losses. Cognitive skills as well as competency in the life skills decline. There is loss of intellectual prowess, and the patient experiences language difficulties, memory loss, concentration difficulties, aberrant emotionality, and altered spatial-motor performance. Verbal and nonverbal communication are affected.

Dental care, even in the early stages of dementia, is generally ignored because of the demands on the patient to handle more basic life functions and because of the relative complexity of motion and muscular coordination required in an activity such as toothbrushing. In the early stages of the disease, patients require instruction and, in the later stages, direct intervention by support personnel.[15]

Socioeconomic factors affecting the elderly

The elderly have the lowest median income of any population group. It is conjectured that to maintain a constant standard of living, the retired individual must retain an income that is 75% of preretirement income.[30] In 1980 fewer than one third of retired persons had income other than Social Security. It is estimated that Social Security replaced about 45% of preretirement income for couples and only 30% of income for individuals.

The U.S. Social Security program was established in 1935. Twenty-nine other countries, mostly in Western Europe, established a social security–type system before the United States. All these countries currently contribute a significantly higher percentage of their national resources to these programs.[5] Although the Reagan administration claimed that the Social Security cost-of-living adjustments contributed to the federal deficit, this has not been the case. For the period from 1986 to 1990, income generated by the Social Security tax exceeded total expenditures.[33] Since 1974 the economic status of the elderly has stabilized. This is the result of the cost-of-living increases that have become an integral part of the system. Despite these adjustments, African-American elderly women have continued to experience a high rate of poverty (in 1985, 41.7% had incomes below the poverty level). Among all women, 50% had incomes within $800 of the nationally determined poverty level. Among the elderly population, 20% were below or near the poverty line.

Although a key program, Social Security is not the sole source of income for the retired elderly. Private pension plans contribute at an increasing rate, although they are distributed unevenly throughout the population. Existing plans tend to be more prevalent among high-wage and long-term employees. Women have limited coverage when compared with men, and divorced and widowed women have the least coverage.[29]

The use of dental services is related to the economic status of the users. Although the Social Se-

curity program and private pension plans have contributed to the needs of the elderly, they remain, to some degree, medically and dentally indigent.

Paying for dental care

Out-of-pocket payment remains the dominant method of paying for dental services. Since 1954, dental insurance has grown at an accelerating pace. According to the NIDR survey,[45] 32% of the dentate elderly and 38% of the edentate elderly have some portion of their dental expenses covered by insurance. Another study reported that, by age, there was a descending rate of dental insurance coverage among the elderly, that is, 36% in the 60- to 64-year age group and only 7% in the 80 and older age group. [33] Approximately 58% of the working adults had coverage.[45] The differential in coverage between employed adults and the elderly has occurred as the elderly have become less of a factor in the work force. In 1980 only 20% of men over the age of 65 were employed.[29] For those elderly who qualify for public assistance and who live in states with dental Medicaid programs, there is the possibility of seeking services under this program.

Medicaid, or Title 19 of the Social Security Act, enacted in 1965, provided federal funds to be distributed among the state public assistance programs. The intent of the program was to provide health benefits to the indigent. Eligibility was limited to those eligible for public assistance, and in some states the benefits were extended to those categorized as medically indigent. They were thought to be individuals who could afford to support themselves except for health care. Some services were required under this program; however, dentistry was not one. Where dentistry was included, it was usually underfunded; where the elderly were included, they accounted for a disproportionate amount of the expenditures for dental care.

Medicare, or Title 18 of the Social Security Act, also enacted in 1965, was a program intended to provide health insurance for those over age 65. The program was to pay for hospital and physician services. Dental services, unless provided under special circumstances, were not to be included.

Medicare, under part A, provides for hospital inpatient care, posthospital extended care, and home health visits by nurses. Part B pays for physician services, outpatient hospital services, and outpatient physical therapy.[6] The patient is responsible for deductibles under part A, and there are premiums and co-insurance provisions under part B. Medicare pays for about 44% of the health care costs of the elderly. Dental care may be provided only under specified conditions of hospitalization; for the most part, this involves oral surgical services. When a dentist provides services that are equivalent to those provided by a physician, such as the treatment of an oral lesion or the treatment of an oral infection (for example, candidiasis), the dentist may bill Medicare. Although this regulation is clearly defined, dentists rarely use it.[24]

Over the past decade there have been initiatives to expand coverage for the elderly. One proposal would have expanded Medicare to cover other outpatient services, including dentistry. An auto manufacturer has proposed that, upon retirement, workers should retain their coverage.[42] Private plans, however, are unlikely to assume programs for the elderly for the following reasons: (1) the uncertainty of cost as a result of inflation increases the insurer's risk, and there is fear of dollar losses; (2) administrative costs are high, especially if only a fraction of the population is involved; (3) current programs, such as Medicaid and Medicare, would undercut the market for these programs; and (4) adverse selection, that is, the purchase of insurance by high-risk groups, would drive premiums up and low-income individuals out.[22] Private insurance companies have sponsored programs that supplement Medicare coverage. A persistent social and medical problem has been the inability to develop feasible programs for long-term care coverage.

Mobile dental care

Dentists have been providing dental services to homebound or institutionalized patients for several years. Recent sensitization of dental students to the existence of dental needs among this population has led to efforts by younger dentists to implement mobile systems.[46] These dentists have seen the treatment of this group as a potential source of income. Federal and state laws have mandated levels of dental services for institutionalized patients. In 1974 the federal government required skilled nursing facilities to retain an advisory dentist. Medi-

care funds were made available for reimbursement of authorized dental consultants.[29] They were to be reimbursed for consultation services only. Some states have strengthened the federal statutes by requiring that recently admitted patients receive an oral examination and thereafter be examined at least once each year. The dental consultants supply the following services: provide inservice education for the nursing home staff, devise strategies for oral hygiene programs, recommend policies for emergency care, and assist patients who seek dental care. Although these policies have existed for many years, there are no funding mechanisms or enforcement procedures that ensure dental care for nursing home patients.[38]

An anecdotal account of a long-standing (22 years) private mobile dental program reports the need for trained dentists and several support personnel. Although general practitioners provide adequate services to the well elderly, the dependent elderly require specially trained practitioners. The specially designed vehicle transports teams of dental practitioners consisting of one dentist and two dental auxiliaries. Backup personnel include a full-time administrator, a laboratory technician, and a full-time coordinator.[41] Coordination of this project is exceedingly complex. Persons who need to be consulted or informed during the treatment process include intraoffice personnel, nursing home personnel, the patient, the patient's family, the physician and the physician's staff, government agencies, and third-party payers.

The treatment of the older adult is a time-consuming process. The complexity of the operation is not limited to medical and dental considerations but extends into social, economic, and management areas. Treatment of the elderly requires consultation at all levels and the team approach, involving several disciplines, to provide the necessary support. Although dental hygiene education has only recently begun to increase the sophistication of its geriatric curriculum, dental hygienists are well educated to contribute to the care of institutionalized patients, as well as older adults who seek care in a private practice.[8]

Special roles for the dental hygienist. Institutionalized patients tend to suffer from poor oral hygiene. This condition relates to the aging process and to the infirmities that affect these individuals.

Nursing home personnel, from nurses to nurses' aides, are assigned to assist with the personal oral hygiene of their patients. Generally, nondental personnel are not capable of mounting an effective oral hygiene program. Dental hygienists are the ideal professionals to be program planners, program initiators and implementers, and health educators and practitioners. A dental program in a nursing home consists of four major components: (1) a preventive program, (2) a treatment program, (3) an administrative procedure for coping with emergencies, and (4) program coordination.

The preventive program begins with periodic oral examinations (phase one). These examinations require a tongue blade survey. Their purpose is to determine the general state of oral health, the presence of pathologic conditions, the state of patient oral comfort, and the degree of personal hygiene achieved by the patient. When necessary, the patient may be referred to a dentist. Phase two of the preventive program should include review of the oral health of the edentulous patients. The oral cavity should be surveyed for oral pathologic states and denture sores. All dentures must be labeled to avoid the commonplace loss of dentures. Phase three should include the implementation of personal care strategies. It involves patient education but also in-service education for the nursing home staff. The staff should be taught to construct the adaptive devices that enable the patients to care for themselves.

Treatment that requires the services of a dentist is generally achieved by taking the patient to a practitioner in the community. Because this effort is often of great inconvenience and expense to the patient, other delivery systems are being explored. The role of the nursing home dental auxiliary is to confirm the need for a dentist and, wherever possible, identify situations that may be remedied by the dentist visiting the nursing home. A reline of an old denture, for example, may be handled through a brief visit by the dentist to the institution.

Dental emergencies arise because of toothaches or postoperative bleeding after dental extractions. The dental hygienist may be able to minister to some instances of bleeding but, more important, will be able to identify situations that require the services of a dentist.

The administrator of the dental program has two major functions: (1) to coordinate all personnel who are involved in the oral health care of the elderly and (2) to attend to the massive, bureaucratic paperwork that accompanies all institutional care. The most important paper management challenge is proposed by the patient chart. The chart contains information that includes the following: a list of the various ailments, a list of drugs being taken by the patient, and a description of orthopedic appliances (for example, hip implants require that the patient receive antibiotic therapy prior to dental extractions). Other paper transactions include the third-party forms that need to be processed and the written referrals that need to be formulated.[16]

The need for dental personnel in nursing homes is well documented. The boxes on pages 117 and 118 list the tasks of dental hygienists according to the views of older adults and of dental hygienists themselves.

The portable delivery of dental services, especially to institutions that are domiciliary for groups of elderly, has some cost-containment and convenience advantages. This system simplifies the procedure for obtaining care for dependent individuals. Because of dental hygienists' training, they are invaluable assets for such programs. The functions of the hygienist would be divided into two phases: (1) those performed prior to the arrival of the ser-

---

TASKS FOR THE DENTAL HYGIENIST IDENTIFIED BY OLDER ADULTS (IN ORDER OF IMPORTANCE)

Noninstitutionalized
1. Teach how to keep one's breath fresh
2. Discuss nutritional needs
3. Teach how to care for false teeth
4. Teach how to brush and floss
5. Teach how to retain one's teeth
6. Teach preventive dentistry
7. Check dentures for proper fit
8. Perform oral examinations
9. Clean teeth

From Marinelli RD: Oral health care for the elderly patient: the role of dental hygienists, *Dent Hyg* 57:10, 1983. (Copyright by the American Dental Association. Reprinted by permission.)

vice delivery team and (2) those provided as a member of the visiting team. During the first phase, the dental hygienist screens patients to identify those with oral disease and determine the order of treatment. Coordination and administrative tasks are accomplished. A health history is compiled from information provided by the patient and from available sources. Financial arrangements are negotiated, and the sources of payments are determined. Potential payers aside from the patient are the family, Medicaid, and Medicare. After the arrival of the team that includes a dentist and perhaps one other auxiliary, the hygienist provides clinical hygiene services.[15]

Private practice

The aging of the U.S. population will have a significant economic impact on private dental practice. A survey of dental practices in five states determined that the percentage of patient visits by older adults exceeded their proportion in the population. For each of the practices surveyed the proportion of revenues attributed to the group of patients 60 years of age and older exceeded their proportion of dental visits. It was also discovered that the elderly paid their dental bills out of pocket, through Medicaid, and through private insurance; those who paid through dental insurance tended to have larger dental bills.[33]

Dental patients over the age of 65 represent one fourth of all dental patients.[38] The proportion of elderly who seek dental care promises to grow. More practice time will be dedicated to care of the elderly, and because care to the older adult is more time-consuming, the dentist will need to organize personnel to optimize the patient visit. One potential strategy is to use auxiliaries who are trained in geriatric dentistry. These auxiliaries would conduct health interviews and preliminary examinations. Medications would be reviewed, perhaps with the assistance of a computerized summary of medications and their actions. Performance of these tasks during the intake process would free dentists to concentrate their efforts on diagnosis, treatment planning, and the delivery of services.

An auxiliary involved as described in oral health assessment and interviewing and review of pharmacologic and medical histories of the elderly suggests the need for dental personnel with additional training. A dental hygienist trained to assess the health status of elderly dental patients would save the dentist time and ultimately contribute to the quality of services provided. The box below lists some suggestions for treating the handicapped and the elderly.

TASKS FOR THE DENTAL HYGIENIST IN THE TREATMENT OF THE ELDERLY PATIENT, IDENTIFIED BY DENTAL HYGIENISTS (IN ORDER OF IMPORTANCE)

1. Patient education
2. Oral examination
3. Perform oral prophylaxis
4. Teach oral examinations to staff
5. In-service training
6. Humanistic oral care
7. Nutrition counseling
8. Radiographic survey
9. Institutional oral screening
10. Bedside prophylaxis

From Marinelli RD: Oral health care for the elderly patient: the role of dental hygienists, *Dent Hyg* 57:10, 1983. (Copyright by the American Dental Association. Reprinted by permission.)

SOME RECOMMENDATIONS FOR TREATMENT OF THE HANDICAPPED AND THE ELDERLY IN PRIVATE PRACTICE

1. There must be special emphasis on history-taking, including a review of the patient's drug regimen and history of cardiovascular disease.
2. Patient must be questioned regarding episodes of syncope, especially upon awakening or sitting up.
3. Background noise should be minimized during interview sessions.
4. Avoid supine positions and bring dental chair to the vertical position slowly.
5. Appointments should be arranged to meet the needs of the patients: cardiac and kidney disease patients are better seen in the morning. Arthritic patients are better seen in afternoon.

From Ettinger RL, Beck JD, Glenn RE: Eliminating office architectural barriers to dental care of the elderly and handicapped, *J Am Dent Assoc* 98:398, 1979. (Copyright by the American Dental Association. Reprinted by permission.)

The clinical treatment of the geriatric patient requires a philosophy of care that emphasizes humanism and directs the practitioner to adjust the style of practice to accommodate the needs of the elderly. The practitioner must develop a "sensitivity to the patient's and family's legitimate goals and objectives and to the legal and other requirements of practice in the long-term care system, the acute care hospital, and the patient's home."[4]

The provision of dental care to the elderly patient is basically the same as the care provided to other segments of the population, "yet the effects of aging on normal laboratory values, clinical presentation, and complexities of care management—plus the present reimbursement morass—clearly indicate that this is a different mode of practice."[4] As these factors become clearer, the dental profession will recognize that geriatric dentistry is "not just special, it is different."[4]

REFERENCES

1. ADA Council on Dental Health and Health Planning: *Oral health care in the long-term care facility,* Chicago, 1983, American Dental Association.
2. Antezak AA, Branch LG: Perceived barriers to the use of dental services by the elderly, *Gerodontics* 1:194, 1985.
3. Beck JD: *Dentists and the elderly: attitude and behaviors.* In Chauncey HH and others, editors: *Clinical geriatric dentistry: biomedical and psychosocial aspects,* Chicago, 1985, American Dental Association.
4. Blandford G: Is geriatric clinical practice different? *Center on Aging* 2:1, 1986
5. Butler RN: *Why survive? Being old in America,* New York, 1975, Harper & Row.
6. Butler RN: An overview of research on aging and the status of gerontology, *Milbank Memorial Fund Q; Health Society* 61:351, 1983.
7. Cohen D, Kennedy G, Eisdorfer C: Phases of change in the patient with Alzheimer's dementia: a conceptual dimension for defining health care management, *J Am Geriatr Soc* 32:11, 1954.
8. Cohen L, Labelle A, Singer J: Educational preparation of hygienists working with special populations in non-traditional settings, *J Dent Educ* 49:592, 1985.
9. Council on Dental Health and Health Planning: Oral health status of Vermont nursing home residents, *J Am Dent Assoc* 104:68, 1982.
10. Epstein CF: Enhancing the dental office environment for the elderly, *Dent Clin North Am* 33:43,1989.
11. Ettinger RL, Beck JD: The new elderly: what can the dental profession expect? *Spec Care Dentist* 2:62, 1982.
12. Ettinger RL, Beck JD: Geriatric dental curriculum and the needs of the elderly, *Spec Care Dentist* 4:207, 1984.
13. Ettinger RL, Beck JD, Glenn RE: Some considerations in teaching geriatric dentistry, *J Am Soc Geriatr Dent* 13:7, 1978.
14. Ettinger RL, Beck JD, Glenn RE: Eliminating office architectural barriers to dental care of the elderly and handicapped, *J Am Dent Assoc* 98:398, 1979.
15. Ettinger RL, Beck JD, Willard DH: *The role of a mobile dental unit program in geriatric education and dental care delivery.* Paper presented at the American Dental Association Conference on Oral Health Care Needs of the Elderly, Chicago, November 19-20, 1980.
16. Fahs DE: Accessible dental care in an extended care facility, *J Geriatr Nurs* 7:21, 1981.
17. Finkel S: *Senile dementia and dental care.* In Chauncey HH and others, editors: *Clinical geriatric dentistry: biomedical and psychosocial aspects,* Chicago, 1985, American Dental Association.
18. Forsyth Dental Center: *Symposium on root surface caries,* Boston, 1985.
19. Gibson WA: *Age, caries, and periodontal disease.* In Chauncey HH and others, editors: *Clinical geriatric dentistry: biomedical and psychosocial aspects,* Chicago, 1985, American Dental Association.
20. Gigt HC: The elderly population oral health status and utilization of dental services, *J Am Soc Geriatr Dent* 13:9, 1978.
21. Gluck GM, Lakin LB: *Determination of common myths among dental students and dental school faculty,* Unpublished data, 1985.
22. Gluck GM, Lakin LB, Nezu A: The aging population and the private practitioner, *J Dent Pract Admin* 3:31, 1986.
23. Jacobs L: The geriatric patient, *Dialog* 14:10, 1983.
24. Kamen S.: Doctor, don't cheat yourself! *J Am Soc Geriatr Dent* 3:1, 1985 (editorial).
25. Kamen S: *Introduction to geriatric dentistry,* Lecture at St. Joseph's Hospital, Paterson, NJ, 1954.
26. Katz RV: Assessing root caries in populations: the evolution of the root caries index, *J Public Health Dent* 40:7, 1980.
27. Katz RV: Root caries: clinical implications of the current epidemiologic data, *Northwest Dent* 60:306, 1981.
28. Katz RV, and others: Prevalence and intraoral distribution of root caries in an adult population, *Caries Res* 6:265, 1982.
29. Kingson ER, Scheffler RM: Aging: issues and economic trends, *Inquiry* 18:197, 1981.
30. Kiyak HA: *Psychosocial factors and dental needs of the elderly,* Paper presented at the American Dental Association Conference on Oral Health Care Needs of the Elderly, Chicago, November 19-20, 1980.
31. Mandel I: Preventive dentistry for the elderly, *Spec Care Dentist* 3:157, 1983.
32. Mandel I: Preventive dental services for the elderly, *Dent Clin North Am* 33:81, 1989.
33. Meskin LH and others: Economic impact of dental service utilization by older adults, *J Am Dent Assoc* 120:665, 1990.
34. Mulligan R, Weitzel KG: Pretreatment management of the patient receiving anticoagulant drugs. *J Am Dent Assoc* 117:479, 1988.
35. Pollack RF: A wrong way to see the aged, *New York Times,* March 14, 1985.
36. Rowe JW: Health care of the elderly, *N Engl J Med* 312:827, 1985.

37. Rozovski SJ: *Nutrition and aging*. In Winick M, editor: *Nutrition in the 20th century,* New York, 1984, John Wiley & Sons.
38. Shaver RO: Dentistry for the homebound, institutionalized and elderly, Lakewood, Colo, 1982, Portable Dentistry.
39. Ship JA, Ship II: Trends in oral health in the aging population, *Dent Clin North Am* 33:33, 1989.
40. Schuman SK: A physician's guide to coordinating oral health and primary care, *Geriatrics* 45:47, 1990.
41. Sinykin S: *Meeting the patient's needs*. Paper presented at Chicago Symposium on Clinical Geriatric Dentistry, June 3, 1983.
42. Starr P: *The social transformation of American medicine,* New York, 1982, Basic.
43. Tryon A: *Organization and methods of delivering geriatric oral health care*. In Chauncey HH and others, editors: *Clinical geriatric dentistry: biomedical and psychosocial aspects,* Chicago, 1985, American Dental Association.
44. United States Bureau of the Census: *Projections of the population of the United States by age, sex and race: 1988 to 2080,* by Gregory Spencer, Current population reports, series p-25, No 1018, Washington, D.C., 1989, US Government Printing Office.
45. United States Department of Health and Human Services, National Institute of Dental Research: *Oral health of United States adults, the national survey of oral health in U.S. employed adults and seniors: 1985-1986,* NIH Pub No 87-2868.
46. United States Public Health Service: *National interview survey, 1981,* Washington, DC.
47. US Senate Special Committee on Aging: *America in transition: an aging society,* 1984-85 ed, Washington, DC, 1985, US Government Printing Office.
48. Wescott WB: Current and future considerations for a geriatric population, *J Prosthet Dent* 49:113, 1983.
49. Yellowitz JA and others: The Minnesota dental insurance program for senior citizens: two year results for the utilization of dental services, *J Am Dent Assoc* 104:453, 1982.

6 Financing Dental Care

The dental care delivery sector of the U.S. economy is currently in the process of diversification and organizational restructuring. The market forces affecting dentistry in today's economy reflect trends that are shaping all health care delivery in the United States. One such development is the change of payment from a purely private out-of-pocket transaction between dentist and patient into a layered group financing of dental care through various types of third parties. This segmentation of payment is a relatively recent phenomenon, recent at least when compared with the growth of hospitalization insurance that has its roots in the 1920s and 1930s. The economic consequences of this trend are just beginning to be felt in dentistry but have been at work in medical care for the past three decades.

Other trends with economic consequences are unique to dentistry. One is the dramatic decline in dental caries in the United States, which has implications for the future of dental care delivery in terms of both the demand and the supply of dental services in the marketplace.

MARKET FORCES: THE DEMAND SIDE

The major forces today in dental care demand can be summarized by two words: *insurance* and *caries,* more specifically, the increase of insurance and the decline of dental caries. Note that the 1970s were the decade of dental insurance. In fact, one review reports that during one 6-year period (1970-76) private-sector dental insurance grew 500%, from 4.8 to 23.1 million persons covered. Dental insurance payments by all insurers in 1981 were approximately $5.81 billion or 34% of all dental health care expenses. The latest figures for total enrollment provided by Delta Dental Plans is that in 1991 more than 100 million Americans were covered by dental insurance plans.

Dental insurance is currently considered one of the most desirable employee benefits available. It is estimated that approximately one of every three Americans is covered by some type of dental insurance plan. In the past 10 years there has been a tremendous growth of such programs. In 1965, 2 million Americans were covered by dental insurance, whereas 148 million had medical insurance coverage. Since then, dental plan offerings by U.S. firms has steadily increased to such a point that a 1990 survey of 944 major employers indicated that 92% offered dental plans.

The influx of third-party dollars in the marketplace can act as a stimulus to increase the consumption of dental care. With dental care insurance subsidizing the market price for dental services, the consumer demand function tends to seek a new equilibrium with the market supply function. This is based on the assumption that a reduction in price to the consumer increases the demand for services.

The more dramatic result of growth of dental insurance is that payment for dental care is consolidating through control by administrators of employee benefit packages. Private industry—management and labor—will play a multidimensional, complex role in health care. Data for listings shown here are from the American Dental Association, Council on Dental Care Programs, 1985. As a consumer of health care whose potential influence derives in part from the massive numbers of workers, industry will become more intimately involved in finding equitable ways to allocate limited resources and improve the quality of the dental care delivery system.

A dramatic decrease in the incidence of dental caries is a countervailing force in the marketplace that might result in a reduction in the use of dental services. Whereas most studies before 1977 showed an average incidence rate of two new cavities per child per year, recent investigations no longer support this data. The 1983 National Preventive Dentistry Demonstration Program, funded by the Robert Wood Johnson Foundation, indicated significant findings of less decay than previously reported. This 4-year national study evaluated preventive dental procedures throughout the United States, starting in the fall of 1977. Results showed that the long-standing pattern of two new cavities per child per year was no longer true.

In December 1981 the National Institute for Dental Research pointed to this lower caries incidence rate. Their study showed tooth decay in children ages 5 to 17 had dropped about 33% from rates reported in Health Examination Surveys of 1963-65 and 1966-70. In the early 1970s, only 28% of children ages 5 to 17 were caries-free, yet by 1981 the number had increased to 37%. Over the last 30 years, caries reduction as great as 60% has been observed.

Comparisons of decayed, missing, and filled surfaces (DMFS) data from four national surveys conducted between 1961 and 1980 in the United States also indicate a substantial decrease in dental caries prevalence and an increase in the number of caries-free children ages 5 to 17 during the last decade. In fact, a substantial proportion of children have no caries at all, although 20% of children account for 60% of all decay. Available literature indicates that this overall decline in dental caries is most likely the result of the increased use of fluoride supplements and fluoridated water supplies.

However, a reduction in dental caries has also been observed in nonfluoridated areas. A countrywide survey conducted in 1970 showed a definite improvement in the dental health of patients regardless of fluoride in their water supply. A 1979 study reported a 17.5% reduction in decay in Columbus, Ohio, which has a nonfluoridated water system. This statistic can most likely be attributed to the use of fluoridated water in processed foods and beverages.

The trend of caries reduction in nonfluoridated areas has also been noted in Massachusetts. Data collected between 1958 and 1978 in some Dedham and Norwood neighborhood schools seem to follow national patterns, although community and school water fluoridation was not a factor during this study period. Both towns showed a marked reduction in the number of decayed and filled surfaces, as well as surfaces both decayed and filled.

In 1951 the average 16-year-old in the United States had 15 teeth affected by decay with 2 extractions. In 1981 the average is 8 affected teeth with virtually no extractions.

The issue, then, is how does the reduction of dental caries translate into changes in demand for dental services? This type of data is usually difficult to obtain and often must be inferred. Dental practice revenue has traditionally been generated by treating the effects of dental caries. A 1977 review of dental care expenditures is presented in Table 6-1. Data for 1977 are shown as a reflection of the income distribution for the typical general dental practice just prior to the observation by epidemiologists of a pronounced decrease in dental caries among children. As Table 6-1 points out, in 1977, operative and endodontic procedures, services to treat the effect of dental caries, accounted for 34.3% of general practice revenue. Generally, fixed prosthetic services are also rendered to treat the effect of dental caries. Therefore a very conservative conclusion is that more than 50% of the income of a general dental practice in 1977 was earned from the treatment of dental caries.

Market forces interplay

In the dental care delivery sector of the U.S. economy there are two trends: one in the direction of increased use of dental services and the other to-

Table 6-1 Percent and expenditures by dental service type for U.S. general practice in 1977

Service	Expenditure %	$ millions
Fixed prosthetics	34.51	3,458
Operative	27.85	2,791
Removable posthetics	9.63	965
Diagnostic	8.25	826
Preventive	7.67	769
Endodontics	6.35	636
Surgery	3.89	390
Orthodontics	1.07	107
Periodontics	.78	78
TOTALS	100.00	10,020

From Douglass CW, Day JM: Cost and Payment of Dental Services in the U.S., *J Dent Educ* 43:7,1979

ward a net reduction in use. Although the trends seem to be polar opposites, in reality, future demand for services is not all that easy to predict. The trend in dental caries reduction indicates that in another 10 to 20 years the present population of relatively caries-free children will be adult consumers of dental care. Traditional dental practices centering on the treatment of disease will have to face adjustments in finances and focus.

Changes in dental materials technology has led to the ability to offer an increased range of preventive and cosmetic services. As private practitioners adjust to falling volume in their main service line, they will tend to compensate by raising fees, extending the service line, and/or increasing patient volume.

The office of the future may require a different mix of personnel. The dominant providers may be hygienists and other auxiliaries providing preventive and educational services rather than dentists offering highly skilled restorative services. The primary role of the dentist will be as diagnostician, coordinator of care, and provider of the more complex procedures involving both the hard and soft tissues of the oral cavity.

Does this mean less of a demand for dentists in the future? A decrease will depend primarily on overall shifts in consumer demand for dental services. At present most surveys indicate that only 55% of the U.S. population will visit a dentist in any given year, with approximately 30% seeking regular care. If the overall impact of dental insurance is to increase the regular consumption of dental care from, for example, 30% to 70% of the population, then the general effect, even taking into account caries reduction, may be a dramatic increase in dental care demand.

Unfortunately, most of the available actuarial analysis performed for dental insurers in both the public and private sector concludes that the percentage of eligible persons actually seeking care is consistent with overall national statistics. Dental insurance help seems to expand the purchasing power of those individuals who are already predisposed to seek dental care. It has not yet significantly altered the behavior of a large segment of the population that, for reasons often having to do with aversive consequences, decides not to seek regular care. Some such consequences may be treatments to reduce pain and/or infection or injection of local anesthetic to allow cutting of hard and soft tissues.

A recent economic review by Cohen and Roesler tends to substantiate the view that price does not in itself regulate the demand for dental services. They found a highly variable price elasticity of demand for dental services. Price elasticity is an economic measure calculated by dividing percent change in demand for a product or service by the percent change in its price. Price elasticity measures the sensitivity of demand for a product or service against fluctuations in price. The review states that the demand for dental services by children was price elastic, but for adults the price was inelastic. Income was found to be a more consistent predictor of use of dental services. The factor the authors did not consider in this review is price elasticity given the impact of caries reduction.

Perhaps in the future a synergism will develop between caries reduction and increase in dental care insurance coverage. If a positive feeling of well-being can replace the association of aversive experiences, a larger portion of the population will seek dental care on a regular basis. The net impact of reduction of aversive treatments and the increase in purchasing power may lead to increased dental care demand, resulting in higher patient volume.

Dental insurance may also provide the impetus in extending the service line in dental care use. In traditional or pre-insurance private practice, fees could more accurately be described as true market prices or an equilibrium price between market supply and demand functions. Not that long ago, dentists would provide a free examination as a loss leader so that monetary issues would not interfere in establishing good communication with the patient. Once patient rapport was established and a total treatment plan accepted, certain service lines such as dentures would be a "net gain," which would compensate the dentist for the loss leader examination. Most dentists realized that the most important aspect of initial patient contact was to establish rapport and confidence that would eventually lead to patient acceptance of treatment options. The unfortunate consequence of this pricing and consumption pattern was the traditional fee schedule's emphasis on the dentist's role as provider of tangible services such as fillings, dentures, and crowns, rather than as diagnostician.

Dental insurance should influence this traditional use pattern and revenue and service mix. With the advent of partial or full coverage for diagnostic service, there should be an observable yet gradual increase in the percent of dental practice revenue derived from these services. In addition, most dental plans largely, if not fully, cover preventive services; therefore, with the decline of dental caries, a larger percentage of practice revenue should also be derived from preventive services.

Is there any evidence for such revenue shifts? Analysis of the claims and patient copayment experience for six separate union management benefit trust funds involving approximately 100,000 eligible enrollees throughout the Commonwealth of Massachusetts indicates sufficient evidence. Table 6-2 compares the 1977 percent expenditures derived from Table 6-1 with the 1991 percent expenditures as derived from the union claims data for general practitioners.* Although such comparisons are open to charges that the populations are not comparable, the union data reflect the consumption pattern of a professional, skilled, and un-

---

*Claims analysis provided by the author, December 1991.

Table 6-2 Percent expenditure by dental service type comparing 1977 U.S. data with 1991 Massachusetts union data

Service type	% 1977	% 1991	Net Change
Diagnostic	8.2	14.9	+6.7
Preventive	7.7	13.7	+6.0
Restorative	27.9	23.8	−4.1
Fixed prosthetics	34.5	22.9	−11.6
Removable prosthetics	9.6	2.0	+7.6
Endodontics	6.4	8.6	+1.2
Periodontics	0.8	9.7	+8.9
Surgery	3.9	2.4	−1.5
Orthodontics	1.1	2.0	+0.9

From Douglass CW, Day JM: Cost and payment of dental services in the U.S., *J Dent Educ* 43:7, 1979.

skilled labor pool of an industrial Northeastern state. The enrollment base of 100,000 individuals ensures that the consumption pattern observed is unlikely to be grossly atypical or subject to adverse selection.

As Table 6-2 points out, according to the 1991 data, diagnostic and preventive services represent an 12.7% increase as compared with the 1977 percent of revenue. By contrast, operative and fixed prosthodontic services indicate a decline of 15.7% for the general practitioner. The other interesting and not unexpected observation is that in 1977 periodontics was almost a negligible 0.8% of total revenue. The 1991 combined union trust fund data indicate that periodontic services now represent a more respectable 9.7% of total private practitioner revenue. A reasonable conclusion from Table 6-2 is that the countervailing forces of caries reduction and increased dental insurance do appear to have an impact on the service mix of consumer demand.

MARKET FORCES: THE SUPPLY SIDE
Background

As previously discussed, the economics of health care delivery have evolved from a system of private transactions between physician and patient to one involving various third parties. This development certainly will have its impact on the demand side, or consumption of dental services, but what was unforeseen was its impact on the supply of dental services, more specifically, the organization and structure of the financing and delivery of dental services.

The growth of insurance is not the only major force to shape and foster changes in dental care delivery. The other factor is the 1976 Supreme Court decision maintaining that state-organized restrictions on advertising by professions is a violation of the First Amendment.

Dentistry, along with other similar professions, maintains that the doctor-patient relationship is sacrosanct and therefore is separate from other types of economic activity. What is evolving is not a repudiation of this concept but a clearer definition of the doctor-patient relationship that is consistent with economic reality and constitutional law.

When the payment of services was primarily a private transaction between physician and patient, all aspects of the therapy environment were private in nature. In today's economy, dental care payments are becoming benefits derived from an employer. In reality they have become another factor in computing labor costs for the production of goods and services in the U.S. economy. It is unrealistic to believe that industry—both labor and management—will not attempt to use its scarce resources to maximize benefits for its workers. If doing so requires a more active role in the payment and delivery of dental services, it will be pursued. The U.S. economy is now facing aggressive worldwide competition, and it is inevitable that all costs of the factors of production will be periodically reviewed. If, for example, a particular industry finds that by maintaining its own health clinics it can reduce labor costs by a certain amount, the economic choice is clear. Maximize production efficiency so prices are competitive.

Of course, what is evolving is not as simple as industry starting clinics and hiring doctors but payment reimbursement by various types of third parties representing a range of financial arrangements between industry and the health care sector. It should be added that the union or company clinic is an option that some industries have pursued, but the main thrust is not to get involved in the delivery of services but to negotiate an acceptable financing structure. Some of the new third parties in health care are health maintenance organizations (HMOs) and their dental counterpart, the prepaid group dental practice. In this particular arrangement the provider of services and insurer of care are the same organization.

This and other types of arrangements will increase competition in the third-party marketplace. It is in essence this competition between traditional insurance companies and other third-party arrangements that will encourage efficiency in the health care delivery system.

To flourish, these newer organizations must be free to develop marketing strategies that both penetrate the existing dental prepayment market and attract persons now without coverage. However, there has been a good deal of professional resistance to the idea of marketing health services. Until 1976 most state court decisions upheld states' rights to inhibit advertising for professional services. For example, in two court decisions, *People v. Duben* (10 N.E. 2d 809 Ill. 229) and *Cherry v. Board of Regents of the State of New York* (44 N.E. 2d 405 N.Y. 148), the Supreme Court stated and reaffirmed the states' right to limit advertising by physicians and dentists. With this legal precedent, most professional organizations, including dentistry, traditionally restricted professionals from using various forms of advertising.

With the evolution of new third parties who may advertise for plan members, the question that would naturally have arisen concerns the ethics of physicians and dentists who are employed by or contract with organizations who in turn advertise on their behalf. This would have been an area of new litigation, but the Supreme Court in 1976 made it a moot issue. The U.S. Supreme Court decided a case on appeal from the Supreme Court of Arizona, *John R. Bates and Van O'Steen Appellants v. The State Bar of Arizona* (76-316 4873, 4896) and upheld the right of attorneys to advertise their fees for certain services. The state's rule prohibiting this was found to be in violation of the First Amendment. The court considered six arguments for restricting price advertising: (1) the adverse effect on professionalism, (2) the inherently misleading nature of attorney advertising, (3) the adverse effect on the administration of justice, (4) the undesirable economic effects of advertising, (5) the adverse effect of advertising on the quality of service, and (6) the difficulties of enforcement. The court was not persuaded that any of them was an acceptable reason to inhibit attorneys' First Amendment right to announce to the public their prices for basic services. However, the court did not hold that advertising by attorneys may not be regulated in any way.

Given these economic and legal trends, the practitioner-patient relationship should and must be properly defined so that professionalism and quality of care are fostered. How a particular patient seeks and pays for service from a particular health care provider does not affect the ethical responsibility of that provider. Salaried dentists should maintain the same level of professionalism as those who work in the more traditional private practice setting. It is the role of the dental schools and professional organizations to define clearly and promulgate the concept of professional responsibility.

Supply side restructuring. There are several options available to industry relating to the administrative and provider reimbursement structure for various health care benefits, including dentistry. Outlined in this chapter are organizational arrangements defined in a broad generic sense. It is beyond the scope of this discussion to analyze the finer details of specific organizations.

There are choices industry can and will make concerning the financial management structure of health care benefits. At present the three possible basic organizational arrangements are as follows.

1. Indemnification of dental benefits through an insurance carrier
2. Self-indemnification and self-administration of the benefit
3. Self-indemnification but with use of a third party to administer the benefit

Insurance option. To establish the proper framework for analysis a few basic concepts should be discussed. As the list points out, insuring involves several choices, including the indemnification of annual benefit costs through an insurance carrier.

In the attempt to explore the underwriting of health care programs such as dental care through an insurance carrier, there should be a clear idea of the potential benefits to industry and how they can be achieved. The simplistic idea of "let the insurance company handle everything" may in the long run turn out to be more costly to industry.

The use of an insurance carrier to indemnify or protect against possible damage or losses, is at best a short-term risk-ameliorating option. In the long run the insurance company passes all costs on to its customers, in this case, industry. However, there are certain advantages. This type of indemnification makes annual budgeting for benefits much more predictable and efficient, and the technical expertise of insurance underwriters and actuaries can be useful in analyzing a program's economic impacts. The insurance company also takes on the more burdensome operational tasks such as claims processing, thus freeing management to concentrate on long-term strategic planning.

Undeniably, the growth of dental prepayment has been marked by an increasing role of the traditional insurance company in the financing of dental services. The insurance company maintains the appropriate administrative talent and resources to maintain large-scale benefits administration. Certainly, for particular industries this option makes the most sense, and currently most dental benefits are administered under this arrangement.

Self-indemnification and self-administration. Another approach to benefits administration is to self-insure and self-administer the benefit. Usually what is established is a union-management trust fund that pays for care directly rather than paying premiums to an insurance company. In a true self-administered benefit, the trust fund handles all aspects of benefit program administration. There are two main advantages to this approach. The trust fund has complete control of the benefit program from policy initiation to implementation and can invest earmarked benefit dollars to expand the resource base or dollars available for future benefits.

If this type of administrative structure is totally maintained by a particular company or union, the cash flow from benefit dollars will remain in its bank accounts until needed to pay for services and will not automatically be sent to the insurance company in regular premium installments. However, as pointed out previously, there is a price for maintaining this level of control. Industry's management must be responsible not only for long-term policy planning and analysis but also for large-scale day-to-day operational activities. This latter responsibility inhibits policy reformulation and creativity. Once a large-scale initiative has been completed, for example, when a computer data base management system is set up, it becomes very difficult to change direction quickly and consider new economic and benefit policy directions.

Role of the third-party administrator. In the private sector a new type of administrative structure has evolved. Known as third-party administrator (TPA), it attempts to bridge the gap between indemnifying and administering through an insurance carrier and self-indemnification and self-administration. This option has the advantage that ultimate budgetary control is in the hands of those who pay for the services. In the private sector this means that if a company self-indemnifies but contracts with a TPA for claims processing and other program management activities, the money budgeted for health care is still in the control of the company for its own cash flow until services are rendered and claims must be paid. The advantage to industry is that the tedious aspect of program management is contracted out, but the analytical and long-term policy tasks remain the responsibility of industry benefit administrators.

PROVIDER REIMBURSEMENT STRUCTURE
Medical economics and insurance

Once again, we must look to the concept of insurance and what it means for ambulatory care programs such as dental care.

The development of benefit packages and premium calculations for prepaid dental care programs differs greatly from similar work for insurance-type programs. The standard definition of an *insurable risk* contains three essential elements: (1) the loss or incident occurs infrequently, such as a flood; (2) the potential loss is very great, for example, destruction of home by fire; and (3) any single individual cannot affect the risk or frequency of the event in the community. Hospitalization is an insurable risk and meets these three criteria. However, expenditure for dental care, and for that matter most ambulatory care, is not an insurable risk. Dental disease is common. Dental care is not expensive, at least not when compared with the cost of hospitalization, and individuals generally know what their level of need is. This last point is the reason that dental care plans cannot be marketed on an individual basis in the private sector. Adverse selection would result from all those persons with heavy accumulated dental needs joining the plan at the same time that those who have maintained their oral health do not join. This type of adverse selection would eliminate any element of cost-sharing, force premiums up to an unmarketable level, and cause closure of the prepaid plan.

Prepaid dental care plans are essentially a budgeting type of arrangement in which predictable expenditures are planned where groups are large enough. The real economic dilemma occurs when providers, who have considerable leverage over use, have no economic incentive to initiate courses of treatment consistent with budgeted premium dollars. With traditional private sector insurance,

the third party is to assume risk for dental claims, and the role of the consumer and the provider is to maximize benefits derived from the plan.

Changes in the marketplace

The introduction of the concept of risk-sharing in prepaid programs is a product of the past decade. In its purest form, the insurers of care and the providers of services fuse into one umbrella organization. This is the HMO concept in which the provider is also given an incentive to initiate courses of treatment consistent with premium dollars.

Are the same forces at work in the dental care marketplace as in the HMO movement for medical care? Around the country, indemnity dental insurance plans are beginning to lose ground to capitation and other provider-type arrangements as large insurers speculate that the market is on the brink of some major shifts. The nature of the more common arrangements follow:

1. Fee for service (FFS): Open panel
2. Fee for service: Participating provider (no provider restriction)
3. Fee for service: Independent practice association/Preferred provider organization model (selected provider participation)
4. Capitation: staff model groups
5. Capitation: Independent practice association model

Range of choices
Fee-for-service options

Fee-for-service open panel. This is the structure of the typical indemnity commercial insurance plan. The basic contractual arrangement is between the insurance company and the insured, whereby the insurance company indemnifies for losses from dental claims as outlined in the policy's list of coverage. Policyholders are free to select the dentist of their choice and can either pay the dentist directly for services rendered and later collect from the insurance company or assign such payments directly to the dentist. The insurance company in turn reimburses for care based on a table of allowances or usual and customary fees up to the 90th percentile. Dentists are free to collect from the patient any differences between their fee and that allowed under the terms of the insurance policy.

Fee-for-service: participating provider (no provider restriction). This is the structure of the typical professionally sponsored insurance plan, such as the Blue Cross/Blue Shield and Delta plans. The basic contractual arrangement is between the insurance underwriter and the provider of services, in this case the dentist. This type of coverage is usually termed *service benefits,* in contrast to the *indemnity benefits* of the previous commercial insurance structure. With Delta plan as a typical example, providers submit their fee schedule with the carrier and cannot charge the patient more than the agreed-upon fees. Becoming a participating provider usually entails signing a provider agreement with the insurance carrier, locking the provider into an agreed-upon fee schedule that the provider submits. This agreement has caused much controversy because most providers (both dentists and physicians) want the ability to bill patients directly for the difference when their fees exceed the fee schedule of the service-benefit contract. "Balance billing" has been the topic of much litigation and legislation.

At the present time a large percentage of providers have become participating providers, usually with the insurance carriers reducing the reimbursable fee by 5% because of guaranteed payment. This has given the Blue Cross/Blue Shield and Delta plans some leverage in the marketplace, but the commercial carriers have countered this economic advantage by offering a more varied product line and packaging it with other types of insurance.

Fee-for-service: IPA/PPO model. Recently, independent practice association (IPA) or preferred provider organizations (PPO) networks have been observed in the marketplace. These organizations are participating-provider service-benefit insurance arrangements, but with the clear intention of negotiating a reduced fee with the providers. To entice providers to reduce their fees as much as 15% to 20%, the concept of a closed panel is introduced. This means that only a few offices will be selected to participate in any given geographic area, thereby guaranteeing each office a greater volume of patients than would otherwise be obtainable.

FEE-FOR-SERVICE-SPECTRUM. In the spectrum of fee-for-service options, if cost containment becomes of greater importance, the most likely solution is to contain, if not reduce, reimbursable fees. There is simplicity and ease in using this approach. Essentially, the problem is tackled by modifying the structure established long ago with a considerable amount of accumulated experience and professional acceptance in the marketplace today.

However, modifying the structure in this way leaves fee for service intact, and the concept of risk sharing is not used. It has been found that providers in the closed-panel PPO arrangement will keep to contractual fee arrangements, but they are not deterred from trying to expand their service options with the patient or increase fees for noncovered or partially covered services. Once again, the third party is at risk, and the provider and patient have an economic incentive to maximize benefits, in this case dollars from the program.

Risk-sharing options. Dental capitation programs have grown in popularity over the past two decades. Most of the major dental insurers, including companies such as Prudential and Connecticut General, have established capitation programs. These companies would not have ventured into this area of the marketplace if they did not feel that doing so was in their best interests.

The essential feature of capitation is that the provider receives a predetermined fixed revenue and must budget his or her time accordingly. The typical industry standard for rate setting is to budget according to the cost of delivering dental services in the typical office. Fees do not play a role in the pricing mechanism.

Given that a fixed cost-based payment will be received, the provision of preventive and maintenance services is preferable to the more complex rehabilitation services that are usually associated with higher fees in the marketplace. One of the main advantages is that each dentist can base the treatment assessment on his or her own diagnosis, and a prior authorization or review by an insurance carrier consultant becomes superfluous.

The main criticism of this approach is that the provider will not have an incentive to perform needed dental work and may in fact collect the capitation payments without delivering the services. However, with adequate monitoring and utilization review, most providers will follow accepted treatment standards. As with any system of reimbursement, there will be a small percentage who will abuse the system for personal gain.

Capitation: staff model groups. Prepaid capitation group practice is the HMO concept as applied to the delivery of dental services. In one setting the patient can receive all required dental services. The economic incentive of this concept is to improve the oral health status of the enrolled population, and the patient has the advantage of one-stop shopping for dental care.

Although this option is enticing, there is a problem in the widespread application of this approach. Approximately 88% of the delivery of dental services is by solo practitioners. Large multispecialty groups are not the mainstay of dental care delivery, however, with the growth of retail-based dental centers, this is rapidly changing. From the perspective of benefits administrators, there are dental care delivery units that do have the potential for this type of arrangement, such as the growing number of group practice outlets in various shopping malls.

Capitation IPA model. The IPA model has the advantage of fitting the benefits of risk sharing of capitation with the dental care delivery system as it presently exists. At first glance it seems a perfect match; however, it does introduce a few problems. How does one handle the issue of specialist services? Should capitation payments go to the general practitioners, who in turn pay the specialists? Should the specialists be capitated directly, or should they be kept on a closely monitored fee-for-service system? In the private sector there are several variations of this arrangement, and each seems to work as intended.

DENTAL PLAN STANDARDS

Various combinations of financial and provider reimbursement structures for dental plans currently exist in the marketplace, although traditional indemnity fee-for-service plans dominate. The growth and design of individual dental plan products has simply evolved with the purchasing employer group on its own in the selection of a specific plan design. Recently a movement has emerged to establish standards for dental plan coverage. Two national organizations have attempted to establish standards for dental plans. The ADA and Health Policy Agenda have developed dental plan designs for both a limited-cost or basic plan and an expanded plan. The Health Policy Agenda is a coalition of medical, labor, and employer organizations that devises basic benefit packages to serve as benchmarks that employers and subscribers could use to evaluate health insurance plans including dental insurance. The ADA has similarly established standards for dental care plans.

The two organizations have developed coverage standards for four major categories of dental services: (1) diagnostic-preventive, (2) routine, (3) complex, and (4) orthodontic. Both urge that there should be no deductibles or copayments for diagnostic, preventive, and emergency services. According to the Health Policy Agenda, these out-of-pocket expenses tend to discourage the patient from entering the system.

The ADA suggests full coverage for two examinations and prophylaxes per year. Bite-wing radiographs are to be provided annually and complete radiographs are to be provided every 5 years. Topical fluoride treatments twice per year are suggested for patients under age 18; sealants and emergency care should be provided as needed.

The basic and expanded model plans developed by the Health Policy Agenda differ somewhat from the recommendations of the ADA. Under its basic plan, examinations, prophylaxes, and fluoride treatments are allowed annually rather than every 6 months. However, both organizations suggest that as the treatment becomes more complex, patient cost-sharing features should be included. The Health Policy Agenda maintains that cost sharing for complex care should be high enough to motivate employees and their dependents to maintain their oral health.

The model dental plans of the ADA and the Health Policy Agenda may differ in specific coverage details, but their development and promulgation are a natural consequence of changes in the financing of dental care. As third-party participation in dental care increases, two national organizations that have established standards have come to the forefront. These standards are to help guide constituents, whether they are employees, dentists, or consumers, to select from the myriad dental plan products now available.

CONCLUSION

This chapter discussed the factors that have led to changes in dental care delivery and the economics of dental care. We are currently in a period of transition, during which alternative modes of delivery of services and financing of these services will evolve. This chapter also discussed the potential impact of caries reduction in dental care delivery.

The reduction of dental caries and the role of fluorides have been well documented by the dental profession. The first step in its understanding occurred in 1902, when Frederic S. McKay gave systematic attention to the mottling he found in his patients. The unfolding of the fluoride story is a classic case study in chronic disease epidemiology. The dental profession can point with pride to its role in significantly preventing a disease that a few years ago was considered ubiquitous and its treatment an almost insurmountable task.

In this decade dental care delivery is also influenced by the unfolding of historical events that at first appear to have no bearing on current dental practice. The growth of fringe benefits is one such factor. Fringe benefits developed during World War II, when the federal government prohibited nearly all wage increases. War industries attracted workers by offering benefits in addition to wages. For example, many employers paid part of the cost of food served in their cafeterias. Later, companies offered medical insurance, life insurance, and accident and disability insurance. Since then, fringe benefits have grown in importance. Labor and management have introduced new benefits, including dental care and stock purchase plans. Unions often accept fringe benefits instead of higher wages because most benefits are not subject to income tax.

Dental professionals must and will adapt to this changing environment. Our responsibilities will not diminish; instead, we must remain involved to ensure the public of the highest standards of care and professionalism.

Case study. Massachusetts Public Employees Health and Welfare Fund

PART I. ESTABLISHMENT OF THE FUND

The Massachusetts Public Employees Health and Welfare Fund (hereafter, the Fund) was established on January 3, 1984, as a result of collective bargaining between the Commonwealth of Massachusetts and a coalition of trade unions, which at that time represented 36,000 state employees. The unions that participated in the coalition were the American Federation of State, County, and Municipal Employees (AFSCME) Council 93; the Service Employees International Union (SEIU) Locals 254, 285, and 509; and the State Police Association of Massachusetts (SPAM). The unions had seen similar jointly managed funds thrive in states like Pennsylvania and New York and made the creation of a Fund a major issue during contract negotiations with the state. The Commonwealth of Massachusetts, mindful of escalating health care costs, desired a managed approach to health care benefits and endorsed the creation of a trust fund with the goal to self-administer health benefits and not merely purchase various insurance products.

Under the terms of the trust agreement that established the Fund, the labor and management trustees were empowered to provide eligible employees and their dependents with "life insurance, weekly sickness and accident benefits, medical, surgical, hospitalization and similar forms of coverage, including drug prescription coverage, eyeglass benefits, dental care, and Medicare." After much discussion, the trustees decided to implement a dental care program effective on July 1, 1985. The demographic composition of the Fund's membership played a significant role in the design of the dental plan and is worth reviewing at this time.

The five participating unions covered workers with an array of job titles, pay levels, and educational qualifications. Members ranged from employees of the state's Department of Education who had earned doctoral degrees to blue-collar workers employed at one of the state mental hospitals who had less than 8 years of formal schooling. Income levels ranged from around $10,000 to more than $50,000 annually. The trustees operated under the theory that many of the lower-wage workers, particularly those who were recent immigrants to the United States, had a lower overall level of dental health and less disposable income to invest in dental care. Higher-wage workers, who tended also to be better educated, had a higher level of dental hygiene and more disposable income to invest in dental care.

The trustees wanted to design a dental program that would encourage lower-income plan beneficiaries without a history of regular clinical dental care to visit the dentist. After carefully reviewing a variety of dental care plan options available to the Fund, the trustees concluded that the creation of their own preferred provider network would allow them to provide more dental services to eligible members at a lower price and, at the same time, to exert greater influence over the providers of care. Some trustees, particularly those who represented higher-paid state employees, argued that some type of indemnity program would be necessary, if only to serve workers in remote locations. Consequently, the trustees decided to create a fully self-insured, dual-choice program featuring a fixed reimbursement schedule indemnity plan (hereafter, the open plan) and a preferred provider plan (hereafter, the closed plan).

The initial plan of benefits was modest, particularly in the open plan. Individual annual open plan maximums were set at $400 per year, and deductibles of $25 for individuals and $50 for families were established. Participants in the open plan received no coverage for crowns, bridges, or orthodontic treatment.

Closed plan benefits were somewhat more generous, reflecting the trustees' decision to encourage member participation in the preferred provider plan. There were no annual maximums, no yearly deductibles, and only very modest copayments for endodontic, periodontic, prosthetic, and orthodontic services. Fifteen dental offices across the state, almost all of which were very large group practices, participated during the first year.

The benefits offered by both plans have improved significantly since 1985. Open plan participants no longer have any deductibles, and the annual individual maximum has increased to $750. Both orthodontic and prosthetic coverage has been added, and reimbursement levels have increased significantly. In the closed plan, required copayments are generally lower today than they were in 1985, and the preferred provider panel has grown to include more than 200 dental offices across the state.

The out-of-pocket cost impact of each option is carefully explained in the plan booklet that is mailed out by the Fund office to all members on a yearly basis. Table 6-3 shows some examples of costs to members for common dental services under the closed and open dental plans.

Unlike many dental plans that experience a dramatic "spike" in use very early in their existence, the Fund's

dental plan took several years to take off. Several factors affected the slow growth of the Fund's dental plan. First, the state workers were used to receiving information about their employee benefits directly from their personnel offices. Because the Fund was a not-for-profit agency independent of the state's traditional personnel and benefits bureaucracy, local benefit staff were unwilling or unable to inform members about the existence of their plan. Second, as a consequence of the inability of the Fund to piggyback on the state's existing employee benefits communications system, a new system, which relied on union officials, fellow workers, and direct mail had to be developed. Because 10% of eligible workers spoke a primary language other than English and many additional workers were functionally illiterate, the communications task was more difficult.

Eventually, however, employees obtained information about the plan and began to use benefits. A survey of some 9,500 workers in late 1988 indicated that the statistically strongest predictor of dental plan usage was length of service with the Commonwealth, indicating to the trustees that it took repeated mailings, health fairs, and union meetings before eligible workers began to take advantage of the plan. However, by the end of the fifth full plan year, overall plan usage had reached approximately 60% of eligible members and dependents.

The trustees contracted with a survey research firm to determine the needs and expectations of their membership. The membership represented workers with an array of job titles, pay levels, and education qualifications. The membership ranged from employees of the state university system who have earned doctoral degrees to low-skill job employees who had less than 8 years of formal education. How did the membership view its dental plan options, and what were their attitudes toward dental care? Was the plan as designed meeting their needs? Was it necessary to have two options?

A pattern did emerge from the survey. It was found that the typical member of the closed panel, with its much more lucrative dental benefits, was an individual who was lower on the socioeconomic scale and whose basic orientation to dental care was to avoid care unless there was an emergency. Without coverage, a comprehensive approach to dentistry would not be affordable for people in this group.

The typical open plan member, by contrast, tended to be an employee who was at the higher end of the pay scale and who was better educated than the employee enrolled in the closed plan. Based on the survey attitude questions, the open plan member tended to visit the dentist on a regular basis and was oriented toward prevention. This group tended to be at a maintenance level of care and more likely to remain with their own dentist rather than switch to a closed panel provider.

Table 6-3 A comparison of a member's personal cost under each dental plan

Dental treatment plan	Closed plan (fixed cost, $)	Open plan (estimate $)
Two-surface amalgam	0	23
Simple extraction	0	25
Molar root canal	50	195
Complete upper denture	100	342
Porcelain to gold crown	150	350

After much discussion of the survey results, the trustees decided to increase efforts to market the plan to the membership, especially those individuals who were not regular visitors to the dentist. The goal was to improve the dental health status of the membership. It was my responsibility to report back to the trustees and determine from claims data if, indeed, the goals were being met.

PART II: USE OF THE FUND

Since the inception of this dental plan, the trustees received periodic reports of service use on a per patient basis. Since 1986, all dental claims from the beginning of the plan were stored on computer tape at Boston University. The claims data source, which is a service-specific data file, was converted into a patient-specific compilation of claims information. Over the years the trustees had been supplied summary reports of patient-specific dental service use that chronicled plan modifications, including increased coverage for the open and closed plan, reimbursable fees, and the number of offices that participate in the closed plan. Also over the years, the Fund office has expended time and resources to better communicate with the enrollees of this plan.

A. NUMBER OF PATIENTS AND DOLLAR EXPENDITURE *Over*

the past 5 years there has been a considerable increase in the number of patients provided dental services under this dental care program. Figures 6-1 and 6-2 summarize those trends. Both figures chronicle the steady increase in the total number of patients and dollar expenditure the plan has experienced over the past 5 years. The number of patients seen by dentists grew from 20,184 in the first year to 41,331 in the fifth year. Given an estimated eligible base of 70,000 enrollees, this represents an increase of the rate from 25% to 59%. The latter use rate is similar in scope to use rates of comparable dental plans and the overall use of dental services of the U.S. population. This 5-year increase in use was the product of many factors, including coverage increases, fee increases, steady increases in the number of participating closed panel offices, and better marketing and communication of the plan to its members. The plan started out as one that could be characterized as underused. In the fifth year, it could be described as exhibiting a use rate comparable with other dental plans.

B. NUMBER OF PROCEDURES PER PATIENT *One concern of the trustees was whether some of the increases in expenditure could be explained by dentists steadily doing more dental procedures for each patient. In other words, were the dentists doing as many dental proce-*

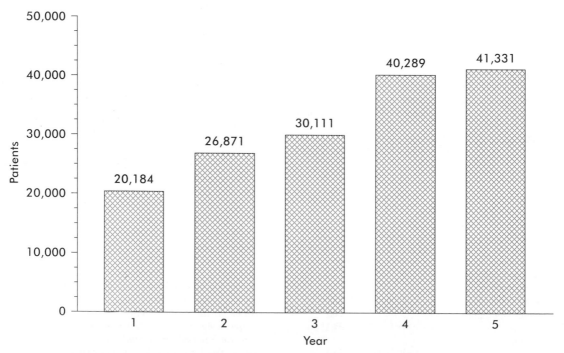

Fig. 6-1 Total number of patients provided dental services under the Massachusetts dental care program.

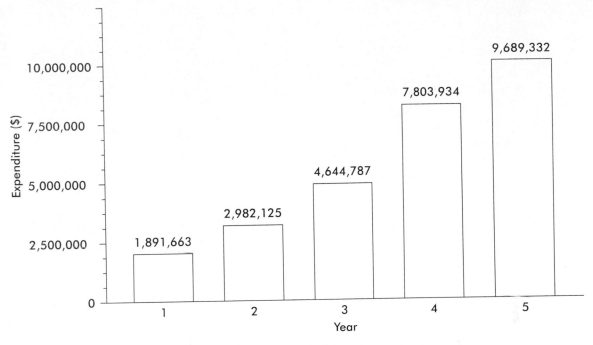

Fig. 6-2 Total paid claims by year under the Massachusetts dental care program.

dures as possible, whether or not they were necessary, to maximize income? Figure 6-3 examines the number of services per patient by year. As Fig. 6-3 points out, the number of dental procedures per patient in fact has remained level over the 5 years of this claim review. It seems that there was no dramatic shift in the number of dental procedures performed per patient.

C. SERVICE MIX TRENDS The most important factor in terms of cost and dental health impact is the 5-year overall trend in the type of service provided to plan members. It is of great importance because it has significance not only in total dollar expenditure but also in the overall health status of the enrolled population. A working hypothesis of dental service use experience is that as more members seek dental care, one would expect a differential in use of specific service types between the open and closed plans. This differential can be explained in part by the difference in coverage between the two plans. A member who requires a more complex and costly treatment plan tends to gravitate toward the closed plan for its more generous benefits, especially when there is a considerable income constraint in the affordability of out-of-pocket expenses. Our demographic analysis had already shown that the closed plan membership consisted of not only lower-

income members, but also members who were not oriented toward preventive dentistry and would exhibit a backlog of unmet dental needs. For this group's claim experience, one should expect to see a service mix with heavy use of rehabilitative services such as bridges, endodontics, and dentures. A different pattern should be exhibited by the open plan group in that it has a higher representation of members of higher incomes and members oriented toward regular dental visits.

To examine this hypothesis the claims were broken into four categories of service type by plan type. The four categories of service expenditure are as follows:

1. Rehabilitative types of services, including dentures, bridges and crowns, root canal, and periodontal therapy; these are the most expensive services to provide
2. Orthodontic services
3. Restorative services such as silver and tooth-colored fillings
4. Diagnostic and preventive services, including radiographs, oral exams, cleaning, and fluoride treatments

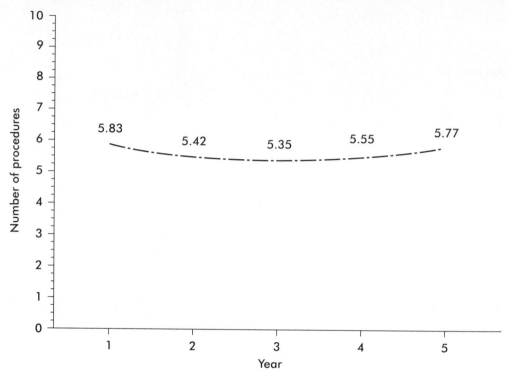

Fig. 6-3 Number of dental procedures per patient per year.

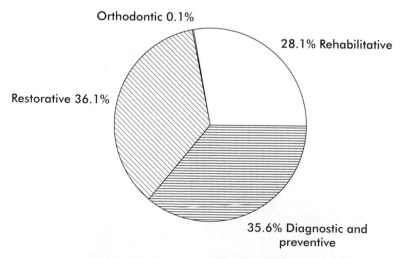

Fig. 6-4 Year one service mix: open plan.

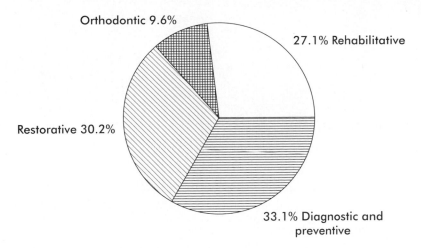

Fig. 6-5 Year five service mix: open plan.

Figures 6-4 through 6-7 examine the mix of service trends as a percentage of total expenditure for both closed and open plans. The service mix for the open plan was relatively constant except for the addition of orthodontic coverage. As expected, the pattern is consistent with a patient pool at or near the maintenance level of dental care. The significant shifts observed were for the closed plan. In year one, rehabilitation services as a total of all services was only 10%. This low percentage represents an underuse of needed services to bring a high-need population to maintenance level. The factors to explain this were alluded to before, but this high-need group required a concerted effort in marketing and out-reach. Another serious constraint in the first year of the plan was that there were only 15 closed plan sites. The percent increase to 45% reflects a greater number of closed plan patients having their backlog of unmet needs cared for. In a few years this group can reach a maintenance level of care, and by most parameters, a higher level of dental health. In this respect the closed plan has been very successful in making inroads to improving the dental health of a population that traditionally has not been active in seeking dental care. The growth in expenditure for dental service is due to more patients seeking care and a backlog of dental needs being met. In this respect the dental care program has been very successful.

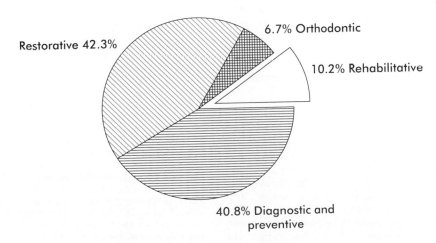

Fig. 6-6 Year one service: closed plan.

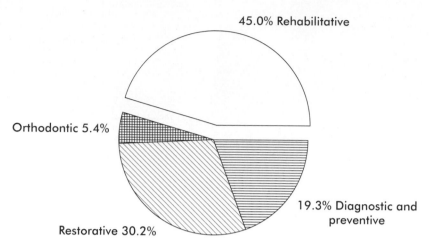

Fig. 6-7 Year five service: closed plan.

EPILOGUE

The data in this case study were presented to the trustees of the Alliance Trust Fund with the intent to follow up with additional reports of the dental care experience of both the open and closed plans. It was hoped that with continuance of the existing plan design a maintenance pattern of service needs would emerge for the closed plan. Since then there has been a dramatic change in the economy of both the United States and Massachusetts. With considerable reduction in the state's work force and budget cuts, the trustees have since been required to cut back on some of the coverage of the closed plan. For the first time since the inception of the plan, a $1,000 maximum has been introduced in the closed plan. Further actuarial analysis will now be confounded with a dramatic modification of plan coverage. This is the reality of the cyclical nature of our economy.

Nevertheless, an unexpected new change has been observed in the enrollment of the closed and open plans. When requested by the trustees to determine the impact of the changes in coverage, a new pattern of enrollment began to emerge. Once a year all plan members are required to re-enroll in either the closed or open plan. Traditionally, when enrollment was examined in relation to job categories and pay scales, a consistent pattern emerged of 70% of the higher-paid employees enrolling in the open plan. That rate has been steadily declining so that as of the writing of this summary, 50% remain in the open plan. More and more of the decision of plan preference seems to be guided by economic considerations. The vision of the original trustees has been borne out. This plan was designed in an era of a thriving economy when it would have been expedient to purchase just dental insurance and not be involved in managed care. The closed plan, with its inherent controls of escalating dental care costs, has been a mechanism to maintain adequate coverage in a time of shrinking resources. The providers of the closed panel are also beneficiaries at a time when many offices are experiencing a reduction in their patient pools. These offices are still experiencing a healthy demand for services from the members of the Alliance Dental Plan, even though the membership is now 30,000, down from a high of 40,000. In the long run, a stable noninflationary dental plan is in the best interest of both the consumer and the dental profession.

BIBLIOGRAPHY

American Dental Association, Council on Dental Care Programs, Chicago, March 1984.

Bell N: Managed care and dentistry: a perfect fit, *Business and Health,* Special report, 1991.

Burnelle J, Carlos J: Changes in the prevalence of dental caries in U.S. school children, 1961-1980, *J Dent Res* 61:1347, 1982.

Cohen DM, Roesler TW: The effect of dental insurance and patient income level on the utilization of dental services and implications for future growth in dentistry, *J Dent Prac Admin* 3:4, 1986.

Douglass CW, Day JM: Cost and payment of dental services in the U.S., *J Dent Educ* 43:7, 1979.

Eilers RD: *Actuarial services for a dental service corporation,* Washington, DC, 1967, US Department of Health, Education and Welfare, Public Health Service.

Glass R: Secular changes in caries prevalence in two Massachusetts towns, *Caries Res* 15:448, 1981.

Leverett P: Fluorides and the changing prevalence of dental caries, *Science* 217:23, July 1982.

Moen B, Poetsch V: Survey of dental services rendered 1969: more preventive less tooth repair, Bureau of Economic Research and Statistics, *J Am Dent Assoc* 81:25, 1970.

Praiss IL and others: Changing patterns and implication for cost and quality of dental care, *Inquiry* 16:131, 1979.

Spencer's Research Reports: *Basic elements of dental plan design as recommended by ADA and health policy agenda,* Chicago, 1991, Spencer's Research Reports.

Weisfeld R: *National preventive dentistry demonstration program, the Robert Wood Johnson demonstration program,* special report No 2, 1983.

SECTION THREE

Dental Disease—Prevalence and Prevention

The prevention of disease of the oral cavity requires a multifaceted approach. It behooves the dental professional to understand the etiology and the prevalence of the disease, as well as specific means for preventing it.

Chapter 7 introduces the concept of the study of dental disease by systematic observation of population groups. The science of epidemiology paved the way for the discovery of fluoride as a caries preventive agent; it allows us to describe the effects of caries and periodontal disease in the population of the United States through the use of indices of disease.

Chapter 8, on the prevention of dental disease, defines prevention and systematically reviews the current approaches to prevention for individuals and groups. A variety of programs such as fluoride mouth rinses, school water fluoridation, and occlusal sealants are described in detail. The cost-effectiveness of these preventive measures is compared, and recommendations for particular approaches are given.

7 Epidemiology of Dental Disease

Epidemiology is a science to which the general practitioner, the specialist, the researcher, and the academician alike can relate. The term itself is derived from the Greek *epidemios,* meaning "prevalent." Epidemiology is the study of the distribution and determinants of disease. Its primary tool is the systematic observation of human beings as they relate to their environment.

Through the brief scenario of modern dentistry, various types of epidemiologic studies have played a leading role in advancing the scientific basis for dental practice. The observational studies by H. Trendley Dean and other dentists in the early to mid-1930s on fluorosis and dental caries identified the association between "Colorado brown stain" or fluorosis and reduced caries incidence.[13,14] The classic studies that followed in the late 1940s through the 1960s in Grand Rapids–Muskegon, Michigan; Newburgh-Kingston, New York; and Evanston–Oak Park, Illinois, are excellent examples of experimental epidemiology.[2,3,5] In these studies fluoride was artificially added to the municipal water supply to raise the levels to optimum in one community, and in the paired community the levels were kept at the lower, naturally occurring level.

Epidemiology can be critically important in identifying the cause or source of an outbreak of an infectious disease, such as hepatitis. Certainly, retrospective follow-up studies are extremely important to dentistry in the 1990s, as the Centers for Disease Control attempts to determine the pathways of transmission of the acquired immunodeficiency syndrome (AIDS) virus relative to dental practice.[8-10] The task of the epidemiologist in the first case of suspected AIDS transmission from health care worker to patients was to trace the source of the virus back from patient to dental office, eliminating all other potential risk factors and sources of the virus along the way. Once it was established that the virus was somehow transmit-

ted during the dental procedure, the issue was to identify the source of the transmission and the mechanism by which it was transmitted. The possibilities for such transmission were myriad, including techniques of the dentist, infection control procedures, and titer of the infecting agent, and the role of the epidemiologist was that of Sherlock Holmes. The conclusions reached through such epidemiologic investigations help the dental profession to learn how best to protect dentist and patient from this deadly disease.

Epidemiology is more than observation and deduction. Although it is a young science, it is firmly founded in medicine, biology, statistics, and the social sciences. More recently, the advances in computer science have enhanced the capabilities of epidemiology. Dentistry is one branch of medicine to which epidemiologic methods are readily adaptable. The oral cavity is continually exposed to a variety of environmental factors that affect its state of health. The quantification of many of these factors and their correlation with the state of oral health in many instances are reasonably straightforward, for example, frequency of sugar consumption and increase in plaque production. In others, suspected causative agents might be more difficult to define, as is the case with aphthous ulcers. Dental epidemiology provides a framework within which we can scrutinize our data to determine whether our theories of cause and effect are valid.

Dental epidemiology is useful in determining the needs of populations. Dental diseases vary greatly from country to country, indeed, from community to community. Through epidemiology we are better able to see how caries rates are falling in the western hemisphere, and how in less developed countries, which previously enjoyed relatively low caries rates, they are now on the rise.[15]

Epidemiology is used to delineate disease patterns in communities. This is of value to dentists involved in program planning for dental care delivery. For example, a survey might disclose that a certain neighborhood is populated by an equal distribution of older adults and young children. The caries rates of the young are low relative to similar neighborhoods because the water in the community was fluoridated many years ago, but a surprisingly high number of adolescents have gingivitis. The survey also shows that among adults 40 to 60 years of age the prevalence of moderate to severe periodontal disease is 35% and that a large number of those over 60 years of age are affected by root surface caries. The program planner may weigh all the findings of the study and decide that, rather than a dental health education program for local schoolchildren, what this population needs most are programs to increase the awareness of the need for periodontal care and a program to provide access to dental care at reasonable fees for working-class families. For more on the use of epidemiologic surveys in planning, see Chapter 10.

Other policy decisions can be aided by epidemiologic studies. The National Institute for Dental Research in 1985-1986 sponsored a major nationwide study, the National Survey of Adult Oral Health of U.S. Adults.[22] This study looked at coronal and root caries, periodontal disease, and a variety of dental pathology in comprehensive examinations of employed adults around the country. The study was cross-sectional by age; that is, it looked at adults selected and stratified according to 5-year age intervals. This sample was scientifically designed so that the 15,000 participants were representative of 100 million working Americans. Among other things, the researchers have been able to develop estimates of the treatment needs of the Americans the sample represents. With information about demand versus need, the researchers were then able to generate projections for personnel needs in periodontics in future years.

THE SCIENCE OF EPIDEMIOLOGY

Epidemiology as a science is organized into three distinct divisions: descriptive, analytical, and experimental. Each branch employs specific methods and measurements and evaluates the disease status of a population from its own perspectives. Any or all may be of value to the health professional, depending on the population and investigation at hand.

Descriptive epidemiology is used to aid in the conceptualization and quantification of the disease status of the community. The major parameters of interest in descriptive epidemiology are incidence and prevalence. These terms are used to describe the extent to which the problem under inquiry exists in the population. *Incidence* is the number of cases that will occur within a population during a specified time period. Incidence is usually expressed as a rate, that is, cases per population per time. It is the result of the force operating on a population over time. For example, the annual death rate in a community is the result of the force of morbidity on the population of that community during the year. Let us say that 60 people in a city of 300,000 died of oral cancer during the year 1992. We could then express the rate of death caused by oral cancer in this population as 60 deaths per 300,000 persons per year.

Now, think of the population as individuals all contributing 1 year of life to a communal concept of living known as *person-years*. Together, these people in 1992 have accumulated 300,000 person-years. We can now express the death rate caused by oral cancer as 60 deaths per 300,000 person years. We can further compress this expression of morbidity and express it by using exponential notation as the rate of 20 deaths per 10^5 person-years. The general form in which incidence rates (IR) are expressed is as follows:

IR = cases/person-time.

The range for incidence rates is from zero to infinity.

Prevalence is the term used to indicate what proportion of a given population is affected by a condition at a given point in time. It is expressed as a percentage of the population, and its range is 0% to 100%.

If we examined 1,000 schoolchildren in September 1992 and found that 200 had gingivitis, we could say that the prevalence of gingivitis in this population in September 1992 was 20%. The general expression for prevalence is as follows:

$$p = \frac{cases}{population} \times 100\%$$

Most dental surveys, such as decayed, missing, and filled (DMF) counts, measure the prevalence of dental disease in populations.

The distinction that must be drawn between incidence and prevalence is one of time. An incidence rate is the expression of an instantaneous force; it is not a period or point in time. Prevalence is an expression of a point estimate. At a given point in time, y number of individuals have a disease. We do not know when the disease first came into being, but we do know that at the time of examination a specific percentage of the population showed signs of having the disease. These cases are the prevalent cases. Their ratio to the total population expressed as a percentage is termed prevalence.

Say we reexamined our schoolchildren in October 1992 and found 16 new cases of gingivitis. We now know that operating under the force we call incidence, etiologic factors have produced 16 incident cases of gingivitis in 1 month. If we consider that each of the previously unaffected 800 children contributed 1 month to the communal concept of person-time, we can compute our incidence rate of 16 cases per 800 person-months. We can further compress this idea by converting this to an annual figure:

$$I = \frac{16 \text{ cases}}{800 \text{ person-months}} \times \frac{12 \text{ months}}{\text{year}} = \frac{.024 \text{ cases}}{\text{person-year}}$$

If our originally affected 200 students still had gingivitis at the October examination, we could compute our prevalence for October as follows:

$$P = \frac{216 \text{ cases}}{1,000 \text{ students}} \times 100\% = 21.6\%$$

When evaluating prevalence and incidence data, the time element must be kept in perspective. With prevalence data, one is probably looking at a disease or condition that is the result of multiple intervening variables, many of which may be unknown, undefined, or uncontrolled, operating over a long period of time. Prevalence data generally have no baseline reference point. In looking at incidence data, there is a baseline reference point, a defined period of time over which the intervening variables were operating, and some definition or quantification of the intervening variables. A good example of an incidence study was done by Hand

and associates,[19] who looked at risk factors for tooth loss in noninstitutionalized elderly living in rural Iowa. This study evaluated tooth loss over a 5-year period. The use of incidence data allowed the researchers to evaluate the more clearly delineated risk factors for tooth loss that were present in late life, that is, during the 5 years of the study, independent of the risk factors that were cumulative during earlier life. Thus factors such as coronal caries, root caries, and periodontal disease could be more clearly evaluated for their contribution to the risk for tooth loss.

Analytical epidemiology is most often used in studies to determine the etiology of a disease. With analytical epidemiology a researcher may attempt to establish that a causal relationship exists between a factor and a disease. In epidemiology causative agents may be considered alone or together with other agents to be necessary or sufficient to cause a disease. A necessary cause is one that must be sustained for a person to get the disease. A sufficient cause is one that is sustained and may cause the disease. There may be more than one necessary or sufficient cause for a disease.

Figure 7-1 illustrates a hypothetical causal theory for periodontal disease. There are two sufficient causes under this theory: sufficient cause 1 accounts for 75% of the cases examined, and sufficient cause 2 gives rise to the remaining 25% of the cases. Factor A is a necessary cause of periodontal disease for both sufficient causes 1 and 2 under this theory. If factor A is not present, the disease will not occur. The presence of factor A alone, however, will not result in the disease state. Factor A, therefore, is a necessary cause but not a sufficient cause.

The remaining factors B, C, and D act together with A to form sufficient causes 1 and 2. Factors B, C, and D, taken individually, are not necessary causes; if any one of them is blocked, the disease can still occur. Separately or together, factors B, C, and D do not constitute a sufficient cause.

The concepts of necessary and sufficient causes are important to a researcher trying to determine the etiologic basis for a disease. If a factor is necessary, and blocking this factor results in 100% of the disease being prevented, this is important information. If the factor is probably necessary but not sufficient, the researcher must look further to

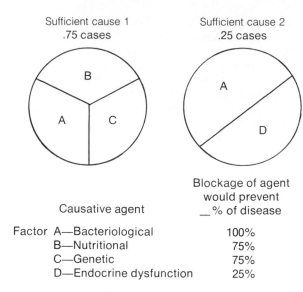

Factor A—Bacteriological   100%
        B—Nutritional   75%
        C—Genetic   75%
        D—Endocrine dysfunction   25%

Fig. 7-1 Periodontal disease: causation in hypothetical population.

unravel the causal web and discover the relationships between all causal factors.

In analytical epidemiology several types of studies are commonly used by researchers to determine the etiology of a disease. Three common study designs are prospective cohort studies, case control studies, and retrospective follow-up studies. Each type has its own strengths and limitations and is suited for specific kinds of research problems.

The prospective cohort study, commonly referred to as a cohort study, is the closest to experimental research in epidemiology. This study is conducted on a general population that is followed through time to see which members develop the disease or outcomes in question. Once this subpopulation is established, the various exposure factors that affected this group are evaluated. This type of study can generate a hypothesis because multiple end points are examined.

Prospective or cohort studies allow an investigator to examine a larger number of hypotheses at one time. The temporal sequence of cause and effect may be clearly seen in a prospective study. A major disadvantage of this type of study is that time must elapse for data to be generated, and often subjects drop out of the study along the way for various reasons. A prospective cohort study can be very expensive because it must be conducted over a fairly long period of time, and the population must be large enough to ensure adequate sample size after attrition. The classic studies by H. Trendley Dean and others[13,14] looking at communities with and without natural fluoride are examples of prospective cohort studies. As in most cohort studies, there were multiple end points to be evaluated in terms of diseases and outcomes—fluorosis and dental caries being of principal interest.

A case control study is conducted by using a population that has a disease and a matching population that does not. Such a study asks the question, "What has been the exposure of the disease group?" In this study a researcher thinks back from effect to cause. Case control studies are especially good for diseases with long induction periods in that a full picture of the etiology may be obtained. A researcher conducting a case control study uses questionnaires and medical histories to review past events and exposures. This type of study is usually relatively inexpensive and requires a fairly short period of time to obtain results. Matching of cases and controls according to factors that may have influenced the course of disease development—for example, race, age, and sex—is important in ensuring the validity of a study. Matching does add to the cost and complexity of a study, however, so it should be done judiciously.

A retrospective follow-up study is used to evaluate the effect that a specific exposure has had on a population. It is commonly used in the area of occupational health hazards. This study starts with an exposure in time past and evaluates the histories of those exposed through to time present. An example of this type of research might be a study of dental assistants who were employed in Anytown, U.S.A., during the period 1940 to 1945 and who were exposed to significant quantities of mercury by mixing amalgam with mortar and pestle. If one could identify this group adequately and follow the health histories of this group through to 1985, various patterns of diseases related to this occupational hazard might emerge. Retrospective follow-up studies are relatively easy and inexpensive, provided that a select exposure group is available and that the follow-up data can be obtained.

Experimental epidemiology is used primarily in intervention studies. Once the etiology of a disease has been established, the researcher may wish to determine the effectiveness of a program of prevention or therapy. One method of doing so is by selecting an experimental population that corresponds to the general population for which the program has been designed. The researcher may then divide the experimental population into two groups, a study group that will receive the preventive or therapeutic treatment and a control group that will not. The researcher must take measures to ensure that these groups are as nearly identical as possible in composition to ensure that the trial will be valid (see Chapter 11 for a discussion of sampling). Measurement of disease incidence in both groups before and after treatment and careful analysis of results provide researchers with information about the effectiveness of the proposed program. They may then extrapolate this information to apply to the general population.

The previously mentioned studies of artificial fluoridation of water supplies are excellent examples of experimental epidemiology. In each situation the artificially fluoridated communities— Grand Rapids, Newburgh, and Evanston—were paired with neighboring communities of Muskegon, Kingston, and Oak Park, respectively, which were comparable on a variety of social and economic variables but had water supplies without artificial fluoride supplementation.[2,3,5] The outcomes of each of these studies were the same: The communities with artificial fluoridation had reduced the caries experience of children in those communities by approximately 50% compared with the children in the control communities where the water was not supplemented with fluoride. This information was certainly extrapolated and applied to the general population in public policy decisions, and now more than 50% of the population in the United States benefits from municipal water that contains fluoride in optimal levels (see Chapter 8).

INDICES IN DENTAL EPIDEMIOLOGY

Researchers in dental epidemiology have found that, to be readily quantified, analyzed, and understood, their observations must be collected and arranged in an orderly manner according to carefully defined criteria and conditions. For this purpose various indices in dental epidemiology have been developed. A dental index is an objective mathe-

matical description of a disease or condition based on carefully determined criteria under specified circumstances. The index should have the properties of validity and reliability. An index is valid when it accurately reflects the extent or degree to which the disease or condition is present; for example, the higher the score, the more severe the disease. To be reliable the index must give the same results, with very limited degrees of tolerance, each time it is applied. That is, if a researcher examined the same patient with the same condition multiple times, each time the results or scores would be the same. Table 7-1 lists various dental indices and their characteristics.

One important way of compensating for the subjectivity of diagnosis is the use of a single examiner or a limited number of examiners who have been calibrated. Calibration is a method of bringing the examiners to a unified diagnostic technique and product. This may be accomplished by having all the examiners work on sample cases, and compare and discuss the findings relative to the specified diagnostic criteria. This process is repeated until the findings of all the examiners concur. Examiners should be checked and recalibrated periodically during a study to ensure uniformity of diagnostic technique and findings. This procedure ensures interexaminer reliability. Individual examiners should also be rechecked periodically to ensure that they have not changed in diagnostic technique over time during the data collection period. This is referred to as "intraexaminer reliability."

Selection of an index

Many well-known indices have been used by researchers and clinicians to describe conditions found in the oral cavity. They include indices to describe caries, periodontal disease, oral hygiene, and orthodontics. The selection of an index is largely determined by the research at hand. What should dental health professionals look for when selecting an index for their research?

The researcher should choose an index that addresses the specific information of interest. For example, an index of periodontal disease is not a direct measure to evaluate the effects of a home care regimen. A plaque or debris index would be more appropriate. The index should be suitable for the

Table 7-1 Characteristics of selected dental indices

	Type of index	Measurement	Administration	Recommendations and comments
Decayed, missing, filled (DMF)	Adult caries	Decayed, missing, and filled teeth	Intraoral exam with mirror and explorer	Decayed, missing, filled surfaces (DMFS) may be more useful in some circumstances; individual components can be manipulated to provide insight into past and present caries experience
Root caries index (RCI)	Root caries	Attack rate of caries on exposed root surfaces.	Intraoral exam with mirror and explorer	More recent modifications include classifications for recurrent decay
Personal hygiene performances index modified (PHP-M)	Oral hygiene	Plaque on five zones of facial and lingual tooth surfaces	Plaque disclosed; all teeth erupted and present are scored	Good measure for intervention studies in smaller populations; may be too time-consuming and detailed for larger surveys
Oral hygiene index simplified (OHI-S)	Oral hygiene	Plaque and calculus on six surfaces of six teeth	Four posterior and two anterior teeth are scored; debris index and calculus index combined into a single score	Good for small and large epidemiologic surveys; well-defined criteria and scoring system
Russell's periodontal index (PI)	Gingivitis and destructive periodontal disease	Gingivitis, loss of epithelial attachment, advanced alveolar bone loss with mobility	All teeth present are examined with a periodontal probe and scored; an average score is obtained	Global index provides rough estimates of extent of disease; modification uses six index teeth for large epidemiologic surveys; newer indices give more detail

Gingival index (GI) (Loe and Silness)	Gingival health	Gingival inflammation and bleeding	Buccal, lingual, mesial, and distal surfaces probed and scored; scores can be computed for selected indicator teeth or whole dentition	Three-point scoring system sometimes difficult diagnostically
NIDR gingival index (NIDR-GI)	Gingival health	Gingival bleeding	NIDR probe placed no more than 2 mm into gingival sulcus at midpoint bucally and carefully swept into mesial interproximal area	Carefully described criteria and scoring make this index easy to train and standardize examiners
Loss of attachment (NIDR)	Periodontal disease	Quantifies loss of attachment in mm	NIDR probe used to measure pocket depth and distance from CEJ to free gingival margin; FGM/CEJ minus FGM/pocket equals loss of attachment	More accurate than pocket depth in estimating disease because it considers recession
Community periodontal index of treatment needs (CPITN)	Periodontal treatment needs	Estimates dental services needed by population	CPITN-E probe used to examine indicator teeth in six segments of mouth; graded scores converted to four-point treatment needs scale	Well defined and tested; designed to estimate treatment needs but not to quantify disease in populations

NIDR, National Institute for Dental Research; *CEJ*, cervico-enamel junction; *FGM*, free gingival margin.

population. An index that uses key teeth to measure periodontal health or half-arch techniques to assess caries experience may be fine in young adult populations. In children with mixed dentitions and in geriatric populations, however, key teeth may be missing, or the attack rate of caries may be different in the right versus the left arch. In choosing an index we must be careful that it will provide valid estimates of disease in the population.

The data should be relatively easy to gather. A caries index requiring bitewing radiographs may be expensive and difficult to carry out in a population of rural Arkansas schoolchildren. The resultant data base may not be worth the added cost of radiographs. A mirror and explorer determination may yield information that gives an adequate indication of the caries activity in that population. Once gathered, the data should be easy to interpret. The simpler the calculations and presentation, the wider the audience on which the study can have an impact. Reproducibility and reliability of data are also important. Uncalibrated examiners and poorly defined examination criteria can undermine an otherwise good project.

A final consideration is the current literature and existing classical studies. Often a study is to be compared with existing work in other populations or to baseline data gathered by another agency. If this is anticipated and comparable criteria are established, the comparison is facilitated and enhanced.

Caries indices

In dentistry the most widely used and best developed in terms of methods and interpretation are the caries indices. The decayed, missing, and filled index is commonly used to measure surfaces (DMFS) affected by dental caries or number of affected teeth (DMFT) in adult populations. In primary dentitions the index usually employed is decayed, extracted, and filled surfaces (DEFS) or teeth (DEFT).

The criteria on which a DMF index is based may vary from study to study, and these must be considered when analyzing data and comparing results of independent investigations. Variations may be found in definitions of what constitutes a carious lesion, the number of teeth at risk, and so on. The

definition must be clear as to what is considered to constitute a filling, and what a missing tooth is. Differences such as 28 teeth at risk rather than 32 will yield considerable disparity in results and thus make comparisons difficult.

The conditions under which the examination is conducted are also of major importance when evaluating study results. For example, given identical surveys, data will vary greatly if one uses bitewing radiographs and the other does not.

The DMF counts provide us with a broad overview of caries activity in a population. More specific information about the population may be garnered by examining the individual components of the index. Figure 7-2 illustrates the use of a graph to display the breakdown of DMF components. The total DMF count of a poor urban population may be identical to one of an affluent suburban population, and yet the oral health status of the groups will probably be dissimilar.

For many purposes, such as determining population needs, DMF data may be used to yield more informative data. An example is the unmet restor-

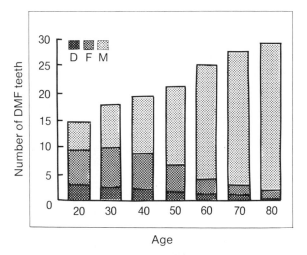

Fig. 7-2 Example illustrates how bar graphs can be used to show breakdown of DMF components. (From National Center for Health Statistics: *Selected dental findings in adults by age, race, and sex: United States, 1960-1962*, PHS Pub No 1000, Series 11, No 7, Washington, DC, 1965, US Government Printing Office.)

Table 7-2 Caries prevalence in permanent teeth before and after 20 years of fluoridation according to sex

	Male		Female		Both	
	1952-53	1972-73	1952-53	1972-73	1952-53	1972-73
Number of children	4,448	2,092	4,405	2,690	8,853	5,592
Caries	11,789*	1,991	12,250	2,037	24,039	4,028
	(2.65)†	(0.69)	(2.78)	(0.76)	(2.72)	(0.72)
Missing	3,177	217	3,317	201	6,494	418
	(0.71)	(0.07)	(0.75)	(0.07)	(0.73)	(0.07)
Filled	6,588	2,156	7,968	2,515	14,556	4,671
	(1.48)	(0.74)	(1.81)	(0.93)	(1.64)	(0.84)
Total DMF‡	21,554	4,364	23,535	4,753	45,089	9,117
% Reduction	69.1		66.9		68.0	

From Yacavone JA, Parente AM: Twenty years of community water fluoridation: the prevalence of dental caries among Providence, Rhode Island school children, *J Rhode Island State Dent Soc* 7:3, 1974.
DMF, decayed, missing, and filled.
*Total number of teeth.
†Mean score.
‡DMF data shows success of water fluridation program in Providence, Rhode Island.

ative treatment needs (UTN) index,[16] which analyzes the needs of the population as follows:

$$UTN = \frac{\text{mean number of decayed teeth}}{\text{mean numbers of decayed teeth and filled teeth}} \times 100$$

This simple yet elegant mathematic manipulation provides us with information about this population that may be readily comprehended by professionals and lay persons alike.

Indices may be used to compare the oral health status of populations following intervention or treatment. An example is a study of the effect of water fluoridation on schoolchildren in Providence, Rhode Island. The water supply of the city was fluoridated in August 1952. In 1953, baseline data were gathered by Clune.[11] In 1972-73 a study was done by Yacavone and Parente[29] using the same techniques and a comparable school-aged population. A reduction of 68% of DMFT was found. Table 7-2 and Fig. 7-3 illustrate how data from such a study may be presented in table or graph form to dramatize the results.

Other reasons why new indices may be developed include population shifts and changes in disease experience. The fastest-growing segment of

our population today is our geriatric population. Because of better dental care, older patients in the United States today are far more likely to keep their teeth throughout their lives than previous generations. This demographic shift and concomitant changes in health care have increased the likelihood that we will see older adults who have root caries. To better understand the etiology of root caries, it is necessary to study populations to determine who is at risk for root caries and to begin to formulate intervention strategies.

The root caries index (RCI) is one that attempts to assess the extent of root caries experience within the context of individual risk for the disease.[21] Katz reasoned that only root surfaces that are exposed to the oral environment are at risk to develop root caries. Those root surfaces where gingival recession has not occurred cannot develop root caries and therefore should not be considered in assessing the attack rate of root caries. The RCI records these data as follows:

$$\frac{(R\text{-}D) + (R\text{-}F)}{(R\text{-}D) + (R\text{-}F) + (R\text{-}N)} \times 100 = RCI$$

where R-D is root surface with decay, R-F is root surface that is filled, and R-N is sound root sur-

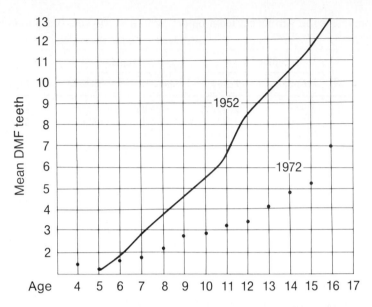

Fig. 7-3 Mean DMF permanent teeth in 1952 (before exposure to fluoridated water) and in 1972 (after 20 years of exposure to fluoridated water). Graph depicts reduction in age-specific DMFT attributable to water fluoridation. (From Yacovone JA, Parente AM: Twenty years of community water fluoridation: the prevalence of dental caries among Providence, Rhode Island school children, *J R I State Dent Soc* 7:3, 1974.)

face. This index was further refined, and a classification of restored root caries with recurrent decay was used in the National Survey of Adult Dental Health.[24]

Plaque and oral hygiene indices

An assessment that is often used to evaluate the need for, or success in, oral hygiene and health education is the measure of oral cleanliness. Of the indices that have been devised to measure oral hygiene, most measure plaque, calculus, or both.

The Personal Hygiene Performance Index (PHP) of Podshadley and Haley, as modified by Martens and Meskin (PHP-M)[25] (Fig. 7-4), is an index that is designed to be repeated following patient oral hygiene education. It may be used both to document and to assist in motivating changes in oral health habits. For this purpose, teeth selected for scoring are recorded and used at subsequent examinations. Each of six selected teeth are divided into five areas, labeled *a, b, c, d,* and *e* on both facial and lingual surfaces. Presence of plaque in lettered areas is noted on the record, and 1 point

is given for each area of plaque. The range of scores is from 0 (best) to 60 (worst). In Fig. 7-5, this index has been used to score the patient before and after oral hygiene instruction and at the follow-up visit.

The recorded information from the examination tells us the total amount of plaque present, as well as which areas in the mouth and which surfaces of the teeth are not adequately cleansed. This can be compiled for all individuals and may be used to analyze and evaluate the effectiveness of home care methods that are being used in the program.

Repetition of this index measures change in individual behavior. In a large population the information is an indication of the amount of change in individual behavior rather than just a change in behavior of the total population. The range of change in individual performance may be used to estimate success and set goals for later in the program or in future programs.

A popular index for clinical epidemiologic research is the Oral Hygiene Index Simplified (OHI-S) of Greene and Vermillion.[17] This index

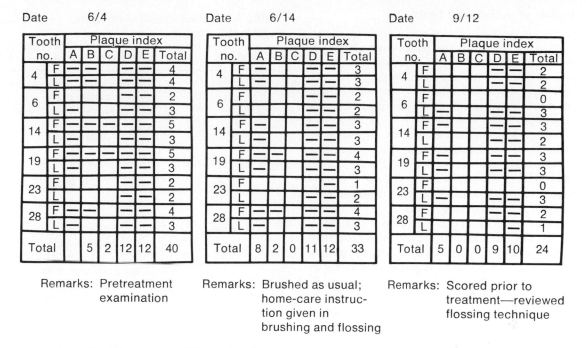

Date 6/4

Tooth no.	A	B	C	D	E	Total
4 F	—	—		—	—	4
4 L	—	—		—	—	4
6 F				—	—	2
6 L	—			—	—	3
14 F	—	—	—	—	—	5
14 L	—			—	—	3
19 F	—	—	—	—	—	5
19 L	—			—	—	3
23 F				—	—	2
23 L				—	—	2
28 F	—	—		—	—	4
28 L	—			—	—	3
Total	5	2	12	12		40

Date 6/14

Tooth no.	A	B	C	D	E	Total
4 F	—			—	—	3
4 L	—			—	—	3
6 F				—	—	2
6 L				—	—	2
14 F	—			—	—	3
14 L	—			—	—	3
19 F	—	—		—	—	4
19 L	—			—	—	3
23 F					—	1
23 L				—	—	2
28 F	—	—		—	—	4
28 L	—			—	—	3
Total	8	2	0	11	12	33

Date 9/12

Tooth no.	A	B	C	D	E	Total
4 F				—	—	2
4 L				—	—	2
6 F						0
6 L	—			—	—	3
14 F	—			—	—	3
14 L				—	—	2
19 F	—			—	—	3
19 L	—			—	—	3
23 F						0
23 L	—			—	—	3
28 F				—	—	2
28 L					—	1
Total	5	0	0	9	10	24

Remarks: Pretreatment examination

Remarks: Brushed as usual; home-care instruction given in brushing and flossing

Remarks: Scored prior to treatment—reviewed flossing technique

Fig. 7-4 Use of modified Podshadley method to evaluate oral hygiene performance.

sets forth a simple method for quantifying the amount of plaque and calculus in its two components, the debris index and the calculus index. These components are added to obtain a single score. This simplified index is based on the six surfaces scored from four posterior and two anterior teeth. Its well-defined criteria for both tooth selection and scoring make it an index that can be determined fairly rapidly and consistently.

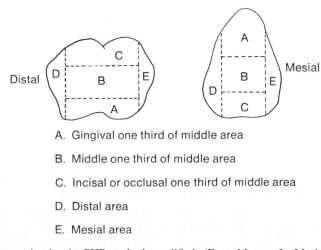

A. Gingival one third of middle area

B. Middle one third of middle area

C. Incisal or occlusal one third of middle area

D. Distal area

E. Mesial area

Fig. 7-5 Plaque scoring by the PHP method, modified. (From Martens L, Meskin L: An innovative technique for assessing oral hygiene, *J Dent Children* 39:12, 1972.)

Indices of periodontal health

There are a number of ways of looking at periodontal health: from the perspective of gingival health, bone loss, mobility, or loss of attachment. A full range of indices have been developed to look at periodontal health from these varied perspectives. A few are described here, and other examples are given in Table 7-1.

One popular index that has been used for many years for gathering and quantifying information about periodontal disease is Russell's Periodontal Index (PI).[28] Russell's index assigns a numeric score to each tooth standing in the mouth and then takes an average of these values for a PI score. The range of the Russell score is from 0 (no inflammation or disease evident) to 8 (advanced destruction with loss of masticatory function), as indicated in Table 7-3. Although the criteria for the Russell examination are fairly well delineated, because of the nature of periodontal diagnostics, evaluation may be subjective. Reproducibility of scores may be more difficult for this PI than for some others.

A commonly used index to evaluate gingival health is the Gingival Index of Loe and Silness.[23,26] This index uses either six indicator teeth or all erupted teeth. Scoring is on a scale of 0 to 3, with 0 being normal tissue and 3 being ulcerated tissue with a tendency toward spontaneous bleeding. Whereas the extremes of 0 and 3 are fairly easy to score, the scores of 1 (mild inflammation) and 2 (moderate inflammation) are sometimes difficult to differentiate, and the presence of bleeding on probing pushes the classification of otherwise mild inflammation into the moderate classification, that is, a score of 2.

As knowledge in dentistry advances, our ways of looking at dental disease change, and so must our ways of measuring the disease experience of our population. In recent years periodontists have shifted their focus of concern from pocket depth to attachment levels. Instead of using simple measurement of pocket depth as the sole indicator of periodontal health and disease, the loss of periodontal attachment is estimated by using a fixed point on the tooth. This measurement is now thought to give a broader picture of the extent of periodontal disease. For the National Survey of Adult Oral Health of U.S. Adults, an index was

Table 7-3 Russell's method of scoring periodontal disease*

Russell score	Criteria for field studies
0 Negative	There is neither obvious inflammation in the gingival epithelium nor loss of function as a result of destruction of supporting tissues.
1 Mild gingivitis	There is an obvious area of inflammation in the free gingiva, but this area does not circumscribe the tooth.
2 Gingivitis	Inflammation completely circumscribes the tooth, but there is no apparent break in the epithelial attachment.
6 Gingivitis with pocket formation	The epithelial attachment has been broken and there is a pocket (not merely a deepened gingival crevice from swelling in the free gingiva). There is no interference with normal masticatory function; the tooth is firm in its socket and has not drifted.
8 Advanced destruction with loss of masticatory function	The tooth may be loose, may have drifted, may sound dull on percussion with a metallic instrument, or may be depressible in its socket.

From Russell AL: A system of classification and scoring for prevalence surveys of periodontal disease, *J Dent Res* 35:350, 1956.
*When in doubt about a given score, assign the lesser score.

devised to record the loss of attachment.[6,22,24] For this index the cervico-enamel junction (CEJ) is used as a reference point, and a special periodontal probe, the NIDR probe, is used. Two measurements are taken: the distance in millimeters from the CEJ to the free gingival margin (FGM), and from the FGM to the base of the pocket. The difference between the two measurements is the loss of attachment:

FGM/CEJ − FGM/pocket = loss of attachment

A similar study, the National Survey of Oral Health in U.S. Schoolchildren, was conducted by the National Institute for Dental Research in 1986-87.[4] In both studies the gingival bleeding was scored by using a gingival index and technique similar to that of Loe and Silness. The primary difference lies in the method of scoring. The NIDR Gingival Index uses a dichotomous scoring system: 0 for no bleeding and 1 for presence of bleeding.

These nationwide studies, with their scientifically selected samples, may well serve as the benchmark for future studies on periodontal health, caries, and other dental diseases in the 1990s. Researchers interested in using these studies as referent populations would do well to note the techniques used.

A periodontal index that has grown in popularity with researchers over the past decade is the Community Periodontal Index of Treatment Needs (CPITN).[1,12] Developed by a joint Fédération Dentaire Internationale/World Health Organization Working Group, the index was designed specifically for epidemiologic surveys of periodontal health. It uses its own probe, the CPITN-E, and 10 index teeth that represent 6 segments of the mouth. The first and second molars are examined in the posterior sextants, and only the worst score of the pair is recorded for the sextant. Thus there are six recordings for each subject. The CPITN assesses pockets, bleeding, and plaque retentive factors (calculus and overhanging restorations). The scoring of the index is on a five-point grading from 0 to 4 in each quadrant, with 0 representing no signs of periodontal disease and 4 representing periodontal pockets of 6 mm or more. These then must be converted into a four-point classification of treatment needs categories, from TN 0, indicating no need for treatment, to TN 3, indicating complex treatment needs that can include surgical procedures, deep scaling, and root planing. An additional four tabulations are designed to provide insight into severity and categories of treatment needs.

For health services planning, especially in countries with socialized health systems, the CPITN has been shown to be useful and valid.[18] In countries without a socialized system of health care, where need and demand may be vastly disparate, the index has considerably less utility.[27] Although there is a version of this index intended for use in the clinical setting, the CPITN is designed to assess periodontal treatment needs rather than periodontal status. Thus its usefulness to the clinician, who may prefer recording actual periodontal disease findings and using direct clinical judgment, is probably limited.

EPIDEMIOLOGY AND DENTAL CARIES

With current scientific knowledge of the causation of dental diseases, why carry out epidemiologic surveys? Certainly needs determination is one reason, and program planning and evaluation another. The distribution of dental caries and the contributing etiologic factors are not a fixed equation. There has been a decrease in caries in Western countries over the past two decades. Less developed countries, which previously had low caries rates, by contrast, have seen significant increases in their caries rates. The etiology of a dental disease may be so complex that the combination of factors contributing to the cause may vary greatly among populations. Thus epidemiologic studies are needed to assist in defining the magnitude of the problem in a particular part of the world and to identify the probable etiology. With this information the intervention methods appropriate to the population and causal agents may be put into place.

The etiologic factors that contribute to any disease are usually divided into three categories: host, agent, and environmental factors. All factors must be present to be sufficient cause for the disease. Table 7-4 illustrates the factors usually recognized as causative in two types of dental caries. Intervention and removal of any necessary factor may prevent all or part of the disease. Examination of a population should include an assessment of host, agent, and environmental factors that may be used to limit the disease.

Worldwide, variations in host, agent, and environmental factors interact to produce a variety of dental diseases at varying rates and intensities. Cultural, genetic, geographic, and other factors all contribute to these variations.[15,20] An understand-

Table 7-4 Etiologic factors contributing to dental caries

Disease entity	Host factors	Agent factors	Environmental factors
Dental caries	Morphology (pits, fissures) Arch form (irregularities)	*Streptococcus mutans* Plaque	Nutrition Oral hygiene Fluoride
Root caries	Decreased salivary flow Gingival recession	*Actinomyces viscosus*	Nutrition Oral hygiene Toothbrush abrasion

ing of these factors is essential if prevention and intervention are to be successful. Local customs, values, dietary habits, and hygiene differ throughout the world. Radical changes in these patterns may not be achievable and, in some cases, may not even be desirable.

A study done in Baja, Hungary, provides an interesting example of how environmental factors can influence the outcome of a disease. In 1955 baseline data were collected in kindergarten children, ages 3 to 6 years, consisting of DMFT counts stratified according to age at last birthday. To assess the results of improved vitamin D prophylaxis that occurred after this time, a second age-specific DMFT was done in the kindergartens in Baja in 1975.[7] Analysis of the data revealed a 10.9% increase in frequency of caries (number of children affected by caries). Intensity of caries experience (mean number of carious lesions per child) increased by 43.5%. Examiners then had to look for factors that might have brought about this unanticipated increase in dental caries. One factor that researchers discussed was the rise in annual sugar consumption from 24.4 kg per person to 37.5 kg per person. Analysis of contributing factors in a case such as this can lead to a shift of priorities in program planning.

THE FUTURE OF DENTAL EPIDEMIOLOGY

With falling caries rates in the United States, is there still work to be done with dental epidemiology? Certainly the problem of dental caries still exists throughout the rest of the world, especially in economically deprived and third world countries. In the United States, periodontal disease will continue to be an important issue for researchers well into the twenty-first century. Other issues of importance to dental health professionals continue to emerge, including the incidence of transmission of AIDS, hepatitis, tuberculosis, and other serious communicable diseases. In all these areas epidemiology and biomedical research will need to work in partnership to isolate causal and transmission mechanisms and to find solutions to the problems of oral disease and dental health care.

REFERENCES

1. Ainamo J and others.: Development of the world health organization (WHO) community periodontal index of treatment needs (CPITN), *Int Dent J* 32:281, 1982.
2. Arnold FA and others: Fifteenth year of the Grand Rapids fluoridation study, *J Am Dent Assoc* 65:780, 1962.
3. Ast DB, Finn SB, McCafferty I: The Newburgh-Kingston caries fluoride study; I, dental findings after three years of water fluoridation, *Am J Public Health* 40:116, 1950.
4. Bhat M: Periodontal health of 14-17-year-old US schoolchildren, *J Public Health Dent* 51(1):5, 1991.
5. Blayney JR, Hill IN: Fluoride and dental caries, *J Am Dent Assoc* 74:233, 1967.
6. Brown LJ, Oliver R, Loe H: Evaluating periodontal status of U.S. employed adults, *J Am Dent Assoc* 121:226, 1990.
7. Bruszt P and others: Caries prevalence of preschool children in Baja, Hungary in 1955 and 1975, *Health Serv Rep* 87:456, 1972.
8. Centers for Disease Control: Possible transmission of human immunodeficiency virus to a patient during an invasive dental procedure, *MMWR* 39:489, 1990.
9. Centers for Disease Control: Update: transmission of HIV infection during an invasive dental procedure—Florida, *MMWR* 40:21, 1991.
10. Centers for Disease Control: Update: transmission of HIV infection during invasive dental procedures—Florida, *MMWR* 40:377, 1991.
11. Clune TW: Prevalence of dental caries on primary and permanent teeth: a study of 8,853 school children, *R I Med J* 36:653, 1954.
12. Cutress TW, Ainamo J, Sardo-Infirri J: The community periodontal index of treatment needs (CPITN) procedure

for populations, groups and individuals, *Int Dent J* 37:222, 1987.

13. Dean HT: Endemic fluorosis and its relation to dental caries, *Public Health Rep* 53:1443, 1938.

14. Dean HT, Arnold FA, Elvove E: Domestic water and dental caries; V, additional studies on the relation of fluoride domestic waters to dental caries experience in 4,425 white children, aged 12 to 14 years, of 13 cities in 4 states, *Public Health Rep* 57:1155, 1942.

15. Glass R: The first international conference on the declining prevalence of dental caries, *J Dent Res* 61:1301, 1982.

16. Gluck GM and others: Dental health of Puerto Rican migrant workers, *Health Serv Rep* 87:456, 1972.

17. Greene JC, Vermillion JR: The simplified oral hygiene index, *J Am Dent Assoc* 68:7, 1964.

18. Grytten J, Holst D, Gjermo P: Validity of CPITN's hierarchical scoring method for describing the prevalence of periodontal conditions, *Community Dent Oral Epidemiol* 17:300, 1989.

19. Hand JS, Hunt R, Kohout FJ: Five-year incidence of tooth loss in Iowans aged 65 and older, *Community Dent Oral Epidemiol* 19:48, 1991.

20. Hunter PB: Risk factors in dental caries, *Int Dent J* 38:211, 1988.

21. Katz RV: Assessing root caries in populations: the evolution of the root caries index, *J Public Health Dent* 40:7, 1980.

22. Loe H: Essential features of the 1985 National Survey of Oral Health of U.S. Adults, *J Public Health Dent* 47:204, 1987.

23. Loe H, Silness J: Periodontal disease in pregnancy, *Acta Odontol Scand* 21:533, 1963.

24. Miller A and others: *Oral health of United States adults: the national survey of oral health in U.S. employed adults and seniors, national findings,* NIDR Publ No 87-2868, Bethesda, MD, 1987.

25. Martens LV, Meskin LH: An innovative technique for assessing oral hygiene, *J Dent Children* 39:12, 1972.

26. Nordstrom NK and others: Testing reliability of plaque and gingival indices: two methods, *J Periodontol* 59:270, 1988.

27. Oliver R, Brown LJ, Loe H: An estimate of periodontal treatment needs in the U.S. based on epidemiological data, *J Periodontol* 60:371, 1989.

28. Russell AL: A system of classification and scoring for prevalence surveys of periodontal disease, *J Dent Res* 35:350, 1956.

29. Yacovone JA, Parente AM: Twenty years of community water fluoridation: the prevalence of dental caries among Providence, Rhode Island, school children, *J R I State Dent Soc* 7:3, 1974.

8 Prevention of Dental Disease

Dentistry has traditionally functioned within the private setting, the one-on-one treatment of the patient by the dental professional. In this century, however, scientific research, technologic advances, and a better understanding of the disease process have contributed to dentistry's emergence from a purely reparative art toward a preventive-oriented science. This emergence encompasses both a greater variety of practice settings and a greater reliance on auxiliary personnel to assist in the provision of services. Significant contributions to the promotion and protection of the public's oral health can now be accomplished by concurrent and cooperative efforts by the dental professional, the individual, and the community.

There has been a dramatic decline in the prevalence of dental caries (dental decay) in this country. The 1979-80 National Institute of Dental Research (NIDR) survey of dental caries in U.S. schoolchildren reported a mean score of decayed, missing, and filled surfaces (DMFS) for 5- to 17-year-olds of 4.77, with approximately 37% of the children being caries-free.[102] A similar survey conducted in 1986-87 by NIDR revealed a mean DMFS of 3.07 and 50% of the same aged children being caries-free.[104] This represents a 36% reduction in the mean DMFS of U.S. schoolchildren in only a 7-year period. Of the disease activity, 58% involved the occlusal surface, 30% the buccal-lingual surfaces, and only 12% the proximal surfaces.

The periodontal health of teenagers was also assessed in the 1986-87 survey.[104] Whereas gingivitis was observed in approximately 60% of the 14- to 17-year-olds, only 6% of the sites examined were affected. A survey of employed adults and seniors conducted by NIDR in 1985-86 has indicated that the prevalence of the more severe levels of periodontal destruction may not be as prevalent as previously believed.[103] Advanced periodontal disease affects fewer than 20% of older adults.

Concomitant with the decline in caries activity has been a reported increase in the prevalence of fluorosis, a developmental defect of the enamel caused by the ingestion of fluoride above what is required for dental health. The increase has been largely in the very mild or mild fluorosis categories, which are usually not a cosmetic problem. Although the consequences of the increase in the milder forms of fluorosis do not appear to have a public health import, public health officials are concerned because an increase in the prevalence of fluorosis can have occurred only as a result of the current generation ingesting more fluoride then previous generations. Fluoride is ubiquitous in nature. Ingested sources include drinking water, bottled beverages, and foods. In addition, dental sources include prescribed fluoride supplements and the inadvertent swallowing of fluoride from mouthrinses, dentifrices, and professional and self-applied topical fluorides.

It is against this backdrop of declined prevalence of oral disease and increased level of fluorosis that this chapter has been written. The purpose is to provide the future dental professionals—that is, dentists, dental hygienists and dental assistants, expanded-function dental auxiliaries, and dental technicians—with highlights and a brief overview of current preventive concepts and their application.

PREVENTIVE DENTISTRY DEFINED

In its broadest sense, preventive dentistry encompasses all aspects of dentistry and those practices by dental professionals, individuals, and communities that affect oral health. In this regard, preventive dentistry has been conceptualized in a number of ways, including a sequence of levels of prevention, a set of priorities, a taxonomy, and a category of services (Table 8-1).[40,87,90,91] Readers should be familiar with these concepts and terms because they are used throughout the dental liter-

Table 8-1 Prevention concepts and the health-disease continuum

Levels of prevention	Primary	Secondary	Tertiary
Prevention concepts			
Priorities of prevention	Prevention of disease initiation	Prevention of disease progression and recurrence	Prevention of loss of function
Taxonomy of prevention	Prepathosis	Intervention	Replacement
Preventive services	Health promotion Specific protection	Early diagnosis and prompt treatment	Disability limitation Rehabilitation
Health-disease continuum	Prepathogenesis	Pathogenesis	

Modified from Dunning JM: *Principles of dental public health,* ed 4, Cambridge, Mass, 1986, Harvard University Press; Leavell HR, Clark EG: *Preventive medicine for the doctor in his community,* ed 3, New York, 1965, McGraw-Hill; Lutz BL: Preventive dentistry: proposal for definition of terms, *J Dent Educ* 37:24, 1973; and Mandel I: What is preventive dentistry? *J Prev Dent* 1:25, 1974.

ature. Each of these concepts commonly looks at preventive dentistry in relation to the oral health-disease continuum. A basic division is made between the prepathogenesis and pathogenesis stages of the disease. Major emphasis is logically placed on those services aimed at the time of the origination and development of the disease, the prepathogenesis stage.

Services directed toward the prepathogenesis stage are referred to as *primary preventive services,* services that prevent the initiation of disease. They are designated as services that provide health promotion and specific protection. Health promotion activities, such as providing instruction in proper plaque removal or daily toothbrushing and flossing, are designed to promote general optimum health, in this case periodontal health. Specific protection activities include services that are designed to protect against disease agents by decreasing the susceptibility of the host or by establishing barriers against agents in the environment. The ingestion of optimally fluoridated water and the application of pit and fissure sealants provide specific protection against caries.

Services directed toward the initial stages of disease pathogenesis are referred to as *secondary preventive services,* that is, those that intervene or prevent the progression and recurrence of disease. They are designated as activities that are aimed at the early diagnosis and prompt treatment of dis-

ease to prevent sequelae. For example, the prompt treatment of a small carious lesion will prevent extended loss of tooth structure.

Finally, services directed toward the end results of disease pathogenesis are referred to as *tertiary preventive* or *replacement services,* those that prevent loss of function. These activities provide disability limitation and rehabilitation. Prosthetic appliances and implants are included in this category.

This global perspective of preventive dentistry is based on the premise that every oral health activity implemented by the individual, the community, or the dental professional is targeted toward the prevention of some aspect of the health-disease continuum. This logic entails the anticipation of disease initiation and its progression or recurrence if appropriate activities are not implemented. Priority is given first to primary preventive services, followed by secondary, and then tertiary services. This reasoning and this methodical selection of priorities and implementation of health-specific and disease-specific measures emerge from this concept of preventive dentistry.

PREVENTIVE DENTISTRY SERVICES

A multitude of preventive dentistry services that can be applied to all levels of prevention are presented in Tables 8-2 through 8-5. Services targeted toward dental caries, periodontal diseases, oral cancer, orofacial defects, malocclusion, and accidents are listed. These tables demonstrate the intricacies of the strategies required to prevent these categories of oral diseases and disorders.

Coordinated efforts by the dental professional, the individual, and the community are needed to attain and maintain optimum oral health because of the complexity of disease etiology. A hypothetical example related to the specific oral disease of dental caries would be an individual who practices excellent oral hygiene, has resided from birth in a community that has optimally fluoridated water, and yet who might develop dental caries on the occlusal surfaces of the teeth. In this example these occlusal lesions can be prevented by application of dental sealants by a dental professional.

A survey of Tables 8-2 through 8-5 shows that most of the individual, community, and professional cooperative efforts are available at the primary prevention level. Beyond that level the dental professional plays a greater role. At the secondary prevention level the individual can use existing dental services, and the community can fund the provision of dental services. Of course, oral diseases and disorders are rarely present at only the prepathogenesis or only the pathogenesis stage. For example, frequently two or more oral diseases may be present and at different stages on the health-disease continuum. An individual may have numerous carious lesions but not periodontal disease, or an individual may have periodontal disease in one quadrant of the oral cavity but not in any of the others. In both cases, primary, secondary, and/or tertiary preventive dental services are needed, and cooperative efforts are still required to attain oral health.

For the delivery of health care services, regardless of whether they are primary, secondary, or tertiary services, considerations must be given to services that are affordable, available, and accessible. A multitude of factors affect health care delivery. Primary preventive dental services address the factors of high cost and labor maldistribution, as most are not costly and many do not require dental personnel for their implementation. Health care services also require complete acceptance and use. These factors are not always easily attained because of variations in the interest, motivation, economic status, and, at times, political inclination of

health care consumers, providers, and administrators. Also, the individual and the community may not be knowledgeable about the necessary procedures. An ideal public health measure should address all these concerns of health care delivery.

Experience with the delivery and use of health services has advanced a philosophy that an "ideal public health measure" should be (1) of proven efficacy in the reduction of the targeted disease; (2) medically and dentally safe; (3) easily and efficiently implemented, using relatively small quantities of materials, supplies, and equipment; (4) readily administered by nondental personnel; (5) attainable by the beneficiaries regardless of their socioeconomic, educational, income, and occupational status; (6) readily available and accessible to large numbers of individuals; (7) inexpensive and therefore affordable by the majority; (8) uncomplicated and easily learned by the users; (9) administered with maximum acceptance on the part of the patient(s); and (10) administered with minimum compliance on the part of the patient(s).*

PRIMARY PREVENTIVE DENTISTRY SERVICES

As mentioned earlier, the main emphasis of preventive dentistry is on selecting priorities for the expenditure of efforts and resources for primary preventive services. Accordingly, the subsequent emphasis of this chapter is in this area. For purposes of brevity, this section addresses only services targeted toward two of the diseases: dental caries and periodontal disease. Each service is defined, and its history, disease prevention effectiveness, implementation and necessary effort, and required patient acceptance and compliance are described. The services are presented in the following outline:

I. Primary preventive services provided in the community
   A. Community water fluoridation
   B. School water fluoridation
   C. Fluoride supplement programs
   D. Fluoride mouthrinse programs
   E. School sealant programs

---

*References 22, 30, 53, 69, 101, 109, 156

Text continued on p. 163.

Table 8-2 Dental caries: individual, community, and dental professional preventive dentistry services

Levels of prevention	Primary		Secondary	Tertiary	
Preventive services	Health promotion	Specific protection	Early diagnosis and prompt treatment	Disability limitation	Rehabilitation
Services provided by the individual	Diet planning; demand for preventive services; periodic visits to the dental office	Appropriate use of fluoride Ingestion of sufficient fluoridated water Appropriate use of fluoride prescriptions Use of a fluoride dentifrice Oral hygiene practices	Self-examination and referral; use of dental services	Use of dental services	Use of dental services
Services provided by the community	Dental health education programs; promotion of research efforts; lobby efforts	Community or school water fluoridation; school fluoride mouth rinse program; school fluoride tablet program; school sealant program	Periodic screening and referral; provision of dental services	Provision of dental services	Provision of dental services
Services provided by the dental professional	Patient education; plaque control program; diet counseling; recall reinforcement; dental caries activity tests	Topical application of fluoride; fluoride rinse supplement/ rinse prescription; pit and fissure sealants	Complete exam; prompt treatment of incipient lesions; preventive resin restorations; simple restorative dentistry; pulp capping	Complex restorative dentistry; pulpotomy; root canal therapy; extractions	Removable and fixed prosthodontics; minor tooth movement; implants

Modified from Dunning JM: *Principles of dental public health*, ed 4, Cambridge, Mass, 1986, Harvard University Press; and Mandel I: What is preventive dentistry? *J Prev Dent* 1:25, 1974.

Table 8-3 Periodontal diseases: individual, community, and dental professional preventive dentistry services

Levels of prevention	Primary		Secondary	Tertiary	
	Health promotion	**Specific protection**	**Early diagnosis and prompt treatment**	**Disability limitation**	**Rehabilitation**
Services provided by the individual	Periodic visits to dental office; demand for preventive services	Oral hygiene practices	Self-examination and referral; use of dental services	Use of dental services	Use of dental services
Services provided by the community	Dental health education programs; promotion of research efforts; provision of oral hygiene aids; lobby efforts	Supervised school brushing programs	Periodic screening and referral; provision of dental services	Provision of dental services	Provision of dental services
Services provided by the dental professional	Patient education; plaque control program; recall reinforcement	Correction of tooth malalignment; prophylaxis	Complete examination; scaling and curettage; corrective, restorative, and occlusal services	Deep curettage; root planing; splinting; periodontal surgery; selective extractions	Removable fixed prosthodontics; minor tooth movement

Modified from Dunning JM: *Principles of dental public health*, ed 4, Cambridge, Mass, 1986, Harvard University Press; and Mandel I: What is preventive dentistry? *J Prev Dent* 1:25, 1974.

Table 8-4 Oral cancer: individual, community, and dental professional preventive dentistry services

Levels of prevention	Primary		Secondary	Tertiary	
Preventive services	**Health promotion**	**Specific protection**	**Early diagnosis and prompt treatment**	**Disability limitation**	**Rehabilitation**
Services provided by the individual	Periodic visits to dental office; demand for preventive services	Avoidance of known irritants	Self-examination and referral; use of dental services	Use of dental services	Use of dental services
Services provided by the community	Dental health education programs; promotion of research efforts; lobby efforts		Periodic screening and referral; provision of dental services	Provision of dental services	Provision of dental services
Services provided by the dental professional	Patient education	Removal of known irritants in oral cavity	Complete examination; biopsy; oral cytology; complete excision	Chemotherapy; radiation therapy; surgery	Maxillofacial and removable prosthodontics; plastic surgery; speech therapy; counseling

Modified from Dunning JM: *Principles of dental public health*, ed 4, Cambridge, Mass, 1986, Harvard University Press; and Mandel I: What is preventive dentistry? *J Prev Dent* 1:25, 1974.

Table 8-5 Orofacial defects, malocclusion, and accidents: individual, community, and dental professional preventive dentistry services

Levels of prevention	Primary		Secondary	Tertiary	
Preventive services	Health promotion	Specific protection	Early diagnosis and prompt treatment	Disability limitation	Rehabilitation
Services provided by the individual		Use of protective devices; habit control	Use of dental services	Use of dental services	Use of dental services
Services provided by the community	Dental health education programs; promotion of protective garb; lobby efforts	Mouthguard program; safety of children's toys; safety of school buildings and playgrounds	Provision of dental services	Provision of dental services	Provision of dental services
Services provided by the dental professional	Patient education	Caries control; space maintainers; genetic counseling; prenatal care; parental counseling	Minor orthodontics	Major orthodontics; surgery	Maxillofacial fixed/removable prosthodontics; plastic surgery; speech therapy; counseling

Modified from Dunning JM: *Principles of dental public health*, ed 4, Cambridge, Mass, 1986, Harvard University Press; and Mandel I: What is preventive dentistry? *J Prev Dent* 1:25, 1974.

II. Primary preventive services provided by the dental professional
   A. Professional topical fluoride applications
   B. Pit and fissure sealants
   C. Diet counseling
   D. Plaque control programs
   E. Dental caries activity tests
III. Primary preventive services provided by the individual
   A. Fluoride dentifrices
   B. Self-applied topical fluoride products
   C. Oral hygiene practices

This outline and the "specific protection" services for dental caries (Table 8-2) highlight the critical role of fluoride in preventive services. Fluoride's effectiveness in caries reduction and its versatility of application cannot be surpassed by any other agent currently available. It can be used systemically, as in community and school water fluoridation and fluoride tablets, and topically, as in solutions, gels, mouthrinses, and dentifrices. Fluoride is effective when incorporated into the enamel structure during tooth maturation, as in systemic use. Topically, it is also incorporated into the outermost surface of the enamel and into incipient carious lesions ("white spots"). Its presence in and on the enamel surface and in the saliva reduces the susceptibility of the tooth surface to dental caries initiation and progression. It has its greatest relative impact on the smooth surfaces of the teeth and can be administered under the auspices of the community, the individual, or the dental professional.

Caries protection of the pit and fissure surfaces can be achieved through the application of dental sealants. In 1983 a National Institutes of Health (NIH) consensus development conference on dental sealants unanimously endorsed the placement of sealants as a highly effective and safe means of preventing pit and fissure caries.[105] Furthermore, the combined use of sealants and fluorides provides optimum caries protection. Because the majority of carious lesions in school-age children involve the pits and fissures, widespread use of sealants will substantially reduce dental caries below the levels that have already been achieved by fluorides and other preventive measures and enable many adolescents to enter adulthood with caries-free dentitions.

When reading the following sections, readers should keep in mind the requisites of an ideal public health measure and refer to Tables 8-2 through 8-5 to attain a relative perspective for each service. Only a few preventive dental services meet this ideal.

PRIMARY PREVENTIVE SERVICES PROVIDED IN THE COMMUNITY

The community-administered services discussed in this chapter involve participation of key community decision makers and the organization of large numbers of people, resources, and commitments for the purpose of preventing dental caries. Other primary preventive community-administered services exist but have not been shown to be as effective and efficient in disease reduction as the following five caries-preventive services.

Community water fluoridation

Fluoridation is the adjustment of the fluoride content of a community's water supply to an optimal level for the prevention of dental caries (tooth decay). The caries-reducing benefits of fluoride in community water were discovered in the process of investigating the cause of "Colorado brown stain," a mottling and staining of the tooth enamel.[94] Today this condition, which is caused by ingestion of excessive amounts of fluoride during the period of tooth development, is more properly known as *enamel fluorosis*. Studies conducted by Dr. H. Trendley Dean[32,33] in areas with naturally occurring fluoride demonstrated a direct relationship between community water fluoride levels and enamel fluorosis and an inverse relationship between dental caries and community water fluoride levels. These studies revealed that in communities with fluoride levels of approximately 1 part per million (ppm), reduction in dental caries experience was substantial, and only 10% of the population had dental fluorosis of the very mildest form (which was not cosmetically detracting). These findings provided the basis for controlled studies of the fluoridation of communal water supplies, and on January 25, 1945, Grand Rapids, Michigan, became the first city in the world to adjust the fluoride content of its water supply to an optimal level for dental health.[5] Soon after, Newburgh, New York; Brantford, Ontario; and

fluoride exposure is generally greater in fluoridated areas; however, there is fluoride exposure in both fluoridated and nonfluoridated areas because of the variety of fluoride sources besides drinking water. Beverages and foods are sources of fluoride, especially if they have been prepared with fluoridated drinking water.

- Optimal fluoridation of drinking water does not pose a detectable cancer risk to humans as evidenced by extensive human epidemiologic data available to date, including the new studies prepared for this report.
- The data available from the two methodologically acceptable studies of the carcinogenicity of fluoride in experimental animals fail to establish an association between fluoride and cancer.
- By comparison with the 1940s, the total prevalence of dental fluorosis has increased in nonfluoridated areas and may have increased in optimally fluoridated areas. Such increases in dental fluorosis in a population signify that total fluoride exposures have increased and may be more than are necessary to prevent dental caries. For this reason, prudent public health practice dictates the reduction of unnecessary and inappropriate fluoride exposure.
- In the 1940s, drinking water and food were the major sources of fluoride exposure. Since then, additional sources of fluoride have become available through the introduction of fluoride-containing dental products. Although the use of these products is likely responsible for some of the declines in caries scores, the inappropriate use of these products has also likely contributed to the observed increases in the prevalence of very mild and mild forms of dental fluorosis.
- Further epidemiologic studies are required to determine whether an association exists between various levels of fluoride in drinking water and bone fractures.
- Crippling skeletal fluorosis is not a public health problem in the United States, as evidenced by the reports of only five cases in 30 years.
- Well-controlled studies have not demonstrated a beneficial effect of the use of high doses of fluoride in reducing osteoporosis and related bone fractures.
- Genotoxicity studies of fluoride, which are highly dependent on the methods used, often show contradictory findings. The most consistent finding is that fluoride has not been shown to be mutagenic in standard tests in bacteria (Ames test). In some studies with different methodologies, fluoride has been reported to induce mutations and chromosome aberrations in cultured rodent and human cells. The genotoxicity of fluoride in humans and animals is unresolved, despite numerous studies.
- Chronic low-level fluoride exposure is not associated with birth defects. Studies also fail to establish an association between fluoride and Down syndrome.
- There is no indication that chronic low-level fluoride exposure of normal individuals presents a problem in other organ systems, such as the gastrointestinal, the genitourinary, and the respiratory systems. The effects of fluoride on the reproductive system merit further investigation in animal and human studies.

As of December 31, 1988, more than 124 million citizens in more than 7,800 communities in the United States were receiving the benefits of optimally adjusted fluoridated water.[24] Additionally, 9 million people residing in 1,846 communities were drinking water with naturally occurring fluorides at levels of 0.7 ppm or higher. Thus more than 53% of the nation's population and almost 61% of those living in areas with public water supplies have access to drinking water with optimal levels of fluoride. Among the 50 largest cities in the United States, 41 have fluoridated water supplies. Only seven states (Connecticut, Georgia, Illinois, Minnesota, Nebraska, Ohio, and South Dakota) currently mandate community water fluoridation.[42]

Community water fluoridation has emerged as one of the most important public health measures of the twentieth century because (1) it is effective in reducing tooth decay in both children and adults; (2) it is safe; (3) its low cost makes it eminently cost-effective; (4) it benefits everyone in the community served by the water supply regardless of socioeconomic status, educational background, or financial ability to seek dental care; and (5) it requires no cooperative effort on the part of individuals other than consuming water regularly. Community water fluoridation must remain the cornerstone of community dental preventive services.

The dental profession plays a crucial role in the recommendation of community water fluoridation as a public health measure.[43] Numerous pamphlets and books have addressed a wide variety of issues regarding the fluoridation controversy. Dental professionals should be aware of these issues, be prepared to use the vast amount of data available, and be cognizant of the political process that is often needed to implement fluoridation at the community level. In addition, it is vital to the support of fluoridation that dental professionals educate their patients on these issues.

School water fluoridation

For the more than 30 million individuals not served by a public water supply, alternative methods of dental caries protection must be used. One method suggested for supplying systemic fluoride to children is fluoridating the individual school water supply. This method was thought particularly suitable in rural schools where kindergarten through grade 12 may attend class in the same or adjacent buildings. In addition to the systemic effects on developing teeth, school water fluoridation, like community water fluoridation, imparts topical effects on erupted teeth.

In 1954 a school water fluoridation pilot study was initiated in St. Thomas, U.S. Virgin Islands, by the U.S. Public Health Service, Division of Dental Health. Because children are exposed to fluoride on school days only, the school water was fluoridated slightly over 3 times the optimum indicated for the community water fluoride. After 8 years, students showed 22% less caries experience than children at schools that were not fluoridating their water supplies.[73]

Subsequent studies were done with increasing and varying amounts of fluoride. In Pike County, Kentucky, the water supplies of two schools were fluoridated at 3.3 times the optimum, and in Elk Lake, Pennsylvania, the water supply of one school was fluoridated at 4.5 times the optimum recommended level for that area. After 8 years the children who had attended the study schools had 32.8% (Pike County) and 33.9% (Elk Lake) less caries experience than students who had attended each school prior to fluoridation.[74]

In Seagrove, North Carolina, after 12 years of school water adjusted at 7 times optimum recommended fluoride level for that locale, the students had an average of 48% fewer DMF surfaces compared with their counterparts at the baseline examinations made before the water was adjusted.[65] Participants in this school water fluoridation study were also examined for dental fluorosis. After 8 years of study in Seagrove, the teeth of 11 of the 134 children examined had questionable fluorosis, although none had definite signs of fluorosis.[66] Even though the results of the Seagrove study showed that dental caries inhibition with a fluoride level of 7 times the optimum level recommended for community fluoridation was somewhat greater than studies using 4.5 times the optimum level, the lower level (4.5 times) is currently recommended for school water fluoridation.[34]

Despite these studies documenting the effectiveness of school water fluoridation in reducing dental decay, it has not been widely implemented. The most recent data on school water fluoridation reveals only 360 participating schools serving 121,223 schoolchildren in this country.[24] These figures are down considerably from the high of 500 schools serving 200,000 students reported earlier. Consolidation of school districts and extensions of community water supplies are probably responsible for these reductions. Because of the national decline in caries that has occurred among U.S. schoolchildren, Horowitz[72] feels the need for initiating school fluoridation programs is less compelling than it once was. However, he further states that discontinuance of these programs would be premature because there are still groups of children with high caries prevalence who could benefit from school fluoridation programs and because little is known about what the effects of cessation on dental health would be.

Fluoride supplement programs

When it is not possible to adjust water fluoride to optimum levels either in the community or in schools, the use of dietary fluoride supplements should be initiated. Fluoride supplements can be administered at home or in community-sponsored school programs, including preschool Head Start programs, and are available in the form of tablets, lozenges, oral rinse supplements, and, for younger children, drops and fluoride-vitamin preparations.

Fluoride supplements function both topically and systemically. The processes of chewing and swishing the tablet or lozenge and of swishing the liquid topically bathe the tooth surfaces. The subsequent swallowing of the supplement leads to the systemic incorporation of fluoride into the developing tooth structure. For younger children who cannot chew, drops or fluoride-vitamin preparations can be added to beverages such as juice or water. The supplements should not be added to milk, which tends to bind fluoride ions and slow absorption.[120]

Current fluoride supplementation recommendations of the American Dental Association (ADA)[30] and the American Academy of Pediatrics[2] are listed in Table 8-7. The fluoride dosage is adjusted according to the age of the child and the fluoride level of the water supply. It should be noted that dietary fluoride is not prescribed when the concentration of fluoride in drinking water is greater than 0.7 ppm or for infants up to 2 years of age when the fluoride level is 0.3 to 0.7 ppm. Because of

the concern of increased fluorosis levels in U.S. schoolchildren, the reader is advised that fluoride supplementation recommendations are under review at the time of this writing. The reader should be alert to any changes in the dosage schedule in the future. It is important for pediatricians and dentists to know the concentration of fluoride in the drinking water of their patients. The local water authority or local or state health department can usually provide accurate information. A careful health history should be taken prior to prescribing dietary fluoride supplements to ascertain if the child is taking other fluoride supplements such as vitamin-fluoride combinations.

The objective of obtaining maximum benefits for both the primary and permanent dentition suggests that supplementation should begin shortly after birth and continue until the eruption of the permanent second molars, which occurs between 12 and 14 years. The ADA's Council on Dental Therapeutics has recommended the continuation of fluoride supplementation until the age of 13; the American Academy of Pediatrics recommends the continuation of supplements to age 16. There is some evidence to indicate that when supplementation is discontinued there is a gradual diminution of protection against caries. Therefore it has been recommended that fluoride treatment should continue after age 13 with various topical programs that are professionally administered or self-applied when indicated for caries-active individuals.[120]

School-based fluoride tablet programs have been successfully and widely practiced. Results of these programs have been reviewed by Mellberg and Ripa.[95] They reported an average reduction in DMFS of 33% with a range of 25% to 64%. Similar to water fluoridation, greater benefits accrue to teeth that erupt after tablet initiation. Dietary fluoride supplements were part of a comprehensive fluoride regimen provided to 5- to 17-year-old schoolchildren in Nelson County, Virginia. Using a retrospective baseline control, investigators reported a 65% lower DMFS prevalence in 6- to 17-year-olds who had participated continuously in the program from 1 to 11 years.[75] In addition to the dietary fluoride supplement, these children were provided with a fluoride-containing dentifrice for use at home and rinsed once a week in school with an 0.2% sodium fluoride solution. In a prospec-

Table 8-7 Dosage schedule for fluoride supplements recommended by the American Dental Association and the American Academy of Pediatrics

Age (years)	Concentration of fluoride in water (ppm)		
	<0.3	0.3-0.7	>0.7
0-2	0.25 mgF/day	0.0 mgF/day	0.0 mgF/day
2-3	0.50	0.25	0.0
3-13*	1.00	0.50	0.0

Data from American Academy of Pediatrics, Committee on Nutrition: Fluoride supplementation, *Pediatrics* 77(5):758, 1986; and American Dental Association, Council on Dental Therapeutics: *Accepted dental therapeutics,* ed 39, Chicago, The Association, 1982. (Reproduced by permission of *Pediatrics.*)
*The American Academy of Pediatrics recommends 16, rather than 13, as the termination age.

tive study, kindergarten and first-grade students in Springfield, Ohio, were assigned to one of three groups that (1) rinsed once a week in school with an 0.2% NaF solution, (2) chewed and swallowed daily in school a 2.2-mg NaF tablet, or (3) followed both procedures.[39] After 8 years on the regimen, DMFS increments of 3.6, 2.8, and 2.4, respectively, for the rinse, tablet, and combined groups were reported. Even though the combined regimen showed increased caries protection, cost considerations and feasibility did not support changes for ongoing programs. Because the direction of the findings on recent programs have favored the tablet over the rinse, the tablet program appears to be the best choice for new programs.

These programs take little time from the academic schedule and are readily integrated into the daily regimen of a school. Generally a school-affiliated dentist has responsibility for prescribing the tablets, yet actual administration of the supplements can be carried out in the classroom by nondental personnel. Tablets are initiated in the earliest grade for maximum effectiveness, generally kindergarten. Garcia[52] has reviewed fluoride supplement programs in terms of 1988 U.S. dollars. She reported a mean cost of $2.53 per child with a range of $0.89 to $5.40. Because of these characteristics, school-based fluoride tablet programs are regarded as appropriate community programs.

School-based fluoride tablet programs require the initial and continued cooperation of school administrators, teachers, students, and volunteers. The reliance and need for sustained motivation, interest, and cooperation on the part of others do not allow school-based fluoride tablet programs to be regarded as an ideal public health activity. However, studies have demonstrated that their use in school programs is both effective and practical.[38,39,75,95]

Dietary fluoride supplements can also be prescribed by a pediatrician or a dentist for use at home. There is an advantage to home administration of dietary fluoride supplements in that supplementation can begin shortly after birth and be given 365 days per year. However, maximum success is dependent on the sustained involvement and motivation of the parents to administer the program daily for 13 years. Continued compliance has been found to be generally poor.[82] Such results

have created the incentive to implement school-based tablet programs. These programs instill a routine and schedule whereby the tablets are ingested more consistently, thus maximizing the likelihood of their effectiveness.

Prescribing fluoride supplements to expectant mothers is currently not recommended.[30] The U.S. Food and Drug Administration[51] ruled in 1966 that the evidence did not support the advertising claim that prenatal administration of fluorides would increase the caries resistance of the child and thus banned such advertisements. The efficacy of prenatal fluorides was examined at the ADA's 1980 annual meeting, and further research to prove clinical effectiveness was recommended.[70] Recently a randomized trial was conducted in which 412 pregnant women were taking 1 mg of fluoride per day, in the form of a 2.2-mg sodium fluoride tablet, and 422 women were taking a placebo tablet, both during the last two trimesters of pregnancy. All offspring in both groups were furnished with dietary fluoride supplements at appropriate dosages. At examination at 5 years of age, the experimental group and the placebo group had mean DFS scores of 0.30 and 0.55, respectively. These differences were not statistically significant. Thus the study did not support the effectiveness of prenatal fluoride in preventing dental caries in the deciduous teeth of offspring.[89]

Fluoride mouthrinse programs

One way in which the topical benefits of fluoride may be attained is by mouthrinsing with a fluoride-containing solution. Many clinical trials have shown that rinsing daily, weekly, or biweekly with dilute solutions of fluoride reduce the incidence of dental caries by approximately 30%.[95,119] Most of these studies have been conducted in nonfluoridated areas and used a neutral sodium fluoride solution. Studies also have shown that in fluoridated areas children who rinse benefit from the procedure.[119]

Fluoride mouthrinses received approval as caries-inhibitory agents by the U.S. Food and Drug Administration in 1974[146] and acceptance by the ADA in 1975.[31] Fluoride mouthrinsing is one of the most widely used caries-preventive public health methods. In the United States it is second only to community water fluoridation. The exact number of American children participating in school-based fluoride mouthrinsing programs is not clear, and the figure has been reported to be as low as 2 to 4 million[145] and as high as 12 million.[99] The availability of over-the-counter products has increased the use of fluoride mouthrinses by children and adults. Several fluoride compounds, fluoride ion concentrations, and rinsing frequencies have been tested in more than three dozen clinical trials.[23,88,95,135] However, two regimens have been adopted as standard for individual programs of patient care or for school-based programs. Respectively, they are a 0.05% NaF rinse (230 ppm F) used daily and a 0.2% NaF rinse (900 ppm F) used weekly or fortnightly.[110] The use of the lower-concentration products for home use is discussed later in this chapter.

A 0.2% sodium fluoride solution may be purchased already prepared or may be mixed at school. If the rinse is to be mixed, premeasured packets of sodium fluoride are purchased, together with plastic containers that are marked at the appropriate water level. The contents of a packet are simply emptied into the container and mixed with tap water to obtain a 0.2% sodium fluoride concentration. In addition to the plastic containers and fluoride packets, other supplies needed to conduct a rinsing program are paper cups and napkins, disposal bags, and calibrated pumps.

If the solution is mixed, it is done on the day of rinsing. Using the calibrated pumps, 5 or 10 ml of solution are placed in the paper cups. Kindergarten children generally rinse with 5 ml and all others with 10 ml. Rinsing is performed for a minute; then the solution is expectorated back into the disposable cups. The children wipe their mouths with napkins and stuff them into the paper cups to absorb the excess liquid. The cups and napkins are collected in a disposal bag. The entire procedure takes about 5 minutes[124] and can be supervised by nondental personnel such as teachers, parents, or school nurses. During a school year, about 30 weekly rinses can be scheduled.

Only children who return a consent form signed by a parent or guardian can participate in a school-based rinse program. Rinsing can be conducted at all grade levels within a school system; however, acceptance of the program is better at the elementary grade level than in junior and senior high school. Perhaps phasing a rinse program into the elementary grades and then gradually extending it into the upper grades as the participants become older may improve the older children's response to the program.

Most North American clinical studies of fluoride mouthrinsing were reported since 1970. Table 8-8 lists studies using the high-concentration fluoride mouthrinses (900 ppm F) with schoolchildren in fluoride-deficient and in fluoridated communities.[119] The caries reductions were determined in each study by comparison with a control group of children who did not use a fluoride mouthrinse.

Studies of fluoride mouthrinsing have given consistently positive results, with few reporting reductions lower than 20%. For the school-based method, using the 0.2% sodium fluoride mouthrinse once a week, caries reductions in fluoride-deficient communities ranged from 16% to 44% with an average of 31% (Table 8-8). In optimally fluoridated communities, except for one study, the results were equally high.

The cost of supplies to conduct a fluoride mouthrinse program range from $0.69 to $1.22 per child per year (in 1988 dollars).[52] The material costs vary depending on how the rinse is dispensed. The least costly method uses pump bottles to dispense the appropriate volume of solution; the most expensive are the already prepared individual packets. In an evaluation of 11 different school-based fluoride mouthrinse programs, the average cost was calculated to be $1.30 per child per year.[52] If volunteers supervise the program, its total cost is low; paid personnel obviously increase the total cost of the program.

Although fluoride mouthrinsing is effective in inhibiting caries in communities with optimal water fluoridation, the initial disease level is low, and therefore the effectiveness in actual tooth surfaces saved from developing caries will also be low. Because of the poor cost-effectiveness ratio in fluoridated communities, school-based mouthrinsing programs are not indicated in these circumstances.[13]

School sealant programs

The application of dental sealants is a highly effective means of preventing pit and fissure caries, the predominant form of caries in U.S. children. As noted earlier, national studies indicate that the

Table 8-8 Effect of mouthrinsing with 900-1,000 ppm sodium fluoride solutions on the permanent teeth of North American children

Study	Compound and F concentration (ppm)	Rinsing frequency	Study duration (months)	% DMFS reduction
Conducted in fluoride-deficient communities				
Horowitz et al, 1971	NaF (900)	Once/week	20	16
	NaF (900)	Once/week	20	44
Packer et al, 1975	APF (1,000)	Once/week	28	41
DePaola et al, 1977	APF (1,000)	Once/day	24	42
Heifetz et al, 1982	NaF (900)	Once/week	36	38*
	NaF (900)	Once/week	36	24*
Ringelberg et al, 1982	NaF (900)	Once/day	18	23
	NaF (900)	Once/week	18	20
Clark et al, 1985	NaF (900)	Once/week	20	34
Brodeur et al, 1988	NaF (900)	Once/week	20	8
Conducted in optimally fluoridated communities				
Laswell et al, 1975	APF (1,000)	Once/week	28	46
Kawall et al, 1981	NaF (900)	Once/week	24	35
Driscoll et al, 1982	NaF (900)	Once/week	30	22*
	NaF (900)	Once/week	30	55*
Bell et al, 1984	NaF (900)	Once/week	42	16†
				0†
				7†
				0†
Brodeur et al, 1988	NaF (900)	Once/week	20	50

Source: Ripa LW: A critique of topical fluoride methods (dentifrices, mouthrinses, operator- and self-applied gels) in an era of decreased caries and increased fluorosis prevalence, *J Public Health Dent* 51:23, 1991.
*Results of two examiners, each examining different children.
†Four different communities.
NaF, neutral sodium fluoride; *APF,* acidulated sodium fluoride with phosphate buffer.

prevalence of smooth-surface caries is declining, caused mainly by the beneficial effect of water fluoridation and other methods of fluoride delivery.[102,104] Although the use of topical and systemic fluorides does provide some protection to the occlusal surfaces, the smooth surfaces generally derive greater benefit from fluorides. As a consequence, since the introduction of fluorides, there has been a relative increase in the proportion of occlusal surface caries, with respect to the total caries experience.

Data from 1971-74 reported that in 5- to 17-year-old children, 24% of the caries occurred on proximal surfaces.[11] This percentage fell to 16% in the NIDR 1979-80 survey and to 12% in the NIDR 1986-87 survey (Table 8-9).[102,104] Conversely, during the same time, the percentage of occlusal, buccal, and lingual caries increased, so

that 88% of all caries in schoolchildren occur on these largely pit and fissure* surfaces.[104] In addition, although caries on all tooth surface types is lower in fluoridated communities compared with nonfluoridated communities, the same high proportion of pit and fissure caries exists in both communities (Table 8-10).[11,121] Therefore caries prevention measures must include the pits and fissures.

In 1983 the NIH Sealant Consensus Panel urged practitioners, dental health directors, and dental educators to incorporate the appropriate use of sealants into their practices and programs.[113] Al-

---

*Buccal and lingual caries in schoolage children principally involves the buccal pits of mandibular molars and lingual fissures (grooves) of maxillary molars.

though dental sealants are more expensive than other primary dental caries prevention methods, their effectiveness and specificity for the surfaces shown to be the most susceptible to dental caries and least responsive to other preventive measures provide strong justification for their inclusion in community-based programs.[34]

Sealants can be practically incorporated into

Table 8-9 Relative (percentage) distribution of caries in specific tooth surfaces of U.S. schoolchildren

Surface	NCHS* survey 1971-74 (%)	NIDR† survey 1979-80 (%)	NIDR† survey 1979-80 (%)
Proximal	24	16	12
Buccolingual	27	30	30
Occlusal	49	54	58
TOTAL	100	100	100

Data from Bohannan HM: Caries distribution and the case for sealants, *J Public Health Dent* 43:200, 1983; Ripa LW and others: *Preventing pit and fissure caries; a guide to sealant use,* Massachusetts Department of Public Health, Massachusetts Health Research Institute, Boston, 1986; National Institute of Dental Research: *Oral health of United States children, the national survey of dental caries in U.S. schoolchildren: 1986-87,* NIH Pub No 88-2869, US Department of Health and Human Services, 1988.
*National Center for Health Statistics.
†National Institute of Dental Research.

Table 8-10 Relative (percentage) distribution of caries in specific tooth surfaces of U.S. schoolchildren from optimally fluoridated and fluoride-deficient communities

Surface	Fluoridated communities	Fluoride- deficient communities
Proximal	6%	11%
Buccolingual	40%	35%
Occlusal	54%	54%

Data from Bohannan HM: Caries distribution and the case for sealants, *J Public Health Dent* 43:200, 1983; and Ripa LW and others: *Preventing pit and fissure caries: a guide to sealant use,* Massachusetts Department of Public Health, Massachusetts Health Research Institute, Boston, 1986.

community-sponsored preventive dentistry programs for schoolchildren. Large-scale school-based sealant programs have been conducted in New Mexico, Tennessee, Minnesota, Kentucky, and Massachusetts.[20,21,35,60]

Because resources are limited, the criteria for participant selection in community sealant programs should incorporate a targeted approach. Criteria for participation in community sealant programs that have been recommended include four levels: community, school, individual, and tooth.[121] Communities with the highest caries levels receive the greatest benefits from school-based preventive dentistry programs, and both fluorides and sealants should be considered. However, the absence of a fluoride program should not preclude the initiation of a sealant program alone (Table 8-10).[121] Lower socioeconomic schools have more children with higher caries incidence and lower treatment levels than higher socioeconomic schools.[12] These schools can be identified by the large number of children on subsidized lunch programs.[26,123] Grade level must also be considered. Given the objective of providing maximum benefit to newly erupted permanent first and second molars, it has been suggested that children in second and sixth grades be included in school sealant programs. These children can be recalled in third and seventh grades to have teeth sealed that were insufficiently erupted in the previous year. Tooth morphology must also be considered. Teeth with deep pits and fissures that tend to catch the point of the explorer should be sealed. Well-coalesced pits and fissures with wide, easily cleaned grooves need not be sealed.

The personnel, schedule, and physical resources of each school must be considered when implementing a school sealant program. Children can walk or be transported to a nearby health department or health center dental clinic to receive their sealant applications. Also, portable dental equipment that is sturdy, yet light enough to be transported between schools, can be used. Portable equipment needed for a school sealant program includes a patient dental chair, operator and assistant stools, extraoral light, portable dental unit with high-volume suction, air compressor, dryer and filter, dry heat sterilizer, and protective glasses if a visible light–cured sealant is used. Both chemically cured and visible light–cured sealants are being used in school sealant program.

Often school sealant programs are conducted with a team approach. Initially, a dentist and recorder using a mirror and explorer examine teeth for caries on the children who returned positive consent forms (in some states, dental hygienists are legally permitted to conduct the examinations). The status of the proximal surfaces must be considered. However, the diagnosis of proximal decay is unlikely because newly erupted teeth are targeted in this approach and thus have not been in the mouth long enough to develop proximal decay. Radiographs are not recommended in school sealant programs. Sealant applications should begin as soon as possible following the screening sessions.

Ideally, the sealant application sessions are conducted by an operator and an assistant. Application of sealants by a dental auxiliary is the least costly method of providing this service (if permitted by the state's practice act). The assistant is chairside during the sealant applications, facilitates the flow of children between the classroom and the treatment room, and maintains records. During the next school year, children who were treated the previous year should be recalled and examined. Sealant should be reapplied to surfaces that have lost their sealant and to eligible teeth that were insufficiently erupted in the previous year.

The cost of sealants in New Mexico's dental disease prevention program was found to be $1.59 per tooth and $7.41 per child.[20] These figures are comparable with the reported costs of $1.20 per tooth and $8.00 per child in a community sealant program in Tennessee.[61] Other programs have reported higher costs, ranging from $12.39 to $36.41 per child.[21,37] More recent cost estimates expressed in terms of 1988 dollars show a similar mean cost of $21.14 per student per year, with a range of $13.03 to $28.23.[52] Factors such as program size, location, available resources, and salary differentials contribute to this variation. Starting a community-based sealant program requires acquisition of new funds or diversion of support from other components of an existing preventive dentistry program. However, the fact that dental caries is now primarily a disease of the pits and fissures is strong justification for the inclusion of sealants in public health programs.

PRIMARY PREVENTIVE SERVICES PROVIDED BY THE DENTAL PROFESSIONAL

The dental profession has the responsibility of supporting, initiating, implementing, and reinforcing community efforts, encouraging, directing, and reinforcing individual efforts, and providing, directly or indirectly, services aimed at preventing oral diseases and promoting oral health. This is a major task, and the following are some of the primary preventive services that can be provided in dental offices.

Professional topical fluoride applications

Professionally applied topical fluoride products are available as solutions, gels, and prophylaxis pastes. Table 8-11 lists the particulars of these products. Topical fluoride solutions were the first to become available to the dental profession. They included a neutral solution of 2% sodium fluoride (9,040 ppm F), an 8% stannous fluoride solution (19,360 ppm F), and an acidulated-buffered solution of sodium fluoride, called acidulated phosphate fluoride (APF), that contains 1.23% fluoride ion (12,300 ppm F). Although the fluoride compounds, pHs, and fluoride concentrations differ among these three agents, Ripa,[111] in a review of 35 clinical trials involving 70 treatment groups, concluded that the caries inhibitions of the permanent teeth of children residing in fluoride-deficient communities from use of these products was similar, approximately 30% (Table 8-12).

Table 8-11 Topical fluoride agents for office use

Vehicle	Application technique	Fluoride compound	Fluoride concentration
Aqueous solutions	Paint on	APF	12,300
		SnF_2	19,360
		NaF	9,040
Gels	Trays	APF	12,300
		NaF	9,040
Prophylaxis pastes*	Rotary Polishers	APF	12,000
		NaF	10,000
			20,000

*Other fluoride compounds and concentrations available.
APF, = acidulated phosphate fluoride; the F ion is derived from NaF.

In recent years, professional topical fluoride solutions have been replaced by fluoride gels. Gels can be applied in mouth trays, compared with solutions that require a paint-on application with cotton-tipped applicator sticks. The more convenient tray application method, coupled with better

patient acceptance and reduced treatment time, has popularized the office use of gels.

Results of clinical trials testing acidulated phosphate fluoride (APF) gels applied in trays at a concentration of 12,300 ppm F are shown in Table 8-13. Most of these studies are positive, indicating that it is an effective anticaries method. Other studies have compared treatments of professionally applied solutions and gels and generally found that the caries inhibitions achieved with gels are similar to solutions.[118]

Recently, 2% neutral NaF gels (9,040 ppm F) have been marketed for professional topical fluoride treatments. These products appeared in response to the concern that the combination of phosphoric acid and sodium fluoride in APF preparations produces hydrofluoric acid (HF), which etches glass filler particles in composite restorations and the surfaces of porcelain crowns.[28] Although it is conceded that there is little danger to the surfaces of composite restorations and porcelain crowns from a single fluoride exposure, the

Table 8-12 Pooled results of clinical trials of professionally applied aqueous solutions of NaF, SnF_2, or APF on the permanent teeth of children residing in fluoride-deficient communities

	Number of treatment groups	% DMFS reduction (averaged results)
NaF	25	29
SnF_2	18	32
APF	27	28

From Ripa LW: Professionally (operator) applied topical fluoride therapy: a critique, *Int Dent J* 31:105, 1981.
APF, acidulated phosphate fluoride; DMFS, decayed, missing, and filled surfaces.

Table 8-13 Caries inhibition from professionally applied APF gel topical treatments

Study	Applications per year	Study duration (years)	% DMFS reduction
Szwejda et al (1967)	1	1	4
Szwejda (1971)	1	2	3
Horowitz (1969)	1	2	22
Horowitz and Doyle (1971)	1	3	24
Bryan and Williams (1968)	1	1	28
Ingraham and Williams (1970)	1	2	41
Cons et al (1970)	1	4	18
Mainwaring and Naylor (1978)	2	3	14
Cobb et al (1980)	2	2	35
Hagen and Bawden (1985)	2	2	30
Horowitz and Kau (1974)	*	5	21
Bryan and Williams (1970)	†	2	37
Shern et al (1976)	5‡	2	+0.5 (DMFT)
DePaola et al (1980)	10§	2	19

From Ripa LW: An evaluation of the use of professional (operator-applied) topical fluorides, *J Dent Res* 69:786, 1990; Ripa LW: A critique of topical fluoride methods (dentifrices, mouthrinses, operator-, and self-applied gels) in an era of decreased caries and increased fluorosis prevalence, *J Public Health Dent* 51:23, 1991.
APF, acidulated phosphate fluoride; DMFS, decayed, missing, and filled surfaces; DMFT, decayed, missing, and filled teeth.
*No additional treatments; examined 2 years after discontinuation of treatment by Horowitz and Doyle (1971).
†No additional treatments; examined 1 year after discontinuation of treatment by Bryan and Williams (1968).
‡Five treatments on consecutive days during first year only.
§10 treatments on consecutive school days during first year only.

cumulative effects of repeated APF treatments could be esthetically damaging; therefore the ADA recommends using a neutral sodium fluoride product when patients have restorations that might be damaged by APF.[28]

Normally, tooth surfaces are coated with pellicle and plaque. Therefore it has been standard to perform a professional prophylaxis before applying fluoride. However, in vivo and in vitro studies have demonstrated that fluoride uptake is not reduced if the teeth remain uncleaned,[112] and four independent clinical studies of professionally-applied APF found that caries inhibition was unaffected when the preliminary professional cleaning step was omitted.[112] Therefore patients may simply rinse with water to remove food particles prior to professional application of fluoride gel. In addition, data from clinical studies do not support the use of fluoride-containing prophylaxis paste alone as an effective caries-preventive regimen.[115] However, a thorough prophylaxis will abrade a thin layer of enamel, resulting in the loss of fluoride from the tooth surface. Thus when a dental abrasive paste is used to clean the teeth, a fluoride-containing prophylaxis paste is indicated in an attempt to replenish the fluoride removed by the abrasive action of the paste.

McCall and associates[93] have shown that a tray's design can affect the distribution of APF gel on teeth, resulting in incomplete coverage and presumably lack of therapeutic effect at uncovered sites. Therefore it is important that the fit of trays be assessed for each patient. Once the correct size is selected, gel is placed in the trays and inserted simultaneously over the maxillary and mandibular teeth. Gel should be applied to air-dried teeth; if they are coated with saliva, dilution will occur. Furthermore, it was reported that when treated with a professional topical fluoride application, 1-minute air-drying will result in significantly more fluoride uptake by the outer enamel.[64] In this study a 2% neutral NaF solution was used, and this effect has yet to be demonstrated with an APF gel.

The gel should be left in contact with the teeth for 4 minutes. Although APF gels are marketed for which manufacturers recommend an application time of 1 minute, this recommendation lacks clinical verification. Wei and co-workers[149,151] have shown that enamel fluoride uptake is significantly less when contact is reduced to 1 minute and rec-

ommend that the clinically proven 4-minute contact be continued.[149,151]

After 4 minutes the tray is removed and the patient is instructed not to rinse, eat, or drink for 30 minutes. Stookey and associates,[141] in an in vivo study, have shown that enamel fluoride uptake by artificially induced incipient lesions is reduced by about half when a patient is allowed to rinse immediately following an APF gel tray treatment.

The routine application of topical fluoride, as part of an office caries-preventive program, should be considered only in countries experiencing high caries rates. Because this description does not fit the United States, where a caries decline of approximately 50% has occurred within the last 20 years, the indication for a professional topical fluoride treatment should be decided on an individual basis. Certainly, the application of topically applied fluoride should not be performed routinely for children who reside in fluoridated communities or who have had maximal exposure to fluoride supplements. There are few clinical data to show that topical fluoride treatments are effective when performed on groups of children in fluoridated communities.[95,148] Nevertheless, for individual children who are exposed to systemic fluoride yet are caries-active, professional topical fluoride treatments should be part of their caries-preventive program. Considering patients' caries activity and exposure to fluoridated drinking water, and recognizing the importance of application frequency on caries inhibition,[59] Ripa and co-workers[120] developed recommendations (listed in Table 8-14) for the use of professional topical fluoride applications for individual patients.

The highest concentrations of fluoride are found in those preparations that are intended for professional use (Table 8-11). One ml of a professional topical fluoride solution or gel contains from 9 to 19 mg F, depending on the product selected. The most commonly used procedure, the APF gel tray technique, uses up to 5 ml of gel (2.5 ml/tray) per treatment, which introduces 61.5 mg F to the mouth. There is the potential that some of the gel can be swallowed, resulting in acute toxic problems.

The most common acute toxic reactions from inadvertent swallowing of professional topical fluoride products is nausea and vomiting.[8,46,128] Recently, however, Spak and co-workers[134] reported

Table 8-14 Application frequency for professionally-applied topical fluoride treatments

Water fluoride status	Caries status		
	Caries-free	Active caries	Rampant caries
F-deficient	2 times/year*	2 times/year	4 times/year
Optimally fluoridated	0	2 times/year	4 times/year

From Ripa LW and others: A guide to the use of fluorides for the prevention of dental caries, ed 2, *J Am Dent Assoc* 113:503, 1986.
*To age 16.

that petechiae and erosions of the gastric mucosa can also occur from swallowing small quantities of fluoride gel. Although in the average patient the significance of this reaction may be minimal, in patients with gastric ulcers the effect may be more profound.

In his review, Ripa[118] cites more than a dozen reports of studies that measured the amount of fluoride retained from a professional topical fluoride application. The range of fluoride retained varied widely, both in volume and as a percentage of the amount introduced into the mouth. For instance, the percentage of the amount of fluoride that was not retrieved when trays were removed from the mouth varied from approximately 10% to 80%.[45,47] However, a number of studies have shown that common-sense precautions can significantly reduce the amount of fluoride gel retained (see Ripa's review[118]). Based on these studies, prudent administration of professional topical fluoride gel in trays requires the following expedients:

1. Seat the patient upright.
2. Use trays with absorptive liners.
3. Limit the amount of gel placed in the trays to no more than 2.5 ml (0.5 teaspoon) per tray.
4. Use suction during and after treatment.
5. Instruct the patient to expectorate after the trays are removed.

Pit and fissure sealants

As already noted in this chapter, as caries prevalence decreased in U.S. schoolchildren, there also was a change in the intraoral caries pattern. Specifically, the percentage of decay occurring on the smooth proximal surfaces was proportionately less, compared with caries of the pits and fissures.

In today's schoolchildren, pit and fissure decay—namely, of the occlusal surfaces and the buccal pits and lingual grooves of molars—accounts for nearly 90% of the total caries prevalence.[104] Although topical fluorides provide some protection against caries of the pits and fissures, sealants are especially meant for this type of caries. Thus all office-based preventive programs should include sealants.

A sealant is a dental resin that is firmly bonded to the enamel surface and isolates the pits and fissures from the caries-producing conditions of the oral environment. There have been many attempts to reduce the rate of occlusal caries, including the elimination of pits and fissures through the physical removal of sound tooth structure. In 1955 Buonocore[17] developed an acid etching technique that enabled dental resins to adhere to tooth surfaces. By applying a weak solution of phosphoric acid to the enamel surface, mineral is removed both at and within the surface to a depth of approximately 25 microns.[68] This exposes the enamel pores and increases the surface area of the enamel. The result is a bonding surface that is at least 100 times stronger than a nonetched surface.[132]

The sealant resin is applied in a viscous, liquid state and enters the micropores, which have been enlarged through acid conditioning. Then the resin hardens because of either a self-hardening catalyst or application of a light source. The extensions of the hardened resin that have penetrated and filled the pores are called tags.[60]

Sealants are classified according to the method by which they are cured or hardened. The first marketed sealant systems, called first-generation sealants, were cured with ultraviolet light. The ul-

Table 8-15 Effectiveness of chemically polymerized sealant systems: averaged results of several clinical studies

Years after sealant placement	Percent retention on completely covered teeth	Percent occlusal caries reduction
1	83	81
2	83	82
3	72	66
4	70	59
5	67	51
6	63	56
7	66	55

From Ripa LW: The current status of pit and fissure sealants: a review, *Can Dent Assoc J* 5:367, 1985.

Table 8-16 Visible light–initiated clinical sealant studies: averaged results of sealant comparisons

Sealant	Number of study groups	Percent retention on completely covered teeth (averaged results)
Visible light initiated	11	79.1
Autopolymerized	8	79.4
Ultraviolet light initiated	3	67.0

traviolet light–cured sealants helped to establish the usefulness of pits and fissure sealants in clinical preventive dentistry,[121] but they have been replaced by more effective systems. Chemically cured sealants, also called autopolymerized sealants, representing second-generation products, surpassed the retention and thus caries-reduction results achieved by ultraviolet light–cured sealants. A rate of 83% complete retention can be expected 1 year after placement of chemically cured sealants, with more than 50% retention after 5 years (Table 8-15).[114] One study reported 66% retention of chemically cured sealant after 7 years.[97] Visible light–cured sealants, the newest type marketed, represent third-generation systems. Several clinical studies of up to 3 years' duration have compared the retention of visible light–cured sealants with chemically polymerized or ultraviolet light–polymerized systems.* As seen in Table 8-16, the visible light–cured and chemically cured systems performed similarly. One study has reported a 5-year comparison between visible light–cured and chemically polymerized systems.[130] This study also found that the clinical retention figures for the two types of sealants were similar. Both chemically cured and visible light–cured sealant systems are currently marketed, and the

---

*References 27,76,125-127,139,143,153,157,158.

ADA has granted full or provisional acceptance to several brands.

The placement of sealants should be limited to previously unrestored pits and fissures. First and second permanent molars are at highest risk to caries and thus benefit the most from sealant application.[12] However, the occlusal surfaces of first and second primary molars, first and second premolars, and third molars are all potential sites for sealants. Sealants should also be considered where other pits and fissures exist, such as the lingual surfaces of permanent maxillary incisors, buccal surfaces of mandibular molars, and lingual surfaces of maxillary molars.[121]

When selecting teeth for sealants in individual patient care programs, the clinician has to consider occlusal morphology and caries pattern.[121] Teeth with steep cuspal inclines and deep fissures, in contrast to those with shallow cusps and highly coalesced pits and fissures, are ideal choices for sealant application. If the occlusal morphology places the tooth at higher risk to caries, the tooth should be sealed as soon as it has erupted sufficiently to allow adequate isolation for the sealant application procedure. If a patient has many proximal lesions, sealants may still be placed on the occlusal surfaces of caries-free teeth; however, fluoride therapy should be initiated to protect the proximal surfaces.

Sometimes it is difficult for a clinician to reach a firm decision that a surface is sound or carious, and the diagnosis of a questionable surface may be made. A surface is questionable when the explorer tip sticks in the tooth surface, but other evidence of caries, such as softness at the tip of the explorer or a white halo of undermining demineralization, is not present.[121] A restoration is not appropriate because the questionable surface has not been diagnosed as carious; however, the area has an increased susceptibility to caries because bacteria and food particles are easily trapped. A questionable surface is an ideal surface for sealing because the sealant will prevent the surface from progressing from a questionable to a carious status.[121]

The effectiveness of sealants appears equal when applied by dentists or dental auxiliaries who have received adequate training (sealant application by dental hygienists and assistants is permitted by at least 32 state practice acts).[58,112] The operator's technique is the primary determinant of a sealant's retention; ideally, sealants should be applied by an operator-assistant team.[121] Maintenance of a dry field and avoidance of contamination of the etched surface by saliva are paramount. Isolation of the site can be achieved by using a rubber dam or a cottonroll retraction system.

The selected tooth surface is first cleansed with a fluoride-free prophylaxis paste and then conditioned with a phosphoric acid etchant. Although etching times of 20 seconds have been reported,[44,138] etching is usually done for 60 seconds. Acid conditioning of the enamel surface produces a marked increase in surface area, which renders the tooth more receptive to bonding. The surface is then washed with water and dried with compressed air. Upon drying, a properly etched surface has a frosty appearance in contrast to the glossy appearance of unetched enamel. Using an applicator, the sealant is then flowed over the dried etched surface. The sealant is allowed to polymerize either by itself or by exposure to a visible light unit. The sealant must remain uncontaminated and undisturbed until it hardens. Setting time varies according to the sealant used. The teeth are inspected visually and with an explorer after polymerization has occurred. If coverage of the pits and fissures is incomplete or if there is a surface air bubble, more sealant can be applied if the tooth has remained uncontaminated. Otherwise, the tooth must be etched again for 10 seconds and washed and dried before additional sealant is added.[68]

Questions regarding the possibility of caries progression beneath properly applied sealants have been answered by clinical studies. The ability of bacteria to survive under sealants is impaired because ingested carbohydrates cannot reach them. Several investigators have found that the number of bacteria in deliberately sealed carious lesions decreases dramatically with time.[55,96] Negative or reduced bacterial cultures have been found several years after sealing, and no studies have identified caries progression beneath an intact sealant.[12,98] Because it is acknowledged that if a carious lesion is sealed the lesion will arrest, the inadvertent sealing of an undiagnosed lesion should not be of concern to clinicians.[54,55,96,98,144]

The last published figures for sealant fees charged by practicing dentists were based upon a 1985 survey conducted by the ADA. Based upon its survey of general practitioners and selected specialists in the United States, the ADA reported the general practitioners' average fee for sealant application was $13.73 per tooth.[18] For pediatric dentists it was $15.90. Office costs for sealants can be minimized by delegating the sealant application procedure to auxiliary personnel where legally permitted, selecting sealant products that have the greatest retention rates, and performing a meticulous application procedure to maximize the sealant's retention.[121]

Educational materials about sealants for patients and parents may be obtained from the ADA, the American Society of Dentistry for Children, and the NIDR. They help inform about the nature, safety, and effectiveness of sealants. The materials can be used with a chairside demonstration of the special vulnerability to decay of pits and fissures along with an explanation of the atraumatic nature of the sealant procedure. Parents and children should be reminded that sealants are one part of a total caries-preventive program that also includes fluorides, brushing and flossing, and a proper diet.

Diet counseling

Diet analysis and counseling have been recommended as methods to control caries for dental patients. An ADA survey[3] found that 89% of dentists provide diet counseling in their offices, but only slightly more than half counsel all of their child patients. Diet instruction may involve a detailed dietary analysis, or it may be limited to warnings about sweet consumption.[3] Considering that half of U.S. schoolchildren are caries-free and the number of lesions or fillings is low and principally limited to the pits and fissures, it is obvious that most children do not require a detailed diet analysis. However, they all should be educated about the basic relationship between diet and dental caries.

All patients should be aware that foods containing sucrose (common table sugar) cause dental decay, that sticky foods that have a prolonged oral clearance time are potentially more cariogenic than sugars in liquid form that quickly leave the mouth, and that the frequency of between-meal snacking of cariogenic foods increases caries risk.[9,107]

Sugar consumption in the United States is approximately 120 pounds per person per year. Although the amount of sucrose consumption is decreasing, total sugar consumption remains the same because the dietary fructose (corn syrup) level has increased, largely because of its replacing sucrose as the sweetener in soft drinks.[19] The replacement of sucrose, glucose, and fructose with artificial sweetening agents, such as aspartame and saccharin, reduces the cariogenicity of a food or renders it noncariogenic.[131] Sorbitol-sweetened chewing gum and candies are much less cariogenic than sucrose- or glucose-sweetened products. "Nonsugar" or sorbitol-containing foods should be encouraged as noncariogenic snack substitutes. Reports of the lowering of the plaque pH by processed cheese[81] and by chewing sorbitol-containing chewing gum,[79,80] and the noncariogenic effects of xylitol, a naturally occurring sugar,[78,129] offer encouragement that non–caries-promoting foods, beverages, and snacks are and will continue to be available as recommended substitutes for more cariogenic fare.

Whereas the caries decline in U.S. schoolchildren has been dramatic, with more than half of U.S. schoolchildren having little or no disease, at the same time a small proportion of children bear a large proportion of the total disease occurrence.[56,57] In one study of schoolchildren conducted in 10 U.S. cities it was found that more than 50% of the caries experience occurred in approximately 20% of the children.[56] In that study, conducted in 1979-80, 16% of the children had DMFT scores of 5 to 8, and 8% had scores of 9

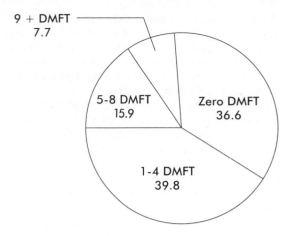

Fig. 8-1 Percent distribution of U.S. schoolchildren (aged 5-17 years) according to DMFT status reported by the National Caries Prevalence Survey 1979-80. Notice that the highest caries levels are borne by slightly more than 20% of the children. (From Graves RC, Stamm JW: Oral health status in the United States: prevalence of dental caries, *J Dent Educ* 49:341, 1985.

or above. The rest had DMFT scores of 4 to 0 (Fig. 8-1). The children with a high caries activity should receive detailed diet analysis and counseling. The basic concept of diet counseling is to assist patients in recognizing cariogenic foods in their diet and to make adjustments in accordance with personal factors that influence patients' food selection. The suggested modifications are decided by the patient with guidance from the dental professional. Investigations undertaken by Bowen and colleagues[14] to assess the cariogenicity potential of foodstuffs should greatly enhance the diet counseling procedure.

There are several methods used for dietary counseling in the dental setting. The most widely used method is that of Nizel.[107] This method adheres to the concept of normal dietary prescriptions with modifications that focus on the patient's problems and are agreeable to the patient. Nizel suggests three rules to adopt when recommending dietary modifications: (1) the prescribed diet should vary from the normal diet as little as possible, (2) the diet should meet the body's requirements for the essential nutrients as generously as the diseased condition can tolerate (for example, rampant dental caries would require a reduction in carbohydrates), and (3) the prescribed diet should take into consideration and accommodate the patient's likes and dislikes, food habits, and other environmental factors as long as it does not interfere with the therapeutic or prophylactic objectives.

Dietary modification and counseling have their greatest success with patients who are motivated and cooperative. Also important are the professional rapport established with the patients, the degree of individualization given to the patients and their problems, and the opportunity for follow-up assessment. Dietary counseling is more efficient when specifically directed to caries-prone patients. Dietary counseling is highly recommended for patients experiencing a high caries rate, including adolescents, who as a group traditionally appear to undergo a high caries attack, and medically compromised adults with salivary disfunction.

Diet counseling is best undertaken in private practices or clinics. It has been taught in elementary schools, but very little impact in terms of disease reduction has been noted. The information presented in a classroom or large group situation cannot focus on an individual's personal problems or provide individualized follow-up assessment. Consequently, diet counseling is not recommended for public health programs.

Plaque control

Regular and thorough removal of plaque by dentists and dental hygienists can successfully control periodontal disease. However, success depends on a high level of personal oral hygiene practiced by the patient. Although it is known that the bacterial agents that cause dental caries are harbored in dental plaque, neither mechanical plaque removal and oral hygiene procedures performed by individuals on themselves nor plaque removal programs conducted in dental office settings have proven effective in caries prevention.[4,115]

Educational programs aimed at enhancing the plaque-removing oral hygiene practices of individual patients can be conducted. A large number of plaque-control programs have been described for use in a dental office setting. Chapter 9 describes several that have been conducted for large groups. The outcomes of these studies show that plaque indices are significantly improved at the end of a program; however, long-range evaluation of these programs have shown a relapse in individual plaque scores to almost baseline levels.

Dental caries activity tests

Dental caries activity tests, often referred to as caries susceptibility tests, are unreliable predictors of future caries experience. Because it is important to identify patients who are at high risk to dental caries, studies that seek to develop a prediction method for high-risk patients are currently underway.[1,36,136] However, to date investigators have not been successful in developing a simple and reliable method for identifying children who will sustain high caries increments.

Although current caries activity tests do not predict future caries susceptibility, they may provide data about the status of microorganisms in the oral environment. In the dental practice setting they are primarily used as motivational tools to educate patients to develop habits conducive to the prevention of dental caries. Generally the tests measure the acid-forming ability of microorganisms present in saliva. Tests are available that examine the pH of dental plaque, the acid-buffering capacity of saliva, and the metabolic activity of acidogenic bacteria. Numerous caries activity tests exist, and selection of the appropriate test is based on clinical judgment.

Detailed information pertaining to caries activity tests can be found in most preventive dentistry or clinical practice textbooks. The use of caries activity tests is feasible in the private practice setting. However, they would not be as effective in public health programs because they require individualized patient follow-up and are time-consuming and costly.

PRIMARY PREVENTIVE SERVICES PROVIDED BY THE INDIVIDUAL

Individuals play a pivotal role in the prevention of their oral disease and promotion of their oral health. The individual acts as both a health care consumer and as a provider. As a consumer, the individual consents to, uses, and demands services. As a provider, the individual self-applies services. To be effective in this dual capacity the individual needs first to be informed as to when, where, why, and how to obtain or apply the necessary services. Second, the individual needs to actively pursue, use, and demand those services. Individually administered services include diet planning and control, self-examination, use of dietary fluoride supplements, application of self-applied fluoride products, oral hygiene practices, and use of fluoride dentifrices. The latter three services are described in this section.

Fluoride dentifrices

Of major interest in preventive dental services is the use of fluoride dentifrices. These products represent a vehicle for topically applying fluoride to teeth that is inexpensive, requires few special instructions for use, and can be obtained without a prescription. Caries reductions of 15% to 30% have been reported following the regular home use of fluoride dentifrices containing stannous fluoride, sodium fluoride, or sodium monofluorophosphate in nonfluoridated communities, regardless of the daily brushing frequency or brushing technique.[95] When recommending a fluoride dentifrice for their patients, dentists should recommend that they purchase one that has the ADA's seal of acceptance, indicating that the ADA recognizes the dentifrice as being therapeutic against caries.

Supported by more than 35 years of research, the benefits of fluoride dentifrices are irrefutable. More recently, however, some attention has been given to the possible risk associated with use of fluoride toothpastes by young children. The fact that the prevalence of the milder forms of enamel fluorosis has increased in the United States indicates that the ingestion of fluoride during the period of tooth development has increased. One possible source of this increased ingestion can be the inadvertent swallowing of toothpaste by young children during the brushing procedure.

Studies have shown that young children may swallow some of their dentifrice.[119] Despite this, most studies attempting to link the use of toothpaste at an early age with fluorosis prevalence have been unsuccessful.[119] Nevertheless, most marketed fluoride dentifrices in the United States have a fluoride concentration of 1,000 to 1,100 ppm. A 1-inch ribbon (1 g) of dentifrice on an adult toothbrush contains approximately 1 mg fluoride. Swallowing even some of this amount will contribute to the total amount of fluoride ingested by chil-

dren. Because enamel fluorosis is principally a cosmetic problem, the incisors are of most concern. These teeth are developing during the preschool period between birth and 6 years, and this is the most susceptible period for fluorosis to occur. Dentists and dental hygienists, therefore, must not only recommend use of a fluoride toothpaste but also teach parents prudent toothbrushing habits for their children. The guidelines for the use of fluoride dentifrices by preschoolers are:[119]

1. Parents should brush preschool children's teeth until they can do it properly themselves.
2. Parents should apply the dentifrice to the toothbrush of preschool children until they can do it properly themselves.
3. Parents should supervise the toothbrushing activity of preschool children.
4. Preschool children should use a child-size toothbrush.
5. Only a pea-size amount of dentifrice should be applied to the toothbrush bristles.
6. Children must be taught to rinse thoroughly after toothbrushing.

High- and low-potency fluoride dentifrices. In addition to the standard dentifrices, which contain 1,000 to 1,100 ppm fluoride, dentifrices containing higher concentrations of fluoride (high-potency dentifrices) and lower concentrations (low-potency dentifrices) have been studied.

High-potency fluoride dentifrices were investigated in the belief that a higher-concentration fluoride product would provide more protection against caries than conventional dentifrices. Toothpastes containing nearly 3,000 ppm F have been clinically tested, and indeed it has been shown that more fluoride provides greater protection against caries.[116] In 1987, following approval by the U.S. Food and Drug Administration and acceptance by the ADA, a high-potency dentifrice containing 1,500 ppm fluoride as sodium monofluorophosphate became available to American consumers for the first time. A high-potency dentifrice should be considered for patients who are experiencing a high caries attack rate or who are deemed to be at high risk. An example of the latter is patients who have salivary gland insufficiency as a result of radiation therapy or for other reasons. Conversely, high-potency dentifrices should not be used by preschool children who, because of their developmental period, are susceptible to enamel fluorosis.

Low-potency dentifrices have been studied because some believe that the availability of a lower-potency dentifrice for young children would reduce their risk of developing enamel fluorosis. However, the therapeutic effectiveness of the dentifrice should not be sacrificed by reducing the fluoride concentration. Although the results are contradictory, the evidence indicates that dentifrices containing 250 ppm F are significantly less effective caries inhibitors than those with conventional fluoride concentrations.[83,100,108] Conversely, in a well-conceived clinical trial using preschool children as the subjects, Winter and co-workers[154] found almost no difference in the caries inhibition to primary teeth of dentifrices containing 550 and 1,055 ppm fluoride. While low-potency dentifrices are available in some countries, there currently is no low-potency fluoride dentifrice on the U.S. market.

Fluoride dentifrices containing anticalculus ingredients. The 1980s saw the sale of fluoride dentifrices that also contain anticalculus agents. Clinical trials of anticalculus dentifrices containing either soluble pyrophosphates or zinc compounds have demonstrated reductions in calculus formation from approximately 10 to 50%,[122] and such dentifrices should be recommended for patients who are heavy calculus formers.

Anticalculus ingredients, such as pyrophosphates, are believed to prevent the calcification of calculus by interfering with calcium and phosphate precipitation from saliva. Conversely, the anticaries action of fluoride in dentifrices is believed to be dependent, in part, upon the promotion of calcium and phosphate precipitation during the remineralization of incipient carious lesions. The question arose, therefore, whether the presence of anticalculus ingredients in dentifrices containing fluoride would compromise their anticaries potential. However, both laboratory and clinical studies indicated that the two ingredients would not act antagonistically.[149] Based on these results, dentists and dental hygienists who recommend dentifrices of proven anticaries formulations that also contain an anticalculus agent can do so with confidence that the anticaries potential is not affected.

Self-applied topical fluoride products

Fluoride mouthrinses. Home use of fluoride mouthrinses is indicated for patients who are caries active; for orthodontic patients with banded, bonded, or removable appliances; and for patients with reduced salivary flow whose teeth are highly susceptible to decay. Patients living in either fluoride-deficient or optimally fluoridated communities can be directed to use a fluoride mouthrinse because, as seen in Table 8-17, the method is effective in both types of communities.

Fluoride mouthrinses used in the home are generally 0.05% neutral sodium fluoride solutions (230 ppm F).[110] Most over-the-counter fluoride mouthrinses are formulated at this concentration and are available without prescription. If an over-the-counter fluoride mouthrinse is indicated, the patient should be advised to buy one that has the ADA's seal of acceptance on its label because all marketed fluoride rinses do not contain the proper fluoride concentration.

The ADA recommends that no more than 264 mg NaF (120 mg F) be dispensed at any one time.[29] A store-purchased 500-ml bottle of a 0.05% NaF rinse solution contains 100 mg F; thus, the packaging of over-the-counter rinses is within the ADA's established safety limits.

Fluoride mouthrinsing is easy to do. The patient is directed to use the solution once a day, usually before bedtime. Either 1 or 2 teaspoonfuls (5 or 10 ml) are recommended, but 1 teaspoon is probably sufficient. The packaging of some commercial fluoride mouthrinses may confine the user to a 10 ml portion. The patient swishes the solution for a minute, applying intermittent pressure with the cheek and lip musculature to force the solution into contact with all the tooth surfaces. The solution is then expectorated. Because young preschool children might swallow rather than expectorate much of the solution,[150] this technique is contraindicated for children younger than 6 years.

As seen in Table 8-17, respectable levels of caries inhibition have been reported from studies of fluoride mouthrinses at concentrations of 200 to 250 ppm F. Fluoride mouthrinses are generally considered to reduce caries by approximately 25% to 30%, in addition to the caries inhibition expected from also using a fluoride dentifrice.

Table 8-17 Effect of mouthrinsing with 200 to 250 ppm F sodium fluoride solutions on the permanent teeth of North American children

Study	Compound and fluoride concentrations (ppm)	Rinsing frequency	Study duration (months)	% DMFS reduction
Conducted in fluoride-deficient communities				
Frankl et al, 1972	APF (200)	1 time/day	24	22
Aasenden et al, 1972	NaF (200)	1 time/day	36	27
	APF (200)	1 time/day	36	30
Packer et al, 1975	APF (200)	1 time/day	28	27
Finn et al, 1975	APF (200)	2 times/day	26	29
Ringelberg et al, 1979	NaF (250)	1 time/day	30	26
DePaola et al, 1980	NaF (230)	1 time/day	24	22
Heifetz et al, 1982	NaF (230)	1 time/day	36	47*
	NaF (230)	1 time/day	36	34*
Ringelberg et al, 1982	NaF (230)	1 time/day	18	28
	NaF (230)	1 time/day	18	17
Conducted in optimally fluoridated communities				
Laswell et al, 1975	APF (200)	1 time/day	28	23
Driscoll et al, 1982	NaF (225)	1 time/day	30	28*
	NaF (225)	1 time/day	30	50*

From Ripa LW: A critique of topical fluoride methods (dentifrices, mouthrinses, operator-, and self-applied gels) in an era of decreased caries and increased fluorosis prevalence, *J Public Health Dent* 51:23, 1991.
DMFS, decayed, missing, and filled surfaces; APF, acidulated phosphate fluoride; the F ion is derived from NaF.
*Results of two examiners, each examining different children.

Fluoride gels. In addition to professional-strength gels for office use, there are also self-applied gels for use in the home. As seen in Table 8-18, the home-use gels include a stannous fluoride gel containing 1,000 ppm F and neutral or acidulated sodium fluoride gels containing 5,000 ppm F. The more concentrated products have been tested in properly designed clinical trials, whereas the stannous fluoride products have been accepted by the ADA because the original Crest toothpaste formulation, which underwent extensive clinical testing, also contained 1,000 ppm F from stannous fluoride.[63,117,119]

Home-use fluoride gels offer the advantage that because they are self-applied, patients can give themselves many more applications than could be accomplished in the dental office. Generally, professionally applied topical fluoride treatments are given twice a year, whereas self-applied fluoride gels can be given 1 or more times a day.

The same indications for recommending fluoride mouthrinsing at home apply to self-applied fluoride gels. Patients who exhibit high caries rates or are at increased caries risk, such as orthodontic patients or medically compromised patients, might benefit from these products. Although some believe the stannous ion has a preferential effect on intraoral bacteria that is useful in preventing gingivitis, in a well-controlled clinical study the only effect on soft tissue parameters of dental health, such as gingivitis, appeared to come only from the mechanical act of brushing and not from the stannous fluoride gel.[155]

Patients brush the stannous fluoride gel on their own teeth. Because there is no abrasive in the gel, it will not clean the teeth; therefore it does not take the place of a fluoride-containing toothpaste, which the patient should continue to use. The 5,000 ppm F gels also can be brushed on the teeth, or they can be applied with custom polyvinyl trays. The trays are vacuum molded in the dental office on plaster casts of the patient's maxillary and man-

Table 8-18 Comparison of topical fluoride gels for office and home use

Fluoride compound	Fluoride concentration %*	ppm F	Application method
Professional application			
APF	1.2	12,300	Mouthtray
NaF	0.9	9,040	Mouthtray
Self-application			
APF	0.5	5,000	Mouthtray
NaF	0.5	5,000	Mouthtray
			Toothbrush
SnF_2	0.1	1,000	Toothbrush

*Percent concentration on a product label may apply to the concentration of either the fluoride ion or the fluoride compound. APF, acidulated phosphate fluoride.

dibular arches. Generally, patients brush their teeth for 1 minute with the gel, or if trays are used, several drops are placed in each tray and held in contact with the teeth for 5 minutes. Patients should be cautioned to expectorate excess gel and not to swallow it. Also, patients should rinse with tap water after brushing or tray application. Because of the potential that young children with developing teeth might swallow some of the gel, home fluoride gels are not recommended for children 6 years and younger.

Oral hygiene practices

Oral hygiene practices involve the thorough daily removal of dental plaque and other debris by toothbrushing and flossing, although mouthrinsing and use of auxiliary aids are also included. Dental caries, gingivitis, and periodontal disease are plaque-mediated conditions. The relationship between oral hygiene and periodontal disease has been both statistically and experimentally established. It has been demonstrated that withholding hygiene procedures results in the onset of initial gingivitis in mouths that may not have registered periodontal problems in the past. However, once adequate hygiene procedures are reinstated, the gingivitis score decreases. The studies conducted on the relationship between dental caries and oral hygiene have demonstrated inconclusive results. Presently,

definitive statements about an association cannot be made.

Toothbrushing. The present concept of toothbrushing evolved around the beginning of the nineteenth century. Prior to that time, wooden "chew-sticks" or a form of toothpicks were used after meals. Apparently the idea of brushing after meals has not changed from earlier times. A thorough once-a-day brushing and flossing are minimally sufficient to disorganize and remove plaque, although brushing after every meal is recommended.

The purpose of toothbrushing is to remove the bacterial plaque from the tooth surfaces without injuring the soft tissues. The recommended method of toothbrushing is determined by the individual patient's manual dexterity, motivation, and oral hygiene. Table 8-19 summarizes the commonly recommended toothbrushing methods.[7,25,50,133,140] There are two basic directions in which a brush is used: horizontal and vertical. Horizontal brushing uses the ends of the bristles, and vertical brushing uses the sides of the bristles. Any other direction in which a brush is used represents a modification of the basic approach. Historically, the most frequently used and recommended method was the roll method. With modifications in technique as an attempt to cleanse the sulcular areas, the Bass method was developed and has become one of the more frequently suggested techniques (Table 8-19).

There are a variety of toothbrushes on the market. They vary in the size of the head of the brush and the length and angulation of the handle. There is no definitive empirical research that statistically or clinically indicates the superiority of one toothbrush over another; however, toothbrush designs are constantly changed in an effort to find the ideal one. There also is no evidence to indicate that a powered toothbrush is superior to a manual or hand brush. The type of toothbrush to recommend primarily depends on the individual patient's manual dexterity. The patient's preference and level of oral hygiene are also to be considered. Currently, a soft, multitufted, round-bristled brush is recommended.

Flossing. Toothbrushing can effectively remove plaque from the smooth tooth surfaces, sulcus, and a portion of the interproximal areas. Flossing is concerned with the removal of plaque

Table 8-19 Summary of methods for brushing

Method	Bristle placement	Motion	Advantages and disadvantages
Bass[7]	Topically, toward gingiva into the gingival sulcus at a 45-degree angle to the tooth surface	Very short back and forth vibratory; bristle ends remain in the sulcus	Removes plaque from cervical areas and sulcus; small area covered at one time; good gingival stimulation; easily learned
Charters[25]	Coronally, with sides of bristles half on teeth and half on gingiva at a 45-degree angle to tooth surface	Small circular with bristle ends remaining stationary	Cleans interproximal but bristly ends do not go into sulcus; hard to learn; hard to position brush in some areas of mouth; excellent gingival stimulation
Fones[50]	Perpendicular to tooth surface	On buccal a wide circular movement to include gingiva and tooth surfaces; on lingual a back-and-forth horizontal motion.	Interproximal areas not cleaned; easy to learn; possible trauma to gingiva
Intrasulcular[25]	Apically, toward gingiva into gingival sulcus at 45-degree angle to the tooth surface or toward gingiva, almost parallel to long axis of the teeth	On buccal and lingual, a very short back-and-forth vibratory or very small circular motion, with bristle tips remaining in the sulcus; then the brush head is rolled toward the occlusal surface; occlusal surfaces cleaned with horizontal stroke	Good interproximal and gingival cleaning; good gingival stimulation; requires moderate dexterity

Continued.

in the remainder of the interproximal areas. There are basically two kinds of floss: waxed and unwaxed. Which to use is a matter of personal preference. Again, no evidence is available concerning the superiority of waxed as compared with unwaxed floss. Also, dental tape, which is a ribbon-like aid, is available. The tape is used like the floss but is wider and bulkier. Generally, floss is recommended over tape because of the ease in usage.

Flossing is recommended on a once-a-day basis. Floss is used by wrapping portions around the index fingers of each hand and by using the thumbs. It is then gently guided interproximally between the contact areas to just beneath the gingival margin, where it is lightly wrapped around the contact surface and the buccal and lingual surfaces. With a back-and-forth motion, it is guided coronally along one interproximal surface to the contact point and then repeated on the adjacent interproximal tooth surface in the same interproximal space. This procedure is carried out throughout the mouth. For those areas that do not allow the floss to pass through the contact points, a variety of floss threaders are available for use on the needle-and-thread principle. The threader is slipped lingually beneath the contact point, and the floss is then employed as usual. Such aids are helpful when the areas beneath a bridge require cleansing.

Mouthrinsing. Mouthrinsing with fluoride-containing mouthrinses, either for home use or in

Table 8-19 Summary of methods for brushing—cont'd

Method	Bristle placement	Motion	Advantages and disadvantages
Physiologic[133]	Coronally and then along and over the tooth surfaces and gingiva	Gentle sweeping that starts on teeth progressing over gingiva	Is "physiologic"; mimics the passage of food over the gingiva; does not emphasize the interproximal or sulcus areas
Roll	Apically, nearly parallel to the tooth surface then in and over tooth surfaces	On buccal and lingual, slight inward pressure at first, then a rolling of the head to sweep bristles over the gingiva and tooth surfaces; occlusal cleaned with horizontal stroke	Does not clean sulcus area; easy to learn; requires moderate dexterity; good gingival stimulation
Stillman[140]	On buccal and lingual, apically at an oblique angle to the long axis of the tooth; ends rest on gingiva and cervical portion of tooth; on occlusal, perpendicular to occlusal surface	On buccal and lingual, slight rotary with bristle ends stationary; on occlusal, horizontal	Excellent gingival stimulation; bristles do not enter sulcus; interproximal area is cleaned when occlusal surfaces are brushed; moderate dexterity required

school-based programs, has already been discussed in this chapter. The acceptance of fluoride rinses as effective against caries ushered in the age of therapeutic mouthrinses. It is recognized that mouthrinses, by becoming vehicles for bringing therapeutic agents into the oral cavity, can provide more than a cosmetic function.

A large number of chemical agents have been studied for their antiplaque and antigingivitis effects. There also are anticalculus mouthrinses. Some antiplaque agents inhibit plaque bacteria for a short time so that they must be used frequently, as often as 6 times a day, to produce measurable changes. These agents include oxygenating compounds (hydrogen peroxide), quaternary ammonium compounds (benzethonium chloride and cetylpyridinium chloride), phenolic compounds (such as found in the commercial product Listerine), and sanguinarine (a benzophenanthradine alkaloid). It has been reported that in appropriate trials frequent use of these agents produced reduc-

tions in plaque and gingivitis scores of 20% to 50%.[84] Antiplaque and antigingivitis agents that produce longer-lasting intraoral effects are chlorhexidine and its analogues.[86] Chlorhexidine gluconate mouthrinse is available upon prescription. If indicated for the treatment of gingivitis, therapy should begin immediately following a dental prophylaxis. Patients rinse for 30 seconds with 1/2 ounce, twice a day. Extrinsic staining of the teeth, composite restorations, and tongue, and a bitter taste are associated with use of a chlorhexidine rinse.

PREVENTIVE DENTISTRY TREATMENT PLANNING

The preceding discussions briefly described some of the currently available primary preventive dental services. The probability of attaining a disease-free oral status is enhanced when any of the previously described efforts are combined. Because a single method of eliminating dental caries or peri-

Problem recognition
by patient/community/dental professional

Problem definition
nature/extent/severity/significance

Problem data collection
host/agent/environmental factors

Problem data analysis

Problem interpretation and presentation

Treatment plan(s) development
goals/priorities/minimum tasks/labor requirements/
cost requirements/constraints identified

Fig. 8-2 Preventive dentistry treatment planning process.

odontal diseases is not yet known, the discriminatory selection of multiple preventive services may result in greater disease reductions. The success of each service alone or of several services together is dependent on appropriate selection and implementation. This is true of all primary, secondary, and tertiary services. The dental profession must be able to recognize the individual patient's or the community's needs and problems and strategically select the most effective and efficient measures and solutions. This is one of the critical skills in dentistry and involves the process of preventive dentistry treatment planning.

The preventive dentistry treatment planning process is shown in Figure 8-2. The first step, problem recognition, has two parts. It entails recognition both by the dental professional and the patient or community. Dual recognition enhances future compliance and acceptance on the part of the patient or community to the professional's recommendations. Problem definition, the next step, helps to delineate the scope of the problem and, eventually, the type of measures to be implemented. This is followed by collection of informa-

tion relevant to the problem. The nature of this data is dependent on what is already known about the disease, its etiology, and its prevention. After sufficient data have been gathered, it is necessary to organize the data for analysis and finally for interpretation or diagnosis. Based on the scientific process, a preventive treatment plan is developed with credence given to (1) the goals to be achieved, necessitating a consideration of what level of effectiveness is desired; (2) the ranking of the goals; (3) the constraints of labor, cost, time, patient acceptance, and patient compliance; and (4) an evaluation of the treatment plan, the achievement of the goals, and the planning process itself.

In an attempt to apply the preventive dentistry treatment planning process in conjunction with an understanding of the disease process and how to prevent it, the following model cases are presented. These two case studies describe situations that may be encountered in professional life.

Case study 1

A 24-year-old male who has just completed radiation therapy for head and neck cancer comes to you with a case of rampant caries on the cervical portion of most of his teeth. He is distressed, has not been eating regular meals, and complains of a "dry mouth." Aesthetics and the retention of his own teeth are very important to this young man, who perceives this problem as monumental at the time you see him.

Case study 2

A recent dental screening of all second-grade children in your community by the U.S. Public Health Service revealed a DMFT index value twice that for the same age group on a national basis. No one in your community seems to be aware of the severity of the problem. The fluoride water level in your community is 0.3 ppm. There are three dentists and two dental hygienists in this community of 13,000 individuals.

In both cases, initially the problem must be recognized. Whether it is dental caries or oral cancer, the problem's existence must be acknowledged in a similar fashion by both the dentist and the patient(s). This may seem simple; however, the recognition of dental caries as a problem varies from individual to individual and from community to community. A dentist should ask, "Who perceives the problem as I do, and who perceives it differently?" The 24-year-old man in Case 1 is definitely concerned. However, the community in Case 2 may be unaware of and/or unable to afford to remedy the problem. Information, grievances, and preferences should be elicited from those experiencing the problem. If this first step is not accomplished, then the success of any treatment is in question.

Once recognized, the problem should be defined. Problem definition involves the preliminary investigation of all aspects of the problem. What is the nature of the patient's or the community's dental caries? Is this a new or an existing problem? What is the extent of the caries? Are the caries on the smooth surfaces only, on the occlusal surfaces only, or everywhere? Are all the children in the community affected or only those in certain residential areas? If so, why? How severe are the caries? Does the patient have active or arrested caries? Are the anterior teeth as affected as the posterior teeth? Is there an aesthetic problem? Will root canal treatment be indicated? What are the individual components of the community's DMFT? Finally, what is the significance of the problem on the community's list of problems and on the patient's priority list of problems? This process may alert the dentist to certain areas that warrant further examination.

The third step is collection of data that relates to the problem. This involves the careful scrutiny of the host, agent, and environmental factors. What are the host factors? Who are the affected persons? What are their ages, genders, races, and socioeconomic, educational, and political backgrounds? How long have they lived in the area? Have they had any recent major changes, for example, medical, nutritional, social? What are the agent factors? Are the plaque indices high? Are the individuals maintaining their oral hygiene practices? What are the environmental factors? What is the fluoride level of the water supply? Are there any dental programs offered in the schools? How many dentists and dental hygienists are there in the area? This process further delineates the investigative process and identifies the areas of concern.

The data collected are then analyzed and interpreted, and the most appropriate treatment plan is developed. All the information gathered in the preceding steps is appropriately filtered and analyzed. The interpretation of the situation is dependent on this analysis and should be supplemented by both an evaluation of the literature and of the dentist's and the patient's (or the community's) previous experience with similar problems. The evaluation of the literature should include what has been done in similar cases, how effective it has been, who has performed the treatment, and the reasons for the successes or failures.

A thorough evaluation of these factors, together with an assessment of the goals of the patient and the community for dealing with this problem, will help the dentist develop a strategy—a preventive dentistry treatment plan. Priorities are established, and questions such as the following are addressed: What are the minimum tasks required for success? What are the labor requirements, both the dentist's and the patient's, to carry out the treatment under consideration? What are the costs? What are the constraints and limitations? How will the treatment plan(s) cope with these barriers? Finally, can the tasks be executed, the labor be mobilized, the costs be met, and the limitations and constraints be managed? In light of the preferred goals and priorities, two or three feasible treatment plans may need to be developed and considered.

The treatment plan for the 24-year-old man would involve professional efforts, including patient education regarding the dental effects of his radiation therapy, dental sealants, professional topical fluoride applications, a rigid plaque-control program, and restorative treatment for the carious lesions. His individual efforts would include stringent oral hygiene practices and daily self-application of either a fluoride rinse or topical fluoride gel. A dentist, a dental auxiliary, and the patient would comprise the essential labor. There are no present constraints in this case study. However, lack of money for treatment, lack of manual dexterity, and lack of motivation may be some of the limitations in similar cases. With these constraints, alternate treatment plans need to be developed. The issue of motivation is a difficult one. In this case it is not a problem. To prevent it from becoming a problem, constant reinforcement is needed. Finally, as a crucial part of this preventive treatment plan, the patient's physicians should be consulted and informed of the dentist's interest in helping with the appropriate dental treatment of future patients prior to their beginning radiation therapy.

The treatment plan for the second-grade children would involve the implementation of some type of fluoride program, such as community water fluoridation or school water fluoridation, or a school fluoride supplement and/or mouthrinse program. Sealants should also be considered. The fulfillment of this treatment plan would require the use of community organization principles, close participation with local government and school personnel, and actions necessary to institute these programs. A fluoride program is indicated because of the cost-benefit ratio, the caries inhibition provided, and the lack of dental personnel in the community. Sealants are indicated because of their effectiveness and specificity for the surfaces shown to be the most vulnerable to caries. In the community described there are limited numbers of dental professionals, and the application of sealants by dental auxiliaries would be highly desirable. Needed restorative services must be provided by dentists.

SUMMARY

This chapter has emphasized the need for cooperative and interrelated efforts between the dental private sector, the public health sector, and individual patients to derive maximum benefits from preventive dentistry initiatives. It is gratifying that at the time of this writing of this third edition of *Community Dental Health,* one of the major dental diseases, dental caries, has shown a dramatic reduction as a result of all the preventive procedures discussed here. Ongoing education by the profession, the patients' acceptance of the responsibility for their own well-being, and the active participation at the community level in preventive programs will ensure a continuation of this trend.

REFERENCES

1. Abernathy JR and others: Development and application of a prediction model for dental caries, *Community Dent Oral Epidemiol* 15:24, 1987.
2. American Academy of Pediatrics, Committee on Nutrition: Fluoride supplementation, *Pediatrics* 77:758, 1986.
3. American Dental Association Health Foundation: Prevention in the dental office: results of a preventive dentistry survey, *J Am Dent Assoc* 108:809, 1984.
4. Andlow RJ: Oral hygiene and dental caries: a review, *Int Dent J* 28:1, 1978.
5. Arnold FA and others: Fifteenth year of the Grand Rapids fluoridation study, *J Am Dent Assoc* 65:780, 1962.
6. Asst DB and others: Newburgh-Kingston caries-fluorine study XIV: combined clinical and roentgenographical dental findings after ten years of fluoride experience, *J Am Dent Assoc* 52:314, 1956.
7. Bass CC: An effective method of personal hygiene, *J La State Med Soc* 106:100, 1954.
8. Beal JF, Rock WP: Fluoride gels: a laboratory and clinical investigation, *Br Dent J* 140:307, 1976.
9. Bibby BG: *Food and the teeth,* New York, 1990, Vantage Press.
10. Blayney JR, Hill IN: Fluorine and dental caries, *J Am Dent Assoc* 74:233, 1967.
11. Bohannan HM: Caries distribution and the case for sealants, *J Public Health Dent* 43:200, 1983.
12. Bohannan HM and others: Indications for sealant use in a community-based preventive dentistry program, *J Dent Educ* 48 (suppl 2):45, 1984.
13. Bohannan HM and others: Fluoride mouthrinse programs in fluoridated communities, *J Am Dent Assoc* 111:783, 1985.
14. Bowen WH and others: A method to assess cariogenic potential of foodstuffs, *J Am Dent Assoc* 100:677, 1980.
15. Brown HK, Poplove M: The Brantford-Sarnia-Stratford fluoridation study: final survey, *Med Serv J Canada* 21:450, 1965.
16. Brunelle JA, Carlos JP: Recent trends in dental caries in U.S. children and the effect of water fluoridation, *J Dent Res* 69(special issue):723, 1990.
17. Buonocore MG: A simple method of increasing the adhesion of acrylic filling materials to enamel surfaces, *J Dent Res* 43:849, 1955.
18. Bureau of Economic and Behavioral Research: Dental fees charged by general practitioners and selected specialists in the United States, 1985, *J Am Dent Assoc* 113:811, 1986.
19. Burt BA: The future of the caries decline, *J Public Health Dent* 45:261, 1985.
20. Calderone JJ, Mueller LA: The cost of sealant application in a state dental disease prevention program, *J Public Health Dent* 43:239, 1983.
21. Callanen VA and others: Developing a sealant program: the Massachusetts approach, *J Public Health Dent* 46:141, 1986.
22. Carlos JP, editor: *Prevention and oral health,* DHEW Pub No (NIH) 74-707, Washington, DC, 1973, US Government Printing Office.
23. Carlos JP: *Fluoride mouthrinses.* In Wei S, editor: *Clinical uses of fluoride,* Philadelphia, 1985, Lea and Febiger.
24. Centers for Disease Control: Fluoridation census 1988—summary, Washington, DC, 1990. US Department of Health and Human Services.
25. Charters WJ: Proper home care of the mouth, J Periodontol 19:136, 1948.
26. Clark BJ and others: Caries and treatment patterns in children related to school lunch program eligibility, *J Public Health Dent* 47:134, 1987.
27. Conti A and others: Evaluation of "ICI" visible light cured dental fissure sealant, *J Dent Res* 62:222, 1983 (abstract).
28. Council on Dental Materials, Instruments and Equipment

and Council on Dental Therapeutics: Status report: effect of acidulated phosphate fluoride on porcelain and composite restorations, *J Am Dent Assoc* 116:115, 1988.

29. Council on Dental Therapeutics: *Accepted dental therapeutics,* ed 38, Chicago, 1979, American Dental Association.

30. Council on Dental Therapeutics: *Accepted dental therapeutics,* ed 39, Chicago, 1982, American Dental Association.

31. Council on Dental Therapeutics: Council classifies fluoride mouthrinses, *J Am Dent Assoc* 91:1250, 1975.

32. Dean HT, Arnold FA, Elvove E: Domestic water and dental caries; V, additional studies on the relation of fluoride domestic waters to dental caries experience in 4,425 white children, aged 12 to 14 years, of 13 cities in 4 states, *Public Health Rep* 57:1155, 1942.

33. Dean HT, Elvove E: Studies on the minimal threshold of the dental signs of chronic endemic fluorosis (mottled enamel), *Public Health Rep* 50:1719, 1935.

34. Dental caries prevention in primary care projects, Washington, DC, 1985, US Department of Health and Human Services, Public Health Service.

35. Disney JA: Personnel and equipment considerations for a community-based sealant program, *J Dent Educ* 48(suppl 2):75, 1984.

36. Disney JA and others: The University of North Carolina caries risk assessment study; II, baseline caries prevalence, *J Public Health Dent* 50:178, 1990.

37. Doherty NJ, Powell AE: Clinical field trial to assess the cost-effectiveness of various caries preventive agents: final report of contract No I DE 52449, Bethesda, MD, 1980, NIDR, NIH.

38. Driscoll WS, Heifetz SB, Brunelle JA: Treatment and post treatment effects of chewable fluoride tablets on dental caries: findings after 7½ years, *J Am Dent Assoc* 99:817, 1979.

39. Driscoll WS and others: Additive effects of fluoride tablets and fluoride mouthrinsing: 8-year findings, *J Dent Res* 67:358, 1991 (abstract).

40. Dunning JM: *Principles of dental public health,* ed 4, Cambridge, 1986, Harvard University Press.

41. Easley MW: The new antifluoridationists: who are they and how do they operate? *J Public Health Dent* 45:133, 1985.

42. Easley MW: The status of community water fluoridation in the United States, *Public Health Rep* 105:348, 1990.

43. Easley MW and others, editors: *Fluoridation: litigation and changing public policy,* Proceedings of a workshop at the University of Michigan, August 9-10, 1983.

44. Eidelman E, Shapira J, Houpt M: The retention of fissure sealants using twenty-second etching time: three-year follow-up, *J Dent Child* 55:119, 1988.

45. Eisen JJ, LeCompte EJ: A comparison of oral fluoride retention following topical treatments with APF gels of varying viscosities, *Pediatr Dent* 7:175, 1985.

46. Ekstrand J, Koch G: Systemic fluoride absorption following fluoride gel application, *J Dent Res* 59:1067, 1980.

47. Ekstrand J and others: Pharmacokinetics of fluoride gels in children and adults, *Caries Res* 15:213, 1981.

48. Erickson JD: Water fluoridation and congenital malfor-

mations: no association, *J Am Dent Assoc* 93:981, 1976.

49. Erickson JD: Mortality in selected cities with fluoridated and nonfluoridated water supplies, *N Engl J Med* 298:1112, 1978.

50. Fones AC: *Mouth hygiene: a textbook for dental hygienists,* Philadelphia, 1934, Lea and Febiger.

51. Food and Drug Administration: Statements of general policy or interpretation, oral prenatal drugs containing fluorides for human use, *Federal Register* 31:13537, 1966.

52. Garcia AI: Caries incidence and costs of prevention programs, *J Public Health Dent* 49:259, 1989.

53. Glossary of evaluative terms in public health, *Am J Public Health* 60:1546, 1970.

54. Going RE: Sealant effect on incipient caries, enamel maturation, and future caries susceptibility, *J Dent Educ* 48(suppl 2):35, 1984.

55. Going RE and others: The viability of microorganisms in carious lesions five years after covering with a fissure sealant, *J Am Dent Assoc* 97:455, 1978.

56. Graves RC, Stamm JW: Oral health status in the United States: prevalence of dental caries, *J Dent Educ* 49:341, 1985.

57. Graves RC and others: Recent dental caries and treatment patterns in U.S. children, *J Public Health Dent* 46:23, 1986.

58. Grol LS: Training and educational needs in pit and fissure sealant application for graduate dental personnel: continuing education and certification courses, *J Dent Educ* 48(suppl 2):66, 1984.

59. Gron P, DePaola PF: Caries prevention in the dental office, *Ala J Med Sci* 5:370, 1968.

60. Gwinnett AJ: *The search for an ideal sealant.* In *Viewpoints of preventive dentistry: the role of pit and fissure sealants,* Johnson & Johnson Co, Woodbridge, NJ, 1978, Medical Education Dynamics.

61. Hardison JR: The use of pit-and-fissure sealants in community public health programs in Tennessee, *J Public Health Dent* 43:233, 1983.

62. Hastreiter RJ: Fluoridation conflict: a history and conceptual basis, *J Am Dent Assoc* 106:468, 1983.

63. Hastreiter RJ: Is 0.4% stannous fluoride gel an effective agent for the prevention of oral disease? *J Am Dent Assoc* 118:205, 1989.

64. Hattab FN: The effect of air-drying on the uptake of fluoride in demineralized or abraded human enamel in vitro, *J Pedod* 11:151, 1987.

65. Heifetz SB, Horowitz HS, Brunelle JA: Effect of school water fluoridation on dental caries: results in Seagove, N.C. after 12 years, *J Am Dent Assoc* 106:334, 1983.

66. Heifetz SB, Horowitz HS, Driscoll WS: Effect of school water fluoridation on dental caries: results in Seagrove, North Carolina, after eight years, *J Am Dent Assoc* 97:193, 1978.

67. Holloway PJ: Public attitudes to fluoridation, *Royal Soc Health J* 97:58, 1977.

68. Hormati AA, Fuller JL, Denehy GE: Effects of contamination and mechanical disturbance on the quality of acid-etched enamel, *J Am Dent Assoc* 100:34, 1980.

69. Horowitz HS: The prevention of dental caries by

mouthrinsing with solutions of neutral sodium fluoride, *Int Dent J* 135:353, 1973.

70. Horowitz HS, moderator: Perspectives on the use of prenatal fluorides: a symposium, presented at the annual session of the American Dental Association, New Orleans, La, Oct 1980, ASDC, *J Dent Child* 48:102, 1981.

71. Horowitz HS: Grand Rapids: the public health story, *J Public Health Dent* 49:62, 1989.

72. Horowitz HS: Effectiveness of school water fluoridation and dietary supplements in school-aged children, *J Public Health Dent* 49(special issue):290, 1989.

73. Horowitz HS, Law FE, Pritzker T: Effect of school water fluoridation on dental caries, St. Thomas, Virgin Islands, *Public Health Rep* 80:381, 1965.

74. Horowitz HS and others: School fluoridation studies in Elk Lake, Pennsylvania, and Pike County, Kentucky; results after eight years, *Am J Public Health* 58:2240, 1968.

75. Horowitz HS and others: Combined fluoride, school-based program in a fluoride-deficient area: results of an 11-year study, *J Am Dent Assoc* 112:621, 1986.

76. Houpt M and others: Autopolymerized versus light-polymerized fissure sealant, *J Am Dent Assoc* 115:55, 1987.

77. Hunt RJ, Eldridge JB, Beck JD: Effect of residence in a fluoridated community on the incidence of coronal and root caries in an older adult population, *J Public Health Dent* 49:138, 1989.

78. Isokangas P and others: Xylitol chewing gum in caries prevention: a field study in children, *J Am Dent Assoc* 117:315, 1988.

79. Jensen ME: Responses of interproximal plaque pH to snack foods and effect of chewing sorbitol-containing gum, *J Am Dent Assoc* 113:262, 1986.

80. Jensen ME, Wefel JS: Human plaque pH responses to meals and the effects of chewing gum, *Br Dent J* 167:204, 1989.

81. Jensen ME, Wefel JS: Effects of processed cheese on human plaque pH and demineralization and remineralization, *Am J Dent* 3:217, 1990.

82. Katz S, McDonald JL, Stookey GK: *Preventive dentistry in action*, Upper Montclair, NJ, 1976, Dental Control Products Publishing.

83. Koch G and others: Caries-preventive effect of fluoride dentifrices with and without anticalculus agents: a 3-year controlled clinical trial, *Caries Res* 24:72, 1990.

84. Kornman KS: The role of supragingival plaque in the prevention and treatment of periodontal diseases: a review of current concepts, *J Periodont Res* 21(suppl):5, 1986.

85. Lang P: Analyzing selected criticisms of water fluoridation, *J Can Dent Assoc* 47:3, 1981.

86. Lang NP, Brecx MC: Chlorhexidine digluconate—an agent for chemical plaque control and prevention of gingival inflammation, *J Periodont Res* 21:(suppl):74, 1986.

87. Leavell HR, Clark EG: *Preventive medicine for the doctor in his community*, ed 3, New York, 1965, McGraw-Hill.

88. Leverett DH: Effectiveness of mouthrinsing with fluoride solutions in preventing coronal and root caries, *J Public Health Dent* 49(special issue):310, 1989.

89. Leverett DH: Eastman Dental Center: Personal communication, May 1991.

90. Lutz BL: Preventive dentistry: proposal for definition of terms, *J Dent Educ* 37:24, 1973.

91. Mandel ID: What is preventive dentistry? *J Prev Dent* 1:25, 1974.

92. Margolis FJ, Cohen SN: Successful and unsuccessful experiences in combating the antifluoridationists, *Pediatrics* 76:113, 1985.

93. McCall DR and others: Distribution of APF gel on toothsurfaces, *Br Dent J* 159:82, 1985.

94. McKay FS: Mottled enamel: fundamental problem in dentistry, *Dent Cosmos* 67:847, 1925.

95. Mellberg JR, Ripa LW: *Self-applied topical fluoride*. In *Fluoride in preventive dentistry: theory and clinical application*, Chicago, 1983, Quintessence.

96. Mertz-Fairhurst EJ and others: Clinical progress of sealed and unsealed caries; I, depth changes in bacterial counts, *J Prosthet Dent* 42:521, 1979.

97. Mertz-Fairhurst EJ and others: A comparative clinical study of two pit and fissure sealants: 7-year results in Augusta, GA, *J Am Dent Assoc* 109:252, 1984.

98. Mertz-Fairhurst EJ, Schuster GS, Fairhurst CW: Arresting caries by sealants: results of a clinical study, *J Am Dent Assoc* 112:194, 1986.

99. Miller AJ, Brunelle JA: A summary of the NIDR community caries prevention demonstration program, *J Am Dent Assoc* 107:265, 1983.

100. Mitropoulous CM and others: Relative efficacy of dentifrices containing 250 or 1,000 ppm F in preventing dental caries: report of a 32-month clinical trial, *Community Dent Health* 1:193, 1984.

101. Myers BA, editor: *A guide to medical care administration, vol 1, Concepts and principles*, Washington, DC, 1975, American Public Health Association.

102. National Institute of Dental Research: *The prevalence of dental caries in United States children, 1979-1980, the national dental caries prevalence survey*, NIH Pub No 82-2245, Washington, DC, 1981, US Department of Health and Human Services.

103. National Institute of Dental Research: *Oral health of United States adults, the national survey of oral health in U.S. employed adults and seniors: 1985-1986*, NIH Pub No 88-2869, Washington, DC, 1988, US Department of Health and Human Services.

104. National Institute of Dental Research: *Oral health of United States children, the national survey of dental caries in U.S. school children: 1986-1987*, NIH Pub No 89-2247, Washington, DC, 1989, US Department of Health and Human Services.

105. National Institutes of Health: *Dental sealants in the prevention of tooth decay*, Consensus Development Conference Statement, vol 4, no 11, US Department of Health and Human Services, Public Health Service.

106. Newbrun E: Effectiveness of water fluoridation, *J Public Health Dent* 49(special issue):279, 1989.

107. Nizel AE, Papas AS: *Dietary counseling for the prevention and control of dental caries*. In *Nutrition in clinical dentistry*, ed 3, Philadelphia, 1989, WB Saunders Co.

108. Reed MW: Clinical evaluation of three concentrations of sodium fluoride dentifrices, *J Am Dent Assoc* 87:1401, 1973.

109. Richards ND: *Utilization of dental services.* In Richards ND, and Cohen LK, editors: *Social sciences and dentistry: a critical bibliography,* London, 1971, Federation Dentaire Internationale.

110. Ripa LW: Fluoride rinsing: what dentists should know, *J Am Dent Assoc* 102:477, 1981.

111. Ripa LW: Professionally (operator) applied topical fluoride therapy: a critique, *Int Dent J* 31:105, 1981.

112. Ripa LW: Need for prior toothcleaning when performing a professional topical fluoride application: a review and recommendations for change, *J Am Dent Assoc* 109:281, 1984.

113. Ripa LW: Sealants: training and educational needs for dental students and dental auxiliary students, *J Dent Educ* 48(suppl 2):60, 1984.

114. Ripa LW: The current status of pit and fissure sealants: a review, *Can Dent Assoc J* 5:367, 1985.

115. Ripa LW: *The roles of prophylaxes and dental prophylaxis pastes in caries prevention.* In Wei S, editor: *Clinical uses of fluorides,* Philadelphia, 1985, Lea & Febiger.

116. Ripa LW: Clinical studies of high-potency fluoride dentifrices: a review, *J Am Dent Assoc* 118:85, 1989.

117. Ripa LW: Review of the anticaries effectiveness of professionally applied and self-applied topical fluoride gels, *J Public Health Dent* 49(special issue):297, 1989.

118. Ripa LW: An evaluation of the use of professional (operator-applied) topical fluorides, *J Dent Res* 69(special issue):786, 1990.

119. Ripa LW: A critique of topical fluoride methods (dentifrices, mouthrinses, operator-, and self-applied gels) in a era of decreased caries and increased fluorosis prevalence, *J Public Health Dent* 5l:23, 1991.

120. Ripa LW and others: *A guide to the use of fluorides for the prevention of dental caries,* ed 2, *J Am Dent Assoc* 113:503, 1986.

121. Ripa LW and others: *Preventing pit and fissure caries: a guide to sealant use,* Boston, 1986, Department of Public Health, Massachusetts Health Research Institute.

122. Ripa LW and others: Clinical study of the anticaries efficacy of three fluoride dentifrices containing anticalculus ingredients: three year (final) results, *J Clin Dent* 2:29, 1990.

123. Ripa LW, Leske GS, Kaufman HW: Caries prevalence, treatment level, and sealant use related to school lunch program participation, *J Public Health Dent* 51:1, 1991.

124. Ripa LW, Leske GS, Lowey WG: Fluoride rinsing: a school-based dental preventive program, *J Prev Dent* 4:25, 1977.

125. Rock WP, Evans RIW: A comparative study between a chemically polymerized fissure sealant resin and a light-cured resin, *Br Dent J* 152:232, 1982.

126. Rock WP, Evans RIW: A comparative study between a chemically polymerized fissure sealant resin and a light-cured resin: three-year results, *Br Dent J* 155:344, 1983.

127. Rock WP, Weatherill S, Anderson RJ: Retention of three fissure sealant resins and the effects of etching agent and curing method—1 year results, *J Paediatr Dent* 5:15, 1989.

128. Rubenstein LK, Avent MA: Frequency of undesirable side effects following professionally applied topical fluoride, *J Dent Child* 54:245, 1987.

129. Scheinin A, Makinen KK: Turku sugar studies, *Acta Odontol Scand* 33(suppl 70):1, 1975.

130. Shapira J and others: A comparative clinical study of autopolymerized and light-polymerized fissure sealants: five-year results, *Pediatr Dent* 12:168, 1990.

131. Shaw JH, Roussos GG: *Sweeteners and dental caries,* Washington, DC, 1978, Information Retrieval.

132. Silverstone LM: Fissure sealants: the enamel resin interface, *J Public Health Dent* 43:205, 1983.

133. Smith TS: Anatomic and physiologic conditions governing the use of the toothbrush, *J Am Dent Assoc* 27:874, 1940.

134. Spak C-J and others: Studies of human gastric mucosa after application of 0.42% fluoride gel, *J Dent Res* 69:426, 1990.

135. Stamm JW and others: The efficiency of caries prevention with weekly fluoride mouthrinses, *J Dent Educ* 48:617, 1984.

136. Stamm JW and others: The University of North Carolina caries risk assessment study; I, rationale and content, *J Public Health Dent* 48:225, 1988.

137. Stamm JW, Banting DW, Imrey PB: Adult root caries survey of two similar communities with contrasting natural water fluoride levels, *J Am Dent Assoc* 120:143, 1990.

138. Stephen KW and others: Retention of a filled fissure sealant using reduced etch time: a two-year study in 6 to 8 year old children, *Br Dent J* 153:232, 1982.

139. Stephen KW and others: A two-year visible light/uv light filled sealant study, *Br Dent J* 159:404, 1985.

140. Stillman PR: A philosophy of the treatment of periodontal disease, *Dent Dig* 38:315, 1932.

141. Stookey GK and others: The effect of rinsing with water immediately after a professional fluoride gel application on fluoride uptake in demineralized enamel: an in vivo study, *Pediatr Dent* 8:153, 1986.

142. Subcommittee on Fluoride of the Committee to Coordinate Environmental Health and Related Programs: *Review of fluoride: benefits and risks,* Washington, DC, 1991, US Department of Health and Human Services.

143. Sveen OB, Jensen OE: Two-year clinical evaluation of Delton and Prisma-shield, *Clin Prev Dent* 8:9, 1986.

144. Swift EJ Jr: The effect of sealants on dental caries: a review, *J Am Dent Assoc* 116:700, 1988.

145. Szpunar SM, Burt BA: Fluoride exposure in Michigan schoolchildren, *J Public Health Dent* 50:18, 1990.

146. US Food and Drug Administration: *Federal Register* 39:17, 1974.

147. US Public Health Service: *Public Health Service drinking water standards 1962,* PHS Pub No 956, Washington, DC, 1962, US Government Printing Office.

148. Wei SHY: *The potential benefits to be derived from topical fluorides in fluoridated communities.* In Forrester DJ, Schultz EM, editors: *International workshop on fluorides and dental caries reductions,* Baltimore, 1974, University of Maryland.

149. Wei SHY, Hattab FN: Time dependence of enamel fluo-

ride acquisition from APF gels; I, in vitro study, *Pediatr Dent* 10:168, 1988.

150. Wei SH, Kanellis MJ: Fluoride retention after sodium fluoride mouthrinsing by preschool children, *J Am Dent Assoc* 106:626, 1983.

151. Wei SHY, Lau EWS, Hattab FN: Time dependence of enamel fluoride acquisition from APF gels; II, in vivo study, *Pediatr Dent* 10:173, 1988.

152. White AW, Antczak-Bouckoms AA, Weinstein MC: Issues in the economic evaluation of community water fluoridation, *J Dent Educ* 53:646, 1989.

153. Williams B, Ward R, Winter GB: A two-year clinical trial comparing different resin systems used as fissure sealants, *Br Dent J* 161:367, 1986.

154. Winter GB, Holt RD, Williams BF: Clinical trial of a low-fluoride toothpaste for young children, *Int Dent J* 39:227, 1989.

155. Wolff LF and others: Effect of toothbrushing with 0.4% stannous fluoride and 0.22% sodium fluoride on gingivitis for 18 months, *J Am Dent Assoc* 119:283, 1989.

156. World Health Organization: *Statistical indicators for the planning and evaluation of public health programs,* technical report series No 472, Geneva, 1971, World Health Organization.

157. Wright GZ and others: A comparison between autopolymerizing and visible-light-activated sealants, *Clin Prev Dent* 10:14, 1988.

158. Zack D, Pilgram J: Comparison of sealant retention rates using self cured vs light cured sealants and liquid vs gel etch, *J Dent Res* 65:793, 1986 (abstract).

SECTION FOUR

Community Dental Programs

In 1965, departments of community dentistry responded to President Johnson's "War on Poverty" with new dental programs. Although community-based programs existed long before this time, new impetus was given to these programs with the advent of increased federal funding. This section deals with organized community programs: how they are developed, how effective they are, and the role of the consumer.

Chapter 9 describes programs designed to provide health information or change behavior—dental health education programs. It documents the degree of success of various programs and suggests types of programs that are cost-effective.

Chapter 10, on planning community programs, introduces the planning process and involves the student in the case study of a community project. The multitude of pitfalls in the path of the prospective health planner are clearly documented. Methods to effect meaningful change are examined, and a step-by-step formula for a successful project is provided.

9 Dental Health Education

Dental health education for the community is a process that informs, motivates, and helps persons to adopt and maintain health practices and lifestyles, advocates environmental changes as needed to facilitate this goal, and conducts professional training and research to the same end.* Health education is any combination of learning opportunities designed to facilitate voluntary adaptations of behavior that are conducive to health.[39] Health education programs are not isolated events but educational aspects of any curative, preventive, or promotional health activity. Comprehension of the multifactorial variables in dental disease and their interaction has increased the emphasis now placed on the educational process to assist in achieving desired health outcomes.

It has been well documented in dentistry and other health areas that correct health information or knowledge alone does not necessarily lead to desirable health behaviors.[27] However, knowledge gained may serve as a tool to empower population groups with accurate information about health and health care technologies, enabling them to take action to protect their health.[33] Both internal and external variables influence whether an individual or community will comply with recommended disease prevention, health maintenance, and/or health promotion procedures. Health promotion is any combination of educational, organizational, economic, and environmental supports for behavior conducive to health.[39] Health promotion refers to actions that are intended either to alter the living environment of persons to improve their health, despite individual actions such as community water fluoridation, or to enable and empower individuals to take advantage of preventive procedures or services by reducing or eliminating access barriers. Other actions might include making available—or removing financial barriers to—procedures such as the appropriate use of fluoride supplements, use of dental sealants, supervised removal of dental plaque, and effective referral and follow-up services for children and women who need treatment.[34] "Education" and "promotion" are intertwined to achieve long-term improved health for maternal and child focus populations, as well as for other populations within American society.

"... Procedures implemented through promotion can prevent a given disease or condition, but only education can foster informed decision making and maintenance of needed programs, services or behaviors. Health education and promotion processes permeate all levels of individuals and groups, and may include working with patients, parents, legislators, industry, and all other levels of influential policy makers, including health care providers."[34]

The dental health educator must be cognizant of available resources and demographic changes affecting social, economic, and health services environments. In addition, the educator must weigh internal and external variables in relation to clinical and behavioral research findings when designing a community program that will be effective in achieving long-term results.

Knowledge of program planning and community organization is essential, and skill development in these areas warrants inclusion in the professional preparation of the dentist and dental hygienist. To date, however, development of these skills has received little attention. The American Dental Hygienists Association (ADHA) responded to the expanding role of the dental hygienist by developing an audiocassette self-study continuing education program of courses that present the latest in theories and techniques intrinsic to success-

---

*Modified from the definition of consumer health education adopted by the 1975 NIH Fogarty International Center and American College of Preventive Medicine Task Force on Consumer Health Education.[21,24,79,105,106]

ful dental hygiene practice. In addition, the ADHA offers five self-study materials in workbook format, which may be particularly helpful for dental professionals with a keen interest in community-based programs and alternative practice settings: *The Dental Health Consultant in Community-Based Programs,*[9] *Contracting for Services in Alternative Practice Settings,*[8] *Care for the Homebound Patient,*[7] *Dental Hygiene Care for the Geriatric Patient,*[10] and *Dental Hygiene Care of the Special Needs Patient.*[11] The ADHA also has available for purchase an array of practical guides for helping career-minded individuals and active program planners achieve success through professional development.

Most professional training revolves around learning specific technical procedures and working with patients on a one-to-one basis. In this situation individual patient motivation is the primary objective of dental health education and unfortunately constitutes only a small component of the overall treatment plan.[14] Ideally, this relationship allows the dental practitioner to tailor the preventive prescription to each individual patient's needs, and patients can identify their own short- and long-term dental health goals. Through this process the dental professional is able to help those patients susceptible to prevention to begin, if they do not already, to internalize the value of good oral health and to practice preventive measures. Chambers,[21] however, has concluded that strong evidence suggests that only a limited number of Americans are amenable to an at-home program of controlling plaque. A principal factor suppressing this number is that healthy habits of living are not supported by deep-seated cultural values. The role of health educator becomes an essential component in the management of dental disease and in helping patients assume responsibility for their own oral health maintenance.

In most cases the same skills that were developed in working with patients on a one-to-one basis are carried over to the community setting. As a result, community dental health programs are usually conducted in much the same manner as individual patient education. Specific educational efforts focus on presenting dental health information and on trying to change an individual's attitudes and behaviors with regard to oral hygiene habits and diet rather than on emphasizing an organized community approach to prevention and control of disease. Emphasis is placed on correct brushing and flossing techniques to help prevent, or at least control, periodontal disease and on nutritional counseling, sealants, fluoride therapy for caries control, use of mouthguards in contact sports, and antismoking and anti-smokeless-tobacco education.

Success of these primary health promotion endeavors relies on the individual's development of specific skills and their incorporation into the person's life-style to reduce the prevalence of caries, periodontal disease, oral injuries, and oral cancer. Although popular, this approach to disease prevention alone, however, has experienced limited success in reducing oral disease and is questioned as being an appropriate focus for public health education.* Behavioral theories applicable on an individual level are not directly transferable to solving group and community level health problems.[33,37] Given Winslow's definition of dental public health—the science and art of preventing and controlling dental disease and promoting dental health through organized community efforts—an alternative approach focusing on individual behavior change would be to target health education efforts to community leaders, as suggested by Frazier.[32] This approach would redirect the educational processes to the selection of prevention and control programs that operate at the community level and do not require daily compliance on the part of the individual. Further, Frazier and Horowitz[33] suggest that focusing health education and promotion efforts with a broader range of children and parent subpopulations produces positive potential for major impact on the oral health of future generations of families in different socioeconomic groups. All mothers and infant caretakers—whether male or female, young or old—need to know how to prevent oral diseases. By imparting that knowledge to the children in their care and by reinforcing good daily oral health habits, the oral health of future generations could improve dramatically. School-based health education and promotion activities are viable ways of reinforcing healthy behaviors.

---

*References 34, 45, 47, 62, 66, 77, 90, 91; Winslow CEA: The untilled field of public health, *Mod Med* 2:183, 1920.

The purpose of this chapter is to present an overview of the current concepts in dental health education and to discuss the transition in educational activities from the traditional approach to current and suggested approaches. By examining three ongoing community programs and examples of other organized community efforts, the student should be able to determine which program goals are appropriate for public health education and possible ways to accomplish those goals. In addition, areas of recent and recommended educational research will be highlighted. We hope that previously held beliefs will be challenged and that the extent, complexity, and importance of community dental health education will be better understood.

BASIC CONCEPTS OF DENTAL HEALTH EDUCATION

The content and methodology of health education are derived from the fields of medicine and public health and from the physical, biological, social, and behavioral sciences. Certain concepts and theories developed in these fields have influenced the efforts and practices of health educators. In the area of dental health education, many of the proven theories of behavioral scientists have been either neglected, forgotten, or unaccepted. Given that the goal of dental health education is the prevention and control of dental disease, it would seem apparent that organized efforts aimed at achieving this goal should adhere to the proven theories and concepts relevant to health education activities.

Cognitive model

One central theory is the belief that behavior is learned by individuals, not merely transmitted by one person to another.[105] How individuals learn certain behavior is a complex process that varies with each person. One person may learn a certain dental behavior from a dentist in a one-to-one educational encounter, whereas another person may not. Research has shown that a fundamental error in many dental health education activities is the assumption that increasing a patient's dental health knowledge will help change dental care behavior. This approach, based on a cognitive learning model, assumes the following sequence:

Knowledge→Attitude→Behavior change.

If this relationship were true, every dental health education program that increased the participants' level of dental knowledge would have resulted in a behavioral change that improved their oral health status over a long period of time. To date, no evaluation of a dental health education program has produced such results.*

An error commonly made with this cognitive approach occurs when the educator fails to assess the learners' level of knowledge before the educational encounter and treats the individual as if he or she were void of any knowledge or past experiences at all. As Yacovone[105] notes, it is important to realize "that the person is already 'behaving' when we encounter him—maybe not as we would like him to, but 'behaving.'" To influence a person's behavior through health education activities, an understanding of the dynamics of behavior is paramount.

A person's behavior is the result of both internal and external forces. One's beliefs, attitudes, interests, values, needs, motives, expectations, perceptions, and biologic factors, plus the influence of family, peer groups, and mass economic factors such as occupation, education, and media, shape and affect one's actions.[56] Socioeconomic factors such as occupation, education, and income have also been shown to have a strong influence on dental health practices and should be considered in designing and implementing health education strategies. The interaction of these forces has been illustrated in a dynamic model developed by Young[106] (Fig. 9-1). Considering this model, it becomes evident that a straight-line relationship between the educator's efforts and the learner's behavior usually does not exist. To develop an effective dental health education program, the educator must be aware of the interaction of all the forces on the learner. The educator must first assess the learner or learners to develop and implement a rational educational program that will result in a sustained behavior change.

Behavioral learning model

A second approach to the educational process is based on a behavioral learning model. This methodology relies on changing the learner's behavior

---

*References 21, 24, 77, 79, 86, 105, 106.

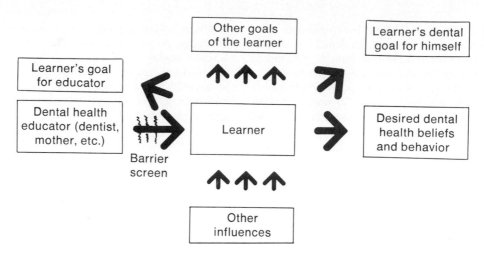

Fig. 9-1 A model of the dental health education process. (Courtesy Young MAC: Dental health education: an overview of selected concepts and principles relevant to programme planning, *Int J Health Educ* 13:2, 1970.)

through prescribed activities that present the appropriate skills, behavior, and knowledge with the hope that the desired attitudes will follow. Programs now focus on having students participate in learning brushing and flossing skills as opposed to just having the teacher demonstrate or lecture on the technique. To be truly effective the educator must assess each learner to prescribe activities that are compatible with that learner's life-style. Individuals will differ in psychomotor development and oral hygiene practices. In some cases it may not be necessary or desirable to try to change an individual's behavior. Once this assessment is completed and the appropriate preventive regimen prescribed when necessary, the learner must be motivated to practice these activities on a daily basis.

Four factors that influence whether an individual practices these preventive dental procedures have been identified in research conducted by Rosenstock[82] and later by Kegeles:[52,53] (1) individuals must feel they are susceptible to dental disease, (2) they must perceive dental disease as a serious consequence, (3) they must believe that dental disease is preventable, and (4) they must attach a certain salience or importance to dental health. If any of these factors is absent, the likelihood of an individual being motivated to adopt and prac-

tice the preventive procedure is significantly reduced.

The major obstacle to prevention of dental disease appears to be the perception that the consequences of dental disease are not serious. In most cases dental disease is not life-threatening, and a large portion of the population functions without their natural teeth. In a 1973 survey conducted by Opinion Research Corporation for the American Dental Association, the public's chief barrier to prevention of dental disease was identified as the low value many Americans place on regular preventive dental care.[5]

Another factor that affects the ultimate outcome of the educational process is how an individual learns. Learning is not an isolated event occurring in formal educational settings, but a continuous process that can be influenced by many uncontrollable variables. An individual is constantly learning about dental health from many informal sources, such as family, peers, and the mass media. Many times the information gained from these sources is misleading, inaccurate, and directly contradictory to the dental health educator's message.[34] Therefore the educator must assess the impact of these informal messages on the learner to develop an appropriate educational program, which should increase the learner's awareness of

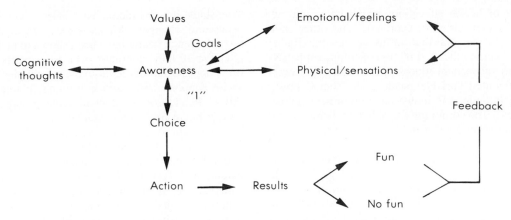

Fig. 9-2 The self-care motivation model. Diagram indicates the key areas of personal growth and awareness associated with an ongoing process of self-care. (From Horowitz LG: The self-care motivation model: theory and practice in human development, *J Sch Health* 55:59, 1985. Copyright, 1985, American School Health Association, Kent, OH 44240.)

these informal messages and teach critical evaluation of their contents.

The self-care motivation model

A third approach to the educational process has been offered by Horowitz and associates.[45] This is a whole-person approach to motivating self-care based on values, awareness, choice, and action. The self-care motivation model (TSCMM) addresses elements and functions common to all individuals and underlying all health behaviors. This model was developed with the specific intention of addressing noncompliance issues in behavior and life-styles that result in negative health consequences. TSCMM makes use of social, psychological, and behavioral science principles to instill a greater sense of personal choice and critical self-governing behavior in patients. Figure 9-2 illustrates the dynamics of this approach. It is widely adaptable, comprehensible, and holds promise for integration by a broad range of age and sociocultural groups.

According to Horowitz, the TSCMM provides an effective framework for patient education efforts and for promoting long-term behavior change among schoolchildren and adults.[45] Instead of concentrating narrowly on each illness or aspect of patient health and trying to alter risk behaviors specific for each illness, TSCMM emphasizes the con-

cept of linking healthy human development and greater self-efficacy to setting personal health goals based on a greater clarity and appreciation for health values. Original in concept, TSCMM is supported by leading behavioral theories and counseling practices as advanced by Assagioli,[12] Rank,[78] Bandura,[13] McClelland and co-workers,[58] Mahoney and Thoreson,[57] Meichenbaum,[61] and Cautella.[18]

Horowitz has also developed related educational curricula to support the dispersal of innovative health education methods and self-care practices in schools and workplaces.[47] The curriculum includes units on stress, relaxation, coping skills, health values clarification, health awareness, self-assessment and self-care, as well as positive life-style choice, positive self-image and self-esteem, and reinforcement.[36] The curriculum emphasizes oral self-care as a starting point within health education. Through exercises in guided imagery the learner participates in covert behavior rehearsal, sensitization, and reinforcement (Fig. 9-2).

Choice making is based on personal awareness of physical, mental, and emotional feedback, which leads to cognitive self-regulation.[48]

Contemporary community health model

The fourth and most current approach is the contemporary community health (or public health) model of health education, which takes into account social, cultural, economic, and other environmental factors that influence health. Rather than "blaming the victim" for noncompliant behavior and subsequent illnesses, the need for changes in influential variables such as the social, political, economic, and industrial environments is recognized. The community health model emphasizes the important role of public involvement in identifying individual and community health problems, setting priorities, and developing solutions to these problems and empowers population groups with accurate information about health and health care technologies. The utility of broad approaches to health education and promotion at the community level has been demonstrated in studies of other health areas.[29,37,38,73] However, with few exceptions, many of the community-level methods employed in these demonstrations have not yet been accepted by dental professionals. The World Health Organization[102,103] has clearly stated the need for using sound community organization and community development principles of working with focus populations, such as sharing in decision making.

The objective of community organization is to create awareness, interest, and desire to solve a problem, while working with others to solve the problem. By involving people in making decisions about regimens or programs to improve their own health, people will tend to unite and maintain the level of commitment to and motivation for carrying out necessary actions to solve the problems.[33,44] Students are encouraged to review the Stanford Five City Project,[29] which describes the communication-change framework; social marketing; the application of formative research in designing, modifying, and distributing printed educational materials; the use of mass media education; program planning; and evaluation. The Stanford Five City Project is an evaluation of a communitywide approach to the control of cardiovascular disease through healthy changes in behavior. This approach may be generalizable to dental disease prevention efforts as we continue to learn to unite a variety of medical, behavioral, communication, and social science theories with demonstrated applications to solve health problems.[37]

Media influence. Silversin and Kornacki[89]

have stated that the media has a role in promoting behavioral change: "Media-based campaigns to promote dental health have been shown to be more effective if they continue over long periods of time, appeal to multiple motives, are coupled with social support, and provide training in requisite skills." In addition, product advertising may influence public opinion and behavior.

Organizations such as Action for Children's Television (ACT),[1] the Center for Science in the Public Interest (CSPI),[19] the National Congress of Parents and Teachers (National PTA),[65] and the American Academy of Pediatrics (AAP)[2,3] have expressed concern about the marketing of relatively nonnutritious foods to children. A nonprofit consumer-advocacy group based in Washington, D.C., CSPI[20] has focused on nutrition and food safety issues since its founding in 1971. It analyzed the advertising that was shown during Saturday morning broadcasts on five television stations, including affiliates of ABC, CBS, NBC, and Fox networks, plus the Nickelodeon cable channel between 8 AM and noon on February 9, 1991. Of the 350 commercials airing, 63.4% were for food. Of the food ads, most were for cereals, followed by restaurants, candy, beverages, cookies, entrees, and chips. There was also one public service announcement on eating. The nutritional value of each food was assessed, giving it a passing score if 25% of its calories came from refined sugar, less than 30% of its calories came from fat, and it contained less than 400 mg sodium. Only 20 of the 222 food commercials passed the test. Dr. Michael F. Jacobson,[19] executive director of CSPI, stated:

While many American adults are waking up to good nutrition, marketers continue to promote lousy eating habits among children. The kind of foods promoted on children's television promote tooth decay, obesity and heart disease. It is shameful that despite years of controversy, broadcasters, the food industry, and government have failed to develop any kind of meaningful nutrition-education campaign for children.

In 1991 U.S. Congressman Ron Wyden[104] of Oregon spearheaded a campaign to demand a greater show of responsibility from the appropriate parties. Specifically targeted were "television broadcasters, food producers and their advertising agencies, and the key government regulatory agencies who can demand that this junk food wasteland be reseeded and nurtured with reasonable nutritional messages for our nation's youngsters." He recommended that the Federal Communications Commission (FCC) formulate an agreement with broadcasters and advertisers to air during Saturday morning—children's prime time—more public service announcements or programming that will encourage children to build their diets around fruit, grains, vegetables, lean poultry and meat, and low-fat milk. Besides the FCC, he contacted the Federal Trade Commission, the Department of Health and Human Services, and the U.S. Surgeon General to demand a call for action.

On June 3, 1991, the National PTA[65] released a policy statement supporting

. . . Rep. Wyden's effort to subject food advertising on children's television to renewed scrutiny. It's ironic that our society spends billions of dollars a year on medical wizardry—heart transplants, CAT-scans, and new pharmaceuticals—to cure diseases, but doesn't take the simplest steps to promote lifelong, health-promoting habits beginning in childhood. Children's television is the place to start.

The AAP, an organization of 41,000 pediatricians, is dedicated to the health, safety, and well-being of infants, children, adolescents, and young adults. On July 23, 1991, at the AAP's conference for media,[2] "Children: Our Future," the AAP released a policy statement, "The Commercialization of Children's Television." In it AAP states that the primary goal of commercial children's television is to sell products to children and that young children cannot distinguish between programs and commercials. Further, the use of commercials and programs to sell products now forms a tight ring of commercialism around children's television from which young viewers cannot escape. Former secretary of the Department of Health and Human Services Dr. Louis Sullivan[93] spoke to the media at this conference:

Children are unprepared to make appropriate food choices. We must be their guardians. We must make sure that the information they receive from television promotes health and well-being . . . not blind consumerism. As the media, you have a responsibility to see that our children are exposed to appropriate, health-promoting programming.

The Children's Television Act of 1990, which took effect in 1992, limits the number of ads allowed during children's shows and mandates that all broadcasters carry children's educational or instructional programming as a condition for license renewal by the FCC. However, the FCC has concluded that this requirement can be met by citing public service announcements or short vignettes in fulfillment of the programming requirement. The academy emphasizes that local oversight will be necessary to monitor how stations meet these guidelines. The academy urged parents to take an active role in educating their children to become responsible and informed consumers and noted that media literacy should be taught to children in schools and in a variety of other settings.[2,3]

Budgets for preventive dental health interventions cannot compete with budgets to promote products that are pushed and pulled into the marketplace with huge sums of money. The success of product advertising is based on linking personal satisfaction or enhanced self-esteem with the use of a product. Thus far dental health promotion has not succeeded in linking preventive dental behaviors with motives other than health.[89]

Parents and school programs. Rubinson[85] has identified parents as the most pervasive intervening variable in school dental health programs. Frequently program developers and evaluators do not consider enlisting the cooperation of parents. Rubinson further states that "the parents will certainly have a direct influence on dental health habits and should be involved with programmatic efforts."[85] The evaluation of dental health programs should be redirected to focus on efforts stressing skill acquisition and reduction of behavioral risk factors through an evaluation plan that is both plausible and realistic in the school setting. Perry and associates[73] have demonstrated the effectiveness of combined school, parent, and community approaches to child health behavior in the Minnesota Home Team project. This case demonstrated how sharing responsibility can be accomplished and established the superior impact of shared responsibility between the school and the home on children's knowledge, skills, and practices with respect to dietary intake of more healthful foods.[37]

The School Health Education Evaluation (SHEE), conducted in collaboration with the U.S.

Centers for Disease Control (CDC),[98] from 1982 through 1984 suggests that exposure to health education curricula in schools can result in substantial changes in students' knowledge, attitudes, and self-reported practices.

The SHEE has provided evidence that school health education curricula can effect changes in health-related knowledge, practices, and attitudes and that such changes increase with the amount of instruction. The potential impact of these changes is significant.[98] In response to this study, many school systems are reevaluating their health curricula and considering increased integration of health messages throughout the curriculum. Teachers will require additional training to develop greater competency on health issues. In view of budgeting limitations, teachers will continue to be the primary source for the dissemination of health education in our schools, with the assistance of health professionals in the community. Students are encouraged to review the 10 basic elements that constitute comprehensive school health education as defined in the SHEE study.[25]

The complexity of the variables that must be taken into account in designing a dental health education program to motivate behavioral change for an individual has been briefly discussed. Greater detail and step-by-step procedures can be found in books devoted solely to the techniques of behavior modification and to the social sciences in dentistry.[27,75,100]

HEALTH EDUCATION IN TRANSITION

Dental health education programs for the community have gone through, and will continue to undergo, periods of transition as further study reveals educational methods that will produce desired preventive practices. Research has shown that behavior is not transmitted; behavior is learned. In health care, learning requires active participation on the part of the learner. For this reason the primary objective of most dental health education programs is to motivate individual students to seek the goal of disease prevention and tooth conservation.

Historically, dental health education for children has been a priority for the dental profession because of the high prevalence of dental caries in this age group. As a result, the school system has emerged as the most logical and practical setting to implement large-scale dental health education programs.[76] The school-based dental health program provides an opportunity to reach the largest number of children during early stages of development when habit patterns can more easily be modified or changed. The school setting also provides an environment conducive to learning and reinforcement for a considerable period of time and allows the teachers to use various strategies for inducing children to participate in appropriate preventive dental health actions.[40]

Early school-based dental health programs based on the cognitive learning model primarily consisted of dental professionals and students participating in short-term projects such as National Children's Dental Health Week, high school career days, and one-time visits to elementary and secondary school classrooms. These projects did not seek to incorporate dental health into the school curriculum; they were (and are where they still exist) seen as an "add-on" activity. Administratively, one-time visits present little difficulty and are often welcomed by the teacher and administration; however, reinforcement or evaluation of the dental health lesson is not usually part of the activity. Most reports on dental health education in the classroom agree that the most effective situation is when the classroom teacher works closely with the dental professional. So, regardless of who actually makes the presentation, the teacher can augment and reinforce oral health concepts and practices. The most significant behavior for the teacher is to be an effective role model of good oral health practices.[77]

Although public interest may be aroused and dentistry's image enhanced, the early school programs, passive and cognitive in nature, were not found to motivate changes in oral health attitudes and behavior.* According to Raynor and Cohen,[80] research in the dental health area suggests that

There must be something more than motivation per se to establish oral hygiene behavior as a habit. Learning oral hygiene must involve the acquisition of a value, or a change in a value. . . . For adults, this involves change in cognitive structure, but for children, cognitive learning is secondary to motivational learning.

---

*References 21, 42, 76, 77, 87, 101.

As a consequence of this realization, the "show and tell" approach has now evolved into programs of "show and do."

A survey of state school health programs by the American School Health Association revealed that only seven states mandate the teaching of dental health and oral hygiene.[17] Unfortunately, even in those seven states requiring instruction on specific health content areas, dental health is given a low priority on the list of required subjects. If dental health education is more than rhetoric and teachers are expected to include it in the curriculum, then adequate teacher training programs are prerequisite.[94] Dental health professionals in the community can serve as valuable resources to the school. Dental health education should be an integral component of all school health education curricula. Regrettably, the majority of dental health education programs were supported through grant funds, and many were terminated when funding expired.[63] Unless a strong constituency supports dental health programs, continued efforts may be stunted as a result of budgeting constraints.

An interesting by-product of school-based dental health education programs may be the "spread effect"[23] or the "ripple effect."[51] These terms have been used to describe the impact of school-based health education programs upon parents. Croucher and colleagues[23] conducted an investigation to assess the possible indirect influence of "Natural Noshers" (a school-based dental health education program that emphasizes home activities for skill development) on the dental behavior and knowledge of other family members. "Natural Noshers" contains two distinct dental health messages, one relating to the prevention of gum disease and the other to dental decay. Take-home literature and supplies emphasize these messages. The results of this study indicate that the parents of children who had been taught "Natural Noshers" had reported new dental information more often than the parents in the control group.[23]

In another project a group of health educators at the University of Maine at Farmington developed a series of health-related games, the "Healthway Arcade."[51] The games were used primarily for an audience of kindergarten through third grade and were structured to address several health issues. "Floss Is the Boss" was a popular follow-along story that used repetition, funny sounds, and a variety of motions to cleverly state the importance of flossing one's teeth. Parental feedback indicated that this live arts format was well received and that many youngsters insisted on reciting parts of the story at home for the family. This ripple effect is another way of getting a message into the home and community.[51]

Some factors may enhance the success of dental health programs in schools: (1) determining who will be responsible for dental health education, (2) involving parents who can provide reinforcement of dental health practices at home, (3) identifying and using community health resources who can contribute their expertise or materials to support dental health education efforts, and (4) evaluating the results of the program.[95]

Three programs, based on both the behavioral and the cognitive learning models, are next described in terms of program development, philosophy and goals, implementation, and evaluation. Findings of formal research investigations as reported in the literature are also presented for review. The student is asked to keep in mind the desired properties of a good oral public health measure and the planning and implementation strategy and criteria for the prevention of dental caries, as outlined in Chapter 8, when critiquing each program in terms of public health planning.

Although all details for each program have not been presented, all major concepts have been included. For further information, contact the individuals in charge of specific programs.

PRESENT APPROACHES
"Learning about Your Oral Health": a prevention-oriented school program

Development. "Learning about Your Oral Health" was developed by the ADA and its consultants in response to a request from the 1971 ADA House of Delegates. The program is available to school systems throughout the United States.[22]

Program philosophy and goals. "Learning about Your Oral Health" is a comprehensive program covering current dental concepts. Materials for preschool, primary, and secondary schools have been developed for educators to facilitate the inclusion of preventive dentistry into school health curricula. The primary goal of the program is to develop the knowledge, skills, and attitudes needed for prevention of dental disease.[6] The first priority of the program is to develop effective plaque-control knowledge and skills. The next consideration is given to increasing knowledge regarding diet and dental health, with an emphasis on understanding the role of sugar and starch. Other areas that are included at all levels in increasing degree of detail are: the significance of fluoride, oral safety, consumer health concepts, the role of dental professionals, oral health in relationship to total health, and community dental programs.

Program implementation. The program format is divided into five levels with specific content defined for each level. The levels are divided by grades: preschool (designed for children too young to read), level I (kindergarten through grade 3), level II (grades 4 through 6), level III (grades 7 through 9), and level IV (grades 10 through 12).

The core material for each of the five levels is self-contained in a teaching packet that allows the classroom teacher to adapt the presentation to the needs of the students. Each packet includes (1) a teacher's self-contained guide on "dental health facts" with a section on handicapped children; (2) a glossary of dental health terms; (3) a curriculum guide featuring content, goals, behavioral objectives, and suggested activities for other classes; (4) five lesson plans for the preschool level and seven or more lesson plans for each of the other levels; (5) four overhead transparencies; (6) 12 spirit masters; and (7) methods and activities for parental involvement.

Supplementary printed material and films coordinated with each level have also been developed. In addition, the ADA, in cooperation with the American Cancer Society, has developed and produced a rock video on the dangers of using smokeless tobacco, which is geared for junior and senior high students, as well as for adult audiences.[4]

Cost of materials. The teaching packet for each level currently costs $8 per level.

Program evaluation. The behavioral objectives provide the basis for evaluating the effectiveness of the lessons at all levels with the exception of levels I and II, which contain pretests and posttests. This program was developed for general use and may be adapted in full or in part to complement another ongoing program.

Formal evaluation. A formal evaluation study of the effectiveness of the ADA's "Learning about Your Oral Health" program was conducted by Dr. Oliver L. Ezell[28] in 1974 and reported during the First National Symposium on Dental Health Education in Schools. The objectives of this study were to determine whether there was an improvement in the oral health behavior and attitudes of junior high school students and whether the ADA's level III program was superior to traditional oral health instruction. The results of the investigation found that the ADA's program (1) more favorably influenced oral health behavior than did the traditional approach to oral health education and (2) effected favorable changes in attitudes toward oral health practices (but not necessarily more so than traditional approaches).[28] The data did not suggest that the ADA's program was effective in improving attitudes toward organized oral health education programs. Ezell noted several factors that could have influenced these results, such as levels of instructor motivation, possible instructor bias, and levels of instructor capability.

In a second investigation by Dr. Donald B. Stone and colleagues,[92] the cognitive aspects of the ADA's level II program were evaluated. The target audience was fifth graders, and the primary focus was determining the value or impact of intensive in-service training for teachers versus a teacher orientation with minimal exposure to curriculum materials. A test was administered to students within 1 week of the program's completion. The results of this study concluded that there was no significant difference between the mean knowledge scores of students taught by teachers who had received intensive training and the scores of students taught by teachers who had received minimal orientation. There was a significant difference between mean knowledge scores of students taught by either of the first two teacher groups and students who had been taught by teachers with no orientation to the program, which may indicate that some teacher orientation to the program is desirable. The Bureau of Health Education and Audiovisual Services revised its program in response to this study to yield the current format.

A third investigation conducted in 1980 by Peterson and Rubinson[74] was reported in the literature in 1982. The objectives of this study were to determine the effects of the ADA level IV school program on the knowledge, attitudes, practices, and dental health status of high school students. The primary instrument employed in this study was the 83-item Dental Knowledge and Attitude Survey, which consisted of three major sections: dental knowledge, dental attitudes, and general health attitudes. The generalizability of the results of this study is limited because this study was confined to a specific geographic area, used a specific educational program, and involved schools that offered a one-semester course in health education to sophomores. The following conclusions are based on the results of this study:

1. The ADA level IV program was effective in improving the oral health knowledge of the secondary school students randomly assigned to the experimental groups of this study.
2. The ADA level IV program produced minor positive changes in dental attitudes, dental locus of control, and health locus of control, none of which was statistically significant.
3. Based on the findings of this study and a review of the literature, high school females generally have higher levels of dental knowledge and more positive attitudes toward dental health than males.
4. The ADA level IV program had a greater impact on the dental knowledge, dental attitudes, dental locus of control, and health locus of control of females than on that of males.
5. There was a low-to-moderate association among secondary students' dental knowledge, dental attitudes, dental locus of control, and health locus of control.
6. The ADA's 1980 Oral Health Teaching and Learning Program for secondary students is an innovative approach to curriculum design and has the potential for contributing to improved dental health teaching and learning.[74]

A fourth investigation was conducted during 1986 to evaluate the effectiveness of the ADA's preschool program. Specifics on this study are currently unavailable.[6]

Texas statewide preventive dentistry program: "Tattletooth II, A New Generation"

Development. The Tattletooth Program was developed in 1974-76 as a cooperative effort between Texas dental health professional organizations, the Texas Education Agency, and the Texas Department of Health through a grant from the Department of Health and Human Services to the Bureau of Dental Health. In its original format this program was used by approximately 500,000 children in Texas per year before the new program was completed in 1989.[97]

In 1985 the Texas legislature mandated that the essential elements for comprehensive health education curricula identified in the School Health Education Evaluation Project[25,98] be incorporated into the curriculum statewide and be taught to the state's more than 3 million schoolchildren. Dental health is one of the required elements. This legislative action stimulated a need for the Tattletooth Program statewide.[95-97]

In May 1987 an advisory committee recommended that a new program be developed to replace the existing Tattletooth Program. The committee developed a model and, with input from the regional staff, formulated a scope and sequence chart and the lesson format. The curriculum was developed according to a systematic process of educational development that began with recognition and analysis of the needs. An educational model was developed, the program was conceptualized, and materials were designed. The new program underwent formative evaluation in the spring of 1988.

In 1989 the Bureau of Dental Health developed a mostly new program, Tattletooth II, A New Generation for Grades K-6, so named because the characters in the artwork for grades kindergarten through second were from the old curriculum. This new curriculum was modified to reflect recommendations obtained from the formative evaluation process. Also, name recognition by the users of the prior program was considered a valuable asset. Separate lesson plans were developed for each grade, and a preschool program is currently under revision. A systems approach was used to develop all educational material.[96]

Three videotapes were produced as part of the teacher training package. The first videotape familiarizes the teachers with the lesson format and content. A second videotape, "Brushing and Flossing," was developed for the dual purpose of teacher training and as an instructional unit to be used by the teacher with the students. A third videotape provides teachers with additional background information as a means of preparing them to teach the lessons. In addition to the curriculum, a public relations plan was formulated, and materials were developed to aid in the implementation of the program. The public relations material consisted of a brochure that provided an overview of the program and a school nurse's brochure. Two news releases were written: one was targeted toward parents and designed for local newspapers; the other was aimed at the readership of professional education journals. A letter to school principals and nurses was sent out as part of a package distributed annually by the Bureau of Maternal and Child Health. A model script for a television interview was another public relations effort. A 2-hour training session using the materials in the new curriculum was televised to the schools via a video network. A brief summary of the new program was run on the computer bulletin board of the Texas Association of School Boards.

Program philosophy and goals. In Texas, dental health education has long been the primary prevention effort of both the private and public dental sectors.[96]

The basic goal of the program is to reduce dental disease and to develop positive dental habits to last a lifetime. The major thrust of Tattletooth is to convince students that preventing dental disease is important and that they can do it.[96,97]

Tattletooth lessons are correlated with the health and science essential elements. The material in the lesson is often related to other subject areas, such as language arts. Both share mutual elements and may fulfill the requirements of the essential elements of both subjects. Some teachers integrate subject matter. References to cultural differences are made throughout each unit, and lessons are currently being translated into Spanish.

To satisfy the legislative requirement that student performance be assessed, the Texas Education Agency requires the Texas Assessment of Academic Skills (TAAS) be given to students in grades 3, 5, 7, 9, and 11. The Tattletooth program is correlated with the objectives and instructional targets of TAAS, thus providing students an opportunity to practice meeting those objectives prior to testing.

Teacher evaluation is done annually by principals and supervisors. Texas teachers are evaluated with a 65-item checklist. The Tattletooth lessons incorporate all the items that could be written into the lessons. A scope and sequence chart shows the teacher what he or she is to teach and what the teacher in the previous grade level should have taught. It also tells the teacher what the students are to learn the next year.

Tattletooth II embraces the six elements of effective lesson design: anticipatory set, setting the objective, input modeling, checking for understanding, guided practice, and independent practice. It emphasizes the important aspects of planning in successful teaching. Teaching decisions fall into three categories:

1. What content to teach next
2. What the student will do to learn
3. What the student will do to prove that learning has occurred

Program implementation. The Texas Department of Health is divided into eight public health regions and employs 16 hygienists in the regions who implement the Tattletooth program. The hygienists instruct teachers using videotapes designed for teacher training and provide them with a copy of the curriculum. In some instances the hygienists are training lead teachers who, in turn, provide training for teachers in their schools.

The bureau provides teachers with a unit overview and a section on organizing dental health lessons. Health promotion activities are encouraged and publicized within the school community. Teachers are encouraged to invite a dental professional to demonstrate brushing and flossing in the classroom. A field trip to a dental office is strongly recommended for kindergarten children. Each unit has a brief introduction that summarizes and gives a theme to the unit. Some units have planning notes that remind the teacher of the need for advance preparations. A unit test is provided so that the teacher will not have to write one. It can also be used as a pretest for diagnostic purposes.

Other resources include bulletin board suggestions, a book list, films, and videotapes available on a free loan for appropriate grade levels, a list of companies providing supplementary classroom resources, and a comprehensive glossary of vocabulary words written for the teacher in English and Spanish that are used in all grade levels.

Topics covered in the curriculum include correct brushing and flossing techniques, awareness of the importance of safety, and factual information relating to dental disease, its causes, and preventive techniques.

In the spring of 1987 the Bureau of Dental Health held a dental health conference for college and university instructors. It is anticipated that these instructors will begin to prepare college students in teacher preparation classes to implement the oral health program. Training students in the 23 college preparatory programs is anticipated to produce less demand for teacher training time and also college students who are motivated and prepared to teach oral health when they get to the classroom.

Cost of program. The Texas Department of Health has no tangible studies to support the cost-effectiveness of the Tattletooth II program in all eight public health regions. In 1990 the regional dental director for Public Health Region Six assessed the cost for program implementation at $289.25 per workshop. Because an average of 953 children benefit from each workshop, the cost per child was estimated at $0.60.

Program evaluation. In the spring of 1988, Tattletooth II underwent formative evaluation by teachers who were selected equally from each of the eight public health regions in Texas. A 19-item questionnaire was developed, consisting of four parts: a set of questions common to each lesson, a set of questions specific to each lesson, a set of questions regarding the lessons as a whole, and a set of questions regarding the teacher's manual. The teachers provided many comments and recommended program modifications. These recommendations were addressed in the second and final draft of the curriculum.

In 1989 a statewide summative evaluation of the seven levels of the Tattletooth II curriculum was conducted. Regional staff received brief training prior to implementing the evaluation. The training and the videotapes were the only things standardized about the teacher training. Bureau staff negotiated scheduling time with each school district and/or school. The amount of time devoted to teacher training varied at each training. The summative evaluation form was the last page of the curriculum. Staff were encouraged to instruct teachers to complete and return the evaluation to the bureau after unit completion during the 1989-90 school year. The evaluation was designed to include a total of 392 teachers: 56 teachers on each grade level and 7 teachers per grade, per region. An estimated 8,624 students were included in the summative evaluation, assuming a class size of 22 students per grade. The 19-item formative evaluation questionnaire was modified and was used as the summative evaluation instrument. A total of 351 of the teachers (89.5%) returned the questionnaire. The rate of returned curriculum evaluations was unevenly distributed among the eight regions.

The results of the Tattletooth II evaluation were positive, with teachers praising the teacher-student interaction that was present as a result of the format. Student responses to the curriculum were positive or very positive. About half the teachers responding had used the previous program, and half the teachers were new to the program. Approximately 94% of the teachers felt that teaching oral health can have a positive effect on children's dental health habits. Most teachers (90%) taught dental health once per year, and the average number of hours in which dental health was taught was 4.2. The bureau states that given teaching requirements, the fact that 88.7% of the teachers spent 45 minutes to 6½ hours teaching "Tattletooth II, A New Generation" is an indication that the curriculum was well received.

The curriculum materials were successful in teaching dental information and in increasing awareness of dental health practices. However, results indicate that the majority of teachers did not provide students with the opportunity to practice the skills of brushing and flossing. Toothbrushes and floss are not readily available because they are no longer provided by the dental program. Although teachers demonstrate dental hygiene skills, students will not master skills unless they are given an opportunity to practice them. Greater efforts need to be made to provide all classroom teachers with an adequate quantity of toothbrushes and dental floss to establish and maintain daily oral care programs.

Parent program

"Dental Health Is a Family Affair" is a slide-tape education program for parents. The program is coordinated by Texas Department of Health's dental hygienists for use with groups such as school parent groups, local health departments, and clinics.

The content covers dental disease problems and their prevention, as well as diet and a section describing characteristics of children's dental development ranging from prenatal to late adolescence. "Dental Health Is a Family Affair" won the ADA Meritorious Award in Community Preventive Dentistry.

Senior citizen program

Four presentations make up the senior citizen's oral health program. The presentations are all geared toward noninstitutionalized senior citizens. The first session provides general oral health information. The second presentation consists of a demonstration of brushing and flossing of natural teeth. The purpose of the third session is to demonstrate the proper method for cleaning partials and dentures. In some regions the dental hygienists clean the dentures in the ultrasonic cleaner and label them. When possible, a fourth session is scheduled, during which a volunteer dentist examines the participants for oral cancer and answers any questions they have.

Prenatal and postnatal program

The prenatal and postnatal program is divided into three parts. The first slide-tape or video presentation, "Mom, It's Up to You! Your Health Depends on You!" focuses on dental diseases and their causes, effective oral hygiene aids, drugs during pregnancy, and proper nutrition. It is followed by a demonstration of brushing. The second presentation, "Mom, It's Up to You! Your Baby Depends on You!" discusses fluoride, aids in relieving teething discomfort, nursing bottle mouth syndrome, and brushing and flossing the baby's teeth. This presentation is followed by a demonstration of flossing. In the presentation "Mom, It's Up to You! Your Toddler Depends on You!" the participant learns about primary and permanent teeth,

dental accidents, and thumbsucking. Each presentation takes about 15 minutes plus demonstration time.[95]

North Carolina statewide dental public health program

Development. North Carolina has a long history of involvement in dental public health and school dental health education. The need for a school dental health education program was realized as early as 1918 when the first scientific paper addressing this subject was presented to the North Carolina Dental Society. Since then, many supportive actions have been initiated, including fluoridation of community water supplies and comprehensive state surveys of the dental disease problems. In 1970 the North Carolina Dental Society passed resolutions advocating a strong preventive dental disease program embracing school and community fluoridation, fluoride treatments for schoolchildren, continuing education on prevention for dental professionals, and plaque-control education in schools and communities.

In 1973 Frank E. Law prepared a report for the North Carolina Dental Society that defined the extent of the dental disease problem and resulted in the initiation of a 10-year program to reduce dental disease. The 10-year preventive dentistry plan had the approval and support of the North Carolina General Assembly. In that same year a coalition of several agencies set up a steering committee that was responsible for developing a practical plan for a program in the schools.[15] This was the first statewide program of its magnitude and remains the largest and most comprehensive of all state public health dental programs. Continuation and expansion of the North Carolina Preventive Dentistry Program for Children (NCPDPC) according to the original plan has been made possible through incremental funding from the state legislature. Initial appropriations in 1974 funded 10% of the program. Under the original plan the program would expand annually by about 10% so that in 10 years the program would include the entire state. A few lean budgetary years hindered progress. Currently the program offers some services to all counties, but the numbers of services provided depends on staff availability.

In addition to funding appropriations from the

state legislature, the North Carolina Division of Dental Health has received funding through grants awarded by the Kate B. Reynolds Health Care Trust. These projects include producing 19 videotapes for classroom teachers in teaching dental health and conducting a statewide oral health survey of a representative sample of North Carolina schoolchildren from kindergarten through grade 12 during the 1986-87 school year.

With the North Carolina Oral Health Survey in 1986, the Division of Dental Health started the process of establishing new long-range goals for the state that reinforce and expand upon those started in 1973.

Program philosophy and goals. The North Carolina Dental Public Health Program is a unique public and private partnership dedicated to the mission of assuring conditions in which North Carolina citizens can achieve optimal oral health. Dental health is considered an important part of general health and can be achieved through the coordinated efforts of individuals, professionals, and community members.[69-72]

The Division of Dental Health's programs are based on prevention and education. The division is organized to provide as many direct services to the citizens of North Carolina as possible. The majority of the staff, public health dentists and dental hygienists, are located in the counties to provide services through local health departments. Primary prevention and education are considered to be the most effective means of decreasing dental disease and promoting dental health. All program activities include educational components to modify the behavior patterns of individuals to improve their oral health habits through dietary change, toothbrushing, and flossing. Young children are the primary focus for education because the earlier a child is reached, the greater the potential for positively affecting the child's attitudes, values, and behaviors. Fluoride is recognized as the most effective public health measure for preventing dental caries.

Objectives that will facilitate attainment of the goals of the division include (1) appropriate use of fluoride, (2) health education in schools and communities, and (3) availability of public health dental staff in all counties.

Program implementation. Dental surveys provide epidemiologic and sociodemographic data useful for program planning, implementation, and evaluation. Dental public health program decisions in North Carolina are founded on statewide, population-based oral health surveys conducted by the Division of Dental Health and the University of North Carolina School of Public Health.[35,49] In the dental health status report presented in 1973, dental disease was found to affect 95% of the total population.[49] Rozier in 1982 stated that the teenage population is at greater risk of developing dental caries than any other age group and that 45% of children and adolescents show evidence of periodontal disease, almost all of which is reversible. According to the 1986-87 North Carolina School Oral Health Survey, 53% of children 5 to 17 years of age have never had a cavity in their permanent teeth.[59]

Disease levels have been going steadily downward since the 1960s. This trend is true for all races and for both the younger and older age groups, but in different degrees of magnitude. There has been a continuing increase in dental care for all children.

The epidemiologic and sociodemographic data from surveys provide needed information for planning, implementing, and evaluating a community-based program. The comprehensive nature of the problem's definition is reflected in the uniqueness of the program, which is designed to reach several segments of the population: young children, parents, teachers, dental professionals, and community leaders. The fiscal year 1990 services delivered through the program included the fluoridation of the water supplies of 130 rural schools; weekly fluoride mouthrinse for more than 416,000 students in 1,051 schools; and screening and referral for more than 339,000 children. Dental health education was presented to 361,000 children and 42,000 adults. More than 33,000 dental sealants were applied.[69]

The coordinated efforts of the staff of dentists, dental hygienists, and health educators is extremely important in program implementation. The activities of the central office consultant staff (made available to all public health dentists and hygienists in the state) provide for continuity in program planning and implementation. With 49 public health dental hygienists and 14 public health dentists working in local programs, it is important that consultation services necessary for program growth be available to them.[59] Also, the consultants serve in a capacity that helps coordinate the individual county programs and needs of staff through statewide conferences, in this way retaining and promoting the philosophy of the statewide preventive dental health program.

To reach children, public health dental staff provide training and consultation to those who work with preschool and school-age children and maternal and child health programs, for example, elementary school teachers, health department staff, and parents. Teachers are believed to be the key in the educational program; to improve their capability for teaching and reinforcement of sound dental principles, they receive preservice, in-service, and follow-up training to cover dental health concepts, practice oral hygiene skills, and integrate dental health into the curriculum.

To help teachers be more effective in their classrooms North Carolina has developed the curriculum "Framework for Dental Health Education," classroom and teacher videos, and teacher guides for kindergarten through grade six, which are integrated with the state-level department of public instruction.

Several additional teaching aids are available for North Carolinians, such as more than 50 different leaflets, worksheets, and handouts on nutrition, fluoride, plaque control, routine dental visits, injury prevention, and smokeless tobacco. In addition, the film library contains some 30 films, videos, and slide sets on dental health, which are free on loan to any school in the state, in addition to the framework videos, which have been distributed to each county. (Note: Because of budget limitations, the materials are made available only to educators and health professionals in North Carolina.)

During 1988 the Division of Dental Health in the North Carolina Department of Environment, Health, and Natural Resources (which was then the Dental Health Section of the North Carolina Department of Human Resources) celebrated the seventieth anniversary of dental public health in the state.

The anniversary theme, "Thanks for the Smiles," and the celebrations were selected to convey appreciation to the countless people who had helped the dental health program over the 70 years. This anniversary celebration was a cooperative venture of citizens, government, private business, and practicing dentists in coordination with the North Carolina Citizens for Public Health, Inc., which is a unique nonprofit corporation for the promotion of public health in North Carolina.

The yearlong anniversary celebration involved three statewide activities in addition to local celebrations in nearly all counties across the state. These celebrations recognized past and current developments and initiated planning for future programs.

A symposium, "Looking to the Future: Exploring Community Approaches to Dental Health," was the final event of this yearlong celebration. The purpose of the symposium was threefold: to provide a forum for exploring the future directions in dental public health, to share ways of enhancing the role of dental public health in the health movement, and to examine methods of coalition building outside health-related fields. Dental public health is more than the prevention and treatment of disease. The social, legal, and ethical issues that affect people's lives must be taken into account. Because the ideas and viewpoints of citizens and representatives from other disciplines must be incorporated in the planning process for dental public health programs, the participants at the symposium included representatives from the private practice of dentistry, dental education, medicine, law, ethics, business and industry, finance, government, and the public at large.

Table 9-1 provides an overview of the total program integrating the three components: education, prevention, and dental care. It also illustrates the focus of education for parents, dental professionals, and community leaders.

North Carolinians believe that one reason their community dental health program has been so successful is the support of the North Carolina Dental Society, which in 1972 went before the legislature to seek funding for the statewide program.

The Division of Dental Health's screening, referral, and follow-up program attempts to maximize the resources available in the private sector and third-party reimbursement. This, most effectively and efficiently, uses the private-practice dentists throughout the state to provide the primary care component of the dental care delivery system.

Program evaluation. Evaluation has been and will continue to be a necessary ongoing process to measure the effectiveness of the dental health program. Some of the evaluations that have been conducted are:[69-72,83,84]

1. The results of a 1968 survey of schoolchildren at the Happy Valley School in Caldwell County, North Carolina, where the school water supply had been fluoridated for 8 years, indicated a 34% reduction in decayed, missing, and filled permanent teeth for children who had 8 years' experience drinking fluoridated water at school.

2. Data collected in the 1976 replication of the 1963 Fulton-Hughes survey were used to evaluate long-range goals and objectives.

3. A 1976 survey of schoolchildren in Asheville, North Carolina, where the community's water supply had been fluoridated for 10 years, revealed a 53% reduction in decayed, missing, and filled permanent teeth for children who had had 10 years' experience drinking fluoridated water.

4. A 1984 survey on the use of sealants in public health dental programs demonstrated an 86% total retention rate after 4 years on permanent teeth.

5. A statewide oral health survey of 7,000 school-age children in 1986-87 had the objectives (1) to describe the oral health status and factors associated with this status by recording the survey participant's DMFTs, DMFSs for primary (deft, dfs) and permanent dentition; number of teeth sealed with dental sealants; extent of gingivitis; and restorative and exodontic treatment needs; (2) to determine the extent, type, and frequency of use of smokeless tobacco products, patterns of use, and knowledge of harmful effects; and (3) to establish a policy advisory committee to the division for Dental Health to the Year 2000. The results of this survey may affect program planning for dental health nationwide.

In addition to these surveys, the effectiveness of the education program in changing knowledge, attitudes, values, and practices of students is evaluated. Effects of the educational program may not become evident for 15 to 20 years; however, the results are expected to be positive (Table 9-2).

SUGGESTED APPROACHES

Each of the community dental health education programs that has been described was chosen for three reasons: first, these programs are some of the most widely known and reported in the literature; second, they represent a variety of approaches to dental health education; third, they illustrate the range of success that can be expected to be achieved, given their programmatic structure and goals. Using the criteria that are presented in Chapters 8 and 10, several issues for discussion should become apparent. For instance, if we assume that the goal for a dental health education program for the community is to reduce the prevalence of dental caries, which of the programs, if any, are using the most cost-effective and clinically proven preventive measures? Which of the programs are using evaluation criteria that will measure caries experience? Which of the programs have determined their priorities based on the collection of data gathered through a formal needs assessment? Which programs are easily implemented and administered?

Answers to these questions begin to identify the inherent weaknesses in the majority of the programs, which to a large extent have lost sight of the goals of disease prevention and tooth conservation. In these cases the primary objectives emphasize motivating a group of students to practice positive health behaviors as if they were individual patients. Success is based on long-term behavior change, which is very difficult to obtain and may not be practical for dental public health.* As concluded at a 1973 conference on prevention and oral health sponsored by the Fogarty International Center for Advanced Study in Health Sciences and the National Institute of Dental Research, "mechanical procedures for plaque prevention do not offer a promising solution to the problem of control of dental diseases for the population at large."[16] In addition, a clear-cut cause-and-effect relationship between dental plaque and caries has

---

References 4, 16, 21, 32, 41, 42.

Table 9-1 Schematic presentation of preventive dental health program in North Carolina

Agencies involved	Target audiences	Approaches
NC Department of Public Instruction NC Department of Environment, Health, and Natural Resources, Division of Dental Health North Carolina Dental Society University of North Carolina School of Dentistry and School of Public Health North Carolina Dental Hygienist's Association North Carolina Dental Assistant's Association North Carolina Association of Local Health Directors	1. Teachers and staff of preschool programs and elementary schools	In-service training for teachers Preservice training in teacher-training institutions Public health dental consultation Provision of educational materials
	2. Students in preschool and elementary grades	Fluoridation of community water supplies Fluoridation of rural school water supplies Fluoride mouthrinse and other topical applications Educational programs and materials for schools Preventive dental services for eligible children
	3. Parents of students	Parent education Education such as agricultural extension clubs, 4-H, civic and community groups Use of mass media for education Partnership with public health personnel such as health educators, nurses, and public health programs such as Maternal and Child Health
	4. Dentists and auxiliaries including students	Representation on advocacy committees for dental public health
	5. Community leaders, official and lay	Professional education

From State of North Carolina, Department of Environment, Health, and Natural Resources Division of Dental Health, Raleigh, NC.

not been clinically proven in human populations. The Research Committee of the American Association of Public Health Dentists in their report "Programs for the Mass Control of Plaque: An Appraisal," states: "On theoretical grounds, it may appear evident that the daily, thorough removal of plaque should have a marked effect on reducing the increment of new carious lesions. As this report attempts to point out, however, this supposition cannot be supported with clinical evidence."[50]

Yacovone[105] has also noted, "Some authorities in community health feel that prevention will only be successful when individual behavior is eliminated." If this is the case, then community educational efforts must focus on those disease-prevention strategies that require the least compliance on the part of the individual. This would require a reorientation to health education and its goal, as well as redirecting the educational efforts to community leaders in an attempt to improve the oral health status through organized community efforts.[32]

This is not to say that school-based educational programs should be eliminated or are not valuable; it does, however, indicate the need for further behavioral research and the need for communities to decide which of the preventive programs and which of the strategies or measures now employed in each program should take priority. If community leaders are expected to make these decisions, then they must be given the tools to do so. This

Table 9-1 Schematic presentation of preventive dental health program in North Carolina—cont'd

Items in dental public health program	Sources of funds

1. Fluoridation of community water supplies
2. Fluoridation of rural school water supplies
3. Appropriate use of fluorides such as mouthrinse, topical applications, and supplements
4. Dental health education in preschools and elementary schools, including preservice and inservice training for teachers and staff
5. Dental education for consumers to include parents and community leaders via agencies such as agricultural extension, industry, civic clubs, and mass media
6. Support services such as:
   Provision of public health dental staff, health educators, maintenance staff
   Provision of supplies and equipment for dental staff
   Production and distribution of educational training aids
7. Coordinated planning among agencies such as the North Carolina Dental Society, North Carolina Committee for Dental Health, and the Division of Dental Health
	Primarily state appropriations for salaries, clinical supplies, office supplies, and educational materials
	Salaries for central office staff include 3 public health dentists, 3 dental health educators, 1 dental hygiene consultant, and other administrative staff to work with 47 field-based public health hygienists and 13 public health dentists as a team for educational and clinical services, as well as other services such as statistical assistance for research, artwork, photography, film rental or purchase
	Six of the 100 counties in NC provide local funding for dental public health programs, including the salaries and supplies for dentists, dental hygienists, and dental assistants; several other counties fund the salaries of dental hygienists and dental assistants; 61 staff are employed full-time by county health departments
	Federal funds augment state funds in the fluoridation of community and rural school water supplies for equipment and training

would necessitate a new role or new responsibilities for the community dental health educator. Frazier states that the appropriate educational methods for this target group are those designed to (1) provide accurate information about the relative merits of various disease prevention and control measures, and (2) stimulate group decision making and action regarding the adoption of effective organized programs.[32]

If these new responsibilities are to be assumed, we must know if community dental health educators are presently prepared and willing to adopt this new role. Hunter's study[50] indicates that dental hygienists feel "capable of providing services for DMF surveys, plaque control programs for community groups and fluoride self-application programs." The dental hygienists surveyed, however, reported lower feelings of competence in areas of health legislation and in serving as an officer or committee member of the national dental hygiene association, both of which require organizational skills and leadership ability.[50] Frazier[31] speaks of the possibility of an alternative educational role in which "the community-based hygienist could become skillful in organizing meetings, conducting seminars and workshops for decision-makers, opinion leaders and community groups." The development of these organizational skills would require appropriate educational experiences, which dental and dental hygiene students presently do not receive as part of their professional training. These skills might best be learned through required field experiences in the community dentistry or public health courses.

Table 9-2 Summary of dental health education programs in terms of development, program philosophy and goals, implementation, costs, and evaluation

	Characteristics of program	
Name of program	Development	Philosophy and goals
Learning about Your Oral Health, ADA	Request for ADA's House of Delegates in 1971 ADA and consultants	Comprehensive program covering preschool, K-12 goal—develop knowledge, skills, and attitudes to prevent disease Priority—plaque-control knowledge and skills
Texas Department of Health, Tattletooth II program, parent program, senior citizen program, prenatal and postnatal program	Texas Department of Health	Goal—reduce dental caries and develop positive dental habits to last a lifetime Program tries to convince students that preventing dental disease is important and they can do it Program focuses on dental health as a part of total health
North Carolina dental public health program	North Carolina Division of Dental Health, dental organizations, Department of Public Instruction, University of North Carolina School of Dentistry and School of Public Health, plus support of General Assembly Based on the documented needs assessment of North Carolina citizens	Prevention and education: prevention and education are the most effective methods to significantly change the prevalence and incidence of dental disease and to promote, protect, and assure oral health for the citizens. Priority—children Mission: assure conditions in which North Carolina citizens can achieve optimal oral health. Long-range plan for continuing the use of dental health materials in the competency-based curriculum "Framework for Dental Health Education"—emphasizes role of classroom elementary teacher for integrating dental health education into curriculum

Although students generally participate in school-based community programs, other types of organized community efforts should serve as viable field experience alternatives. Following are several issues that require professional support and involvement and are currently receiving national attention:

1. Water fluoridation
2. Appropriate use of fluoride mouthrinses, supplements, and topical applications
3. Sealants
4. Frequency of use, types of product used, patterns of use, and knowledge about the harmful effects of smokeless tobacco
5. Efforts by consumer interest and child advocacy groups, such as Action for Children's Television, Center for Science in the Public Interest, and the National Parent and Teachers Congress, and professional organization such as the AAP to monitor and restrict ad-

Table 9-2 Summary of dental health education programs in terms of development, program philosophy and goals, implementation, costs, and evaluation—cont'd

Characteristics of program		
Implementation	**Costs**	**Evaluation**
Five levels with core material for teachers to adapt to needs of students Overheads and spirit masters are included Films and videotapes are available Dental hygienists serve as technical consultants for school districts and promote dental education for expectant women, parents, and senior citizens Supportive materials are available for teachers and program hygienists	$8 for teaching packet Film and videotape rental and sales costs vary	Levels I and II—pretests and posttests Behavioral objectives provide basis for teachers to develop evaluation mechanisms
Statewide implementation plan Teachers are trained to present dental health information for school-age population Priorities are community and rural school water fluoridation and fluoride mouthrinse Public health dental staff provides training and consultative services to teachers, parents, professionals, and community Several teaching adjuncts are available; curriculum videotapes and guides	Estimated at $0.60 per child; state-legislated budget State budget includes salaries	Field testing Statewide continuous monitoring of material use Comprehensive survey of dental disease in 1976 and 1986-87 funded by Kate B. Reynolds Health Care Trust Survey of schoolchildren after 10 years of community water fluoridation and 8 years of rural school water fluoridation

vertising of cariogenic, high-cholesterol, nonnutritious foods directed at children
6. Infection-control measures
7. Healthy People 2000 national health promotion and disease prevention objectives[99]

The need for active participation in these areas cannot be overemphasized. Visible support and action in the community, for instance, can make the difference in whether a referendum for water fluoridation is passed.[26,30,43,60] Two examples illus-

trating this point are the defeat of the referendum to continue water fluoridation in Flagstaff, Arizona, in March 1978 and the passage of the referendum in Seattle, Washington, in 1973.

Fluoridation, in each of these cases and in most cases, has proved to be a highly emotionally charged issue. In Flagstaff, organized opponents to water fluoridation, namely, the National Health Federation (NHF), held public forums and disseminated large amounts of propaganda. The usual tactic was to link fluoridation to cancer. Other arguments—that fluoridation is unconstitutional, fluoridation is a form of medication, and fluoridation is contrary to the right of "free choice of health care"—were also cited.[67] To combat these unscientific charges and the emotional fervor with which they are made it is incumbent on all dental professionals in the community and students during their training to familiarize themselves with the NHF and other antifluoridation groups' strategies and the documented evidence refuting their claims. It is also a professional responsibility to educate voters, community leaders, and agencies regarding the benefits of fluoridation and regarding the movements opposed to fluoridation, which pose a danger to the oral health of the community. In the Flagstaff, Arizona case, an initial survey indicated that the referendum would pass 2 to 1; however, the NHF was able to reverse this prediction by creating an illusion of scientific controversy. Fortunately, in Seattle, Washington, the opposition was not as active or successful. Here the dental profession focused on building a broad base of community support; it educated people to understand the workings of the ballot and on how to vote. Fifteen days before voters went to the poll, dental and dental hygiene students along with community volunteers actively campaigned door-to-door for fluoridation. This successful strategy should be examined by communities where fluoridation is an issue. Success at one point in time does not mean that at some future date the decision could not be reversed, as it was in Flagstaff. Dental professionals must continue to be visible in the community to reinforce the benefits of fluoridation and the decision made by the voters. Dental health education must be provided on a continuous basis if it is to serve as a means for health promotion.

Student activities and the degree of involvement in each of the listed areas may vary from state to state. An examination of existing legislation and accreditation standards for primary and secondary schools can provide students with "ammunition" to assist communities in improving their oral health. Action taken by the Alabama Dental Association to eliminate the sale of sweets in local schools led to their discovery of the Southern Association of Schools' accreditation standard, which prohibits the sale of sweets in schools, and resulted in its enforcement. The standard was not being enforced by the Accrediting Division of the Department of Education because it did not have a working definition of the word *confection*. The Alabama Dental Association and Alabama Nutrition Council were able to provide the needed definition, as well as a list of acceptable snack foods. This effort should serve as an example of what can be accomplished, and it identifies activities in which students can certainly become involved.[88]

Educational experiences in these areas will afford students the opportunity to begin developing necessary organizational and planning skills. Only through working with dental and other professional societies, state and local agencies, and community leaders and decision makers can an organized community effort be effective in preventing and controlling dental disease.

RESEARCH

The most promising avenue to improving oral health lies in the prevention of dental disease.

The National Institute of Dental Research (NIDR) National Caries Program conducted an 11-year study beginning in 1972 to determine the long-term effects of the combination of student-applied fluoride agents (fluoride mouthrinsing, fluoride tablets, and fluoride toothpaste) among schoolchildren living in a rural area with low concentrations of fluoride in the drinking water. In school, participating students ingested a 1-mg fluoride tablet and rinsed weekly with a 0.2% sodium fluoride solution. The children also received fluoride dentifrice and toothbrushes for home use throughout the calendar year. In 1983 dental examinations of study participants aged 6 to 17 years, who had continuously participated in the program for 1 to 11 years, depending on school grade, showed a mean prevalence of 3.12 DMFS, which was 65% lower than the corresponding score of 9.02 DMFS for children of the same ages at the baseline examinations. The preventive program inhibited decay in all types of surfaces: 54% in occlusal surfaces, 59% in buccolingual surfaces, and 90% in mesiodistal surfaces.[46]

In a second study conducted by the NIDR National Caries Program the effects of supervised daily dental plaque removal by children were evaluated for a 3-year period. This study was initiated in 1973 in a rural fluoride-deficient community. Approximately 450 children in grades 5 through 8 were initially included in the study to determine the effect on oral hygiene, gingival inflammation, and dental caries from supervised daily flossing and brushing in school. A fluoride-free dentifrice was used. In June 1976 final examinations were conducted using the same indices and examiners:

In the treatment group, the mean plaque and gingival scores at program completion were 18% and 29% lower, respectively, than at baseline. The differences in plaque and gingival scores were statistically significant. However, differences between groups disappeared during summer vacation. The increment of dental caries was lower in the treatment group but not significant either for teeth or for surfaces.[45]

The National Preventive Dentistry Demonstration Program (NPDDP), carried out between 1976 and 1983, was the largest, most comprehensive school-based preventive dentistry program ever conducted anywhere. Its purpose was to determine the costs and effectiveness of several types and combinations of generally accepted school-based preventive dental procedures to provide the database for developing the most effective modern school-based preventive dental program. The preventive procedures selected included five general categories: (1) fluorides (topical and systemic), (2) sealants, (3) diet regulation, (4) plaque control, and (5) classroom health education. The major findings from this program follow:

1. There was a sharp decline in the prevalence of dental caries from the later 1970s to the early 1980s.
2. The application of dental sealants is the most effective preventive measure of those used in the program.
3. Community water fluoridation is effective in reducing dental caries.
4. Classroom-based preventive measures are ineffective.[54,81]

The study was reviewed and critiqued by a review committee of the American Public Health Association. Although the committee had reservations as to the specific design of the study as well as the analytical methods applied, their general consensus was that the first three findings of the

study appear to be correct. The fourth finding is considered questionable because of possible flaws in study design. Niessen[68] forecasts that health education programs will continue to be an important component of the dental public health program.

The NPDDP suggests several elements of dental research that need improvement or greater emphasis. The profession should adopt a more conservative attitude when projecting the expected benefits from the practical application of preventive measures whose merit is supported by only a few clinical trials conducted by a limited number of investigators. Many clinical trials conducted by totally independent investigators should be mandated before any preventive measure is regarded as safe, effective, and efficient.

It is imprudent to neglect basic research while pushing ahead with practical application. The lack of basic research on the mechanism of fluoride action in the prevention of dental decay and in the production of enamel fluorosis was evident from this study. Several of the modes of application of the agent may have been duplicating rather than reinforcing each other.

Greater attention should be given to monitoring the prevalence of dental diseases so that up-to-date indices are available that will further delineate characteristics of populations to be studied. There is a need for maintenance of an established pool of skilled clinical investigators who would be available to take part in large-scale national clinical trials. Also, there is a need to foster new research leading to improved clinical trial methodology, reduced cost, and possibly the reduction in the size of groups to be studied.

As a result of this study, two additional areas of research have been identified: (1) there is a definite need to develop and apply better outcome measures for the evaluation of the effectiveness of school dental health education programs, and (2) more research is needed to identify the significant characteristics of groups susceptible to dental diseases.[81]

In 1986-87 NIDR[64] conducted the National Survey of Dental Caries in U.S. School Children, which revealed that 53% of children age 6 to 8 years and 78% of 15-year-olds have caries. Further, the proportion of black and Hispanic adolescents with untreated decay is approximately 65%

higher than for the total population. Periodontal disease is also quite prevalent. Results from the North Carolina School Oral Health Survey of 1986-87 referenced earlier parallel much of the data from the NIDR survey.[84]

Given that fluoridation is highly cost-effective and requires no behavior change on the part of the individual to produce its effects, future research should explore strategies for increasing its acceptance.[89] In fluoridated areas, surveys should be conducted to determine if families are consuming fluoridated tap water versus purchased bottled water, which may lack the appropriate fluoride content. Perhaps targeting groups at high risk may be a more effective way to reach individuals affected with caries.[68]

Further details about each of the previously mentioned research projects can be obtained from the organizations involved.

SUMMARY

An analysis of the information presented in this chapter leads to several conclusions regarding the status of and future for community dental health education programs. We have seen that the traditional educational activities based on either the cognitive or behavioral models of learning alone cannot be effective in achieving the goal of disease prevention and control. Techniques developed and refined for educating an individual patient differ from those that should be applied to the community. Behavioral research and expert opinions agree that educational methodologies are now available that can be successfully applied to the community at large, as demonstrated by the Stanford Five City Project and the Minnesota Home Team. Are dental public health professionals ready and willing to use the public health model for contemporary health education and foster community involvement in decision making? Will such community involvement change the perception of dental disease so that persons will seek early detection and treatment for problems? Will financial barriers continue to alienate many subgroups within American society from obtaining desired or needed dental treatment? Are we fostering public-sector and private-sector partnerships to advance health education and health promotion? Are we continuing to build a strong network of support for dental public health by forming coalitions with other health care professionals, industry, legislators, parents, patients, and health advocacy organizations? Are we as health professionals monitoring children's television program advertising to assure that broadcasters carry children's educational or instructional programming that promotes health and well-being? Are we participating in efforts on the state and local community levels to achieve Healthy People 2000 national health promotion and disease prevention objectives?

Dental health education programs for the community should be applicable to all segments of the population and should be developed through appropriate program planning and implementation criteria. A needs assessment should be conducted to define the extent of the problem and serve as baseline data and to determine program objectives and priorities, alternative solutions, and evaluation guidelines. Formative and summative evaluation must be an ongoing and integral component of the plan; it must focus on measuring the program's effectiveness in terms of disease reduction, not merely increased knowledge or improved performance level. Longitudinal behavioral studies should be conducted to validate the cost-benefit and cost-effectiveness ratios of each program.

Existing curricula and field experiences for dental and dental hygiene students must be reexamined and revised in light of the new responsibilities these professionals must assume in the community setting. Students should be educated in community organization, group dynamics, program planning and implementation strategies, effectiveness of community preventive measures, community decision-making processes, and the necessary communication, management, and leadership skills.

Research must continue to develop, test, and evaluate new combinations of preventive programs and to evaluate the effectiveness of any new strategies for community dental health education. More must be known about the relationship between plaque and dental caries and about the acquisition of oral health as a value. Community programs must use the approaches most likely to succeed against known barriers to receiving dental care and maintaining good oral health.

If the success of dental health education programs in schools is judged by effectiveness based on knowledge, attitudes, and skill acquisition, evaluators of such programs must be held accountable for conducting evaluation studies in a manner appropriate to these predetermined general objectives.

Dental health education in schools can be more of a priority, however, that involves the efforts of many people. Universities and colleges charged with the responsibility of preparing school personnel must include dental health as a component of the curriculum. School districts also need to explore ways of including dental health education on a permanent basis. Parents must be encouraged to support dental health activities through reinforcement at home and can also join health professionals in demanding that dental health education be a mandatory component of health education in every curriculum. We also need more professional support for proven effective preventive measures such as water fluoridation, appropriate use of fluoride supplements, and topical applications and sealants.

There are several major changes taking place that will affect the dental profession and the oral health of the public: a reduction in tooth decay, an increased awareness of the prevalence of periodontal disease, infection control and dental treatment phobias associated with contraction of HIV disease, population demographics that may affect the prevalence of root caries, periodontal conditions and oral cancer in association with advancing age, and finally an alarming increase in the use of smokeless tobacco among American youth, as well as the increase in oral cancer associated with tobacco use and alcohol consumption. Future planning in community dental health education will include the targeting of preventive measures for specific subgroups with documented unmet needs within the general population. Innovative programs for persons with developmental disabilities residing in the community and in state institutions, as well as programs for the elderly (ambulatory, homebound, and institutionalized) have been developed. Homeless individuals and families, unemployed or underemployed and uninsured people, and children and adults who have HIV disease have a myriad of unaddressed needs, one of which is professional dental care. Creativity and resourcefulness in future program planning are essential in view of our finite resources, especially funding, which is so crucial to program development, implementation, and evaluation.

REFERENCES

1. Action for Children's Television: News release, Cambridge, Mass, June 3, 1991, The Organization.
2. American Academy of Pediatrics: *Policy statement: the commercialization of childrens' television,* Chicago, 1991, American Academy of Pediatrics.
3. American Academy of Pediatrics: *News release: pediatricians suggest eliminating TV food ads aimed at children, criticize children's television,* Chicago, July 23, 1991, The Academy.
4. American Association of State and Territorial Dental Directors: *Policy statement: resolution on preventive dentistry,* March 1974, The Association.
5. American Dental Association: Ask higher dental priorities at AMA-Kennedy meeting, *ADA Leadership Bull* 7(16), 1978.
6. American Dental Association: *Learning about your oral health: a prevention-oriented school program,* Chicago, 1986, The Association.
7. American Dental Hygienists' Association: *Self-study course: care for the homebound patient,* Chicago, 1983, The Association.
8. American Dental Hygienists' Association: *Self-study course: contracting for services in alternative practice settings,* Chicago, 1986, The Association.
9. American Dental Hygienists' Association: *Self-study course: the dental health consultant in community-based programs,* Chicago, 1983, The Association.
10. American Dental Hygienists' Association: *Self-study course: dental hygiene care for the geriatric patient,* Chicago, 1986, The Association.
11. American Dental Hygienists' Association: *Self-study course: dental hygiene care of the special needs patient,* Chicago, 1983, The Association.
12. Assagioli R: *Psychosynthesis,* New York, 1971, Penguin Books.
13. Bandura A: *Social learning theory,* Englewood Cliffs, NJ, 1977, Prentice Hall.
14. Bandura A, Cervone D: Self-evaluative and self-efficacy mechanisms governing the motivational effects of goal systems, *J Pers Soc Psychol* 45:1017, 1983.
15. Bivins EC: *History and development of dental public health in North Carolina,* report prepared for the North Carolina Department of Human Resources, Division of Health Services, Dental Health Section, 1974.
16. Carlos JP, editor: *Prevention and oral health,* Fogarty International Center Series on Preventive Medicine, vol I, DHEW Pub No NIII 74-707, US Department of Health, Education and Welfare, Public Health Service, National Institute of Health, 1973.
17. Castile AS, Jerrick SJ: *School health in America,* ed 2, Atlanta, 1979, US Department of Health, Education and Welfare, American School Health Association.
18. Cautella JR: Covert reinforcement, *Behav Ther* 1:35, 1970.
19. Center for Science in the Public Interest: *News release: childrens' television called a junk food cafeteria,* Washington, DC, June 3, 1991, The Center.
20. Center for Science in the Public Interest, *Report: content analysis of childrens' television advertisements,* Washington, DC, 1991, The Center.

21. Chambers DW: Susceptibility to preventive dental treatment, *J Public Health Dent* 33:82, 1973.

22. Cozort PJ, Sheffrin S: *Learning about your oral health.* Paper presented at the first national symposium on dental health education in schools, American Dental Association, Bureau of Health Education, Chicago, October 1975.

23. Croucher R and others: The "spread effect" of a school-based dental health education project, *Community Dent Oral Epidemiol* 13:205, 1985.

24. Davis MS: Variations in patients' compliance with doctors' orders: analyses of congruence between survey responses and results of empirical investigations, *J Med Educ* 41:1037, 1966.

25. Davis RL and others: Comprehensive school health education: a practical definition, *J Sch Health* 55:335, 1985.

26. Domoto PK, Faine RC, Rovin S: Seattle fluoridation campaign 1973—prescription of a victory, *J Am Dent Assoc* 91:583, 1975.

27. Dworkin SF, Ference TP, Giddon DB: Behavioral science and dental practice, St. Louis, 1978, Mosby–Year Book.

28. Ezell OL: *Evaluation of the American Dental Association's prevention-oriented program in a school health education setting.* Paper presented at the first national symposium on dental health education in schools, American Dental Association, Bureau of Health Education, Chicago, October 1975.

29. Farquhar JW and others: *The Stanford five city project: an overview.* In Matarazzo JD, Weiss SM, Herd JA, editors: *Behavioral health: a handbook of health enhancement and disease prevention,* New York, 1984, Wiley.

30. Frankel JM, Allukian M: Sixteen referenda on fluoridation in Massachusetts: an analysis, *J Public Health Dent* 33:96, 1973.

31. Frazier PJ: A new look at dental health education in community programs, *Dent Hygiene* 52:535, 1978.

32. Frazier PJ: *The effectiveness and practicality of current dental health education programs from a public health perspective: a conceptual appraisal.* Paper presented at the Dental Health Section Symposium, annual meeting of the American Public Health Association, Miami Beach, October 1976.

33. Frazier PJ, Horowitz AM: Oral health education and promotion in maternal and child health, a position paper, *J Public Health Dent* 50:390, 1990.

34. Frazier PJ and others: Quality of information in mass media: a barrier to the dental health education of the public, *J Public Health Dent* 34:244, 1974.

35. Fulton J, Hughes JT: *The national history of dental disease,* Chapel Hill, NC, 1965 School of Public Health, University of North Carolina.

36. Gravies RC and others: A comparison of effectiveness of the "Toothkeeper" and a traditional dental health education program, *J Public Health Dent* 35:81, 1975.

37. Green LW: Bridging the gap between community health and school health, *Am J Public Health* 78:1149, 1988.

38. Green LW, Anderson CL: *Community health,* St. Louis, 1986, Mosby–Year Book.

39. Green LW, Johnson KW: *Health education and health promotion.* In Mechanic D, editor: *Handbook of health,* healthcare and the health professions, New York, 1983, Wiley.

40. Haefuer DP: School dental health programs, *Health Educ Monogr* 2:212, 1974.

41. Heifetz SB, Suomi JD: The control of dental caries and periodontal disease: a fundamental approach, *J Public Health Dent* 33:2, 1973.

42. Heifetz SB and others: Programs for the mass control of plaque: an appraisal, *J Public Health Dent* 33:91, 1973.

43. Hirakio SS, Foote FM: Statewide fluoridation: how it was done in Connecticut, *J Am Dent Assoc* 75:174, 1967.

44. Hochbaum GM: Interview Godfrey M. Hochbaum, PhD, *Fam Community Health* 12(3) 72:4, 1989.

45. Horowitz AM and others: Effect of supervised daily plaque removal by children: results after third and final year, *J Dent Res* 1977 (abstract).

46. Horowitz HS and others: Combined fluoride, school-based program in a fluoride-deficient area: results of an 11-year study, *J Am Dent Assoc* 112:621, 1986.

47. Horowitz HS and others: Evaluation of a combination of self-administered fluoride procedures for the control of dental caries in a nonfluoride area: findings after four years, *J Am Dent Assoc* 98:219, 1979.

48. Horowitz LG: The self-care motivation model: theory and practice in human development, *J Sch Health* 55:57, 1985.

49. Hughes JT, Rozier RG, Ramsey DL: *Natural history of dental diseases in NC, 1976-1977,* Durham, NC, 1982, Carolina Academic Press.

50. Hunter EL: Volunteerism of dental hygienists, *Dent Hygiene* 52:535, 1978.

51. Kamholtz JD, Wood B: Competing with Ronald McDonald, Cap'n Crunch and the Pepsi Generation, *J Sch Health* 52:17, 1982.

52. Kegeles SS: Why people seek dental care: a review of present knowledge, *Am J Public Health* 51:1306, 1961.

53. Kegeles SS: Why people seek dental care: a test of a conceptual formulation, *J Health Hum Behavior* 4:166, 1963.

54. Klein SP and others: The cost and effectiveness of school-based preventive dental care, *Am J Public Health* 75:382, 1985.

55. Levy GF: A survey of preschool oral health education programs, *J Public Health Dent* 44:10, 1984.

56. Lewin K: *Field theory in social science,* New York, 1951, Harper & Brothers.

57. Mahoney M, Thoreson C: *Self-control: power to the person,* Monterey, Calif, 1974 Brooks/Cole.

58. McClelland DC and others: *The achievement motive,* New York, 1976, Irvington.

59. McMahon EL, Hensey ER: Celebrating 70 years of NC dental public health, *J Public Health Dent* 50, 1990.

60. McNeil DR: Political aspects of fluoridation, *J Am Dent Assoc* 65:659, 1962.

61. Meichenbaum DH: *Cognitive behavior modification,* New York, 1976, Irvington.

62. Meskins HM, Martens LV, Katz BJ: Effectiveness of community preventive programs on improving oral health, *J Public Health Dent* 38:302, 1978.

63. Mulholland DN: A comprehensive dental health education program, *J Sch Health* 48:225, 1978.

64. National Institute of Dental Research: *Oral health of United States children: the national survey of dental caries in U.S. school children, 1986-1987,* DHHS Pub No (PHS) 89-2247, Bethesda, Md, 1989, US Department of Health and Human Services.
65. National PTA Statement: *Concern about T.V. advertising of non-nutritious foods to children,* Washington, DC, June 3, 1991. The Organization.
66. Nasi J: *Stakes of measures to prevent periodontal disease: effectiveness and practicality in community programs.* Paper presented at the annual meeting of the American Public Health Association, Miami Beach, October 1976.
67. National Health Federation: *This is the National Health Federation,* leaflet.
68. Niessen LC: New directions: constituencies and responsibilities, *J Public Health Dent* 50:133, 1990.
69. North Carolina Department of Environment, Health, and Natural Resources, Division of Dental Health: Program plan, May 1991.
70. North Carolina Department of Human Resources, Division of Health Services, Dental Health Section: *A ten-year report,* 1985.
71. North Carolina Department of Human Resources, Division of Health Services, Dental Health Section: *Program report—FY86, program plan—FY87,* 1986.
72. North Carolina Department of Human Resources, Division of Health Services, Dental Health Section: *1986 conjoint report,* 1986.
73. Perry CL and others: Parent involvement with children's health promotion, the Minnesota home team, *Am J Public Health,* 78:1156, 1988.
74. Peterson FL Jr, and Rubinson L: An evaluation of the effects of the American Dental Association's dental health education program on the knowledge, attitudes, and health locus control of high school students, *J Sch Health* 52:63, 1982.
75. Pipe P and others: Developing a plaque control program, Berkeley, Calif, 1972, Praxis.
76. Podshadley AG, Schweikle ES: The effectiveness of two educational programs in changing the performance of oral hygiene by elementary school children, *J Public Health Dent* 30:17, 1970.
77. Podshadley AG, Shannon JH: Oral hygiene performance of elementary school children following dental health education, *J Dent Child* 37:293, 1970.
78. Rank O: Will therapy: the therapeutic applications of will psychology, New York, 1978, W W Norton.
79. Raynor JF, Cohen LK: A position of school dental health education: behavioral influences on oral hygiene practices, *J Prev Dent* 1:11, 1974.
80. Raynor JF, Cohen LK: *School dental health education.* In Richards ND, Cohen LK, editors: *Social sciences and dentistry: a critical bibliography,* London, 1971, Fèdèration Dentaire International.
81. Review of the national preventive dentistry demonstration program, *Am J Public Health* 76:434, 1986.
82. Rosenstock IM: Why people use health services, *Milbank Memorial Fund Q* 44:94, 1966.
83. Rozier RG and others: *Dental health in North Carolina: a chartbook,* Chapel Hill, NC, 1982, Department of Health Policy and Administration School of Public Health, University of North Carolina.
84. Rozier RG, Dudney GC, Spratt CJ: *The 1986-87 NC school oral health survey,* monograph, Raleigh, NC, 1991, NC Department of Environment, Health and Natural Resources, Division of Dental Health.
85. Rubinson L: Evaluating school dental health education programs, *J Sch Health* 52:26, 1982.
86. Sacket DL, Haynes RB: *Compliance with therapeutic regimens,* Baltimore, 1976, Johns Hopkins University Press.
87. Shiller WR, Dittmer JC: An evaluation of some current oral hygiene motivation methods, *J Periodontol* 39:83, 1968.
88. Shorey NL: *Using state policy to affect dental health education: vending.* Paper presented at the second national symposium on dental health education in schools, American Dental Association, Bureau of Health Education, Chicago, October 1977.
89. Silversin J, Kornacki MJ: Acceptance of preventive measures by individuals, institutions, and communities, *Int Dent J* 34:170, 1984.
90. Smith LW and others: Teachers as models in programs for school dental health: an evaluation of "The Toothkeeper," *J Public Health Dent* 35:75, 1975.
91. Stamm JW, Kuo HC, Neil DR: An evaluation of the "Toothkeeper" program in Vermont, *J Public Health Dent* 35:81, 1975.
92. Stone DB, Mortimer RG, Rubinson L: An evaluation of the cognitive aspect of the American Dental Association's learning about your oral health teaching and learning program, level II. Paper presented at the first national symposium on dental health education in schools, American Dental Association, Bureau of Health Education, Chicago, October 1975.
93. Sullivan L: Speech at American Academy of Pediatrics' media conference, Chicago, July 23, 1991.
94. Taub A: Dental health education: rhetoric or reality? *J Sch Health* 52:10, 1982.
95. Texas Department of Health, Bureau of Dental and Chronic Disease Prevention: *Preventive dentistry program,* Austin, 1992, Texas Department of Health.
96. Texas Department of Health, Bureau of Dental and Chronic Disease Prevention: *Summative evaluation report for the Texas Department of Health oral health curriculum, "Tattletooth II, a New Generation,"* Austin, 1990, Texas Department of Health.
97. Texas Department of Health: *Tattletooth program: statewide implementation plan,* Austin, 1986, Texas Department of Health.
98. US Department of Health and Human Services, Public Health Service, Center for Disease Control: *Current trends: the effectiveness of school health education,* MMWR 35:593, 1986.
99. U.S. Department of Health and Human Services, Public Health Service: *Healthy people 2000, national health promotion and disease prevention objectives,* Washington DC, DHHS Pub No (PHS) 91-50213.
100. Weinstein P, Getz T: *Changing human behavior: strategies for preventive dentistry,* Chicago, 1978, Science Research Associates.

101. World Health Organization: *Dental health education,* technical report series No 449, Geneva, 1970, The Organization.

102. World Health Organization: *New Approaches to health education in primary health care,* Geneva, 1983, The Organization.

103. World Health Organization: *Prevention methods and programmes for oral diseases,* Geneva, 1984, The Organization.

104. Wyden R: *Press statement: Saturday morning television ads aimed at kids are "starved" on nutritional value,* Washington, DC, June 3, 1991.

105. Yacovone JA: Translating research in the social and behavioral sciences for more effective use in community dentistry, *J Public Health Dent* 36:155, 1971.

106. Young MAC: Dental health education: an overview of selected concepts and principles relevant to programme planning, *Int J Health Educ* 13:2, 1970.

10 Planning for Community Dental Programs

René Dubos has pointed out that most of human history has been a result of accidents and blind choices. When a crisis occurs, our solutions are immediate and involve piecemeal efforts rather than considered and thoughtful planning. The need to develop our ability to predict, plan, and thus prevent the same crisis from recurring should have the highest priority.[3]

WHY PLAN?

As part of our role as health professionals we will be called on to assist health agencies and organizations in developing plans for obtaining dental care. We now need to develop our own abilities to take our dental expertise and channel it into the areas of policy development, decision making, and program planning in a system more complex than the one with which we are familiar in the private dental office. This complex system may take the form of a community, an organization, a corporation, or an institution. The system can be better understood if we look on it as a patient, possessing certain needs and characteristics. Because we are dealing with more than one individual, planning a program for a community or institution requires a deep understanding and analysis of the system as a whole as well as of the individual members that make up the system.

Planning dental care for the patient

The steps the dentist takes when seeing a patient for the first time can be compared with the steps a planner takes when viewing a system for the first time. A new patient who walks into the dental office is given a complete medical and dental history. This provides background information on the patient's health, history of diseases, and drug reactions, as well as the patient's history of dental care. In addition, information on the patient's ethnic background, degree of education, and financial status may indicate the patient's attitude about dental care, the type of dental care wanted, and how that care will be financed. A clinical examination with the use of radiographs further reveals the type and quality of dental care received and identifies any existing conditions or disease requiring treatment. For the dentist these steps assess the needs of the patient.

The next step is to identify and diagnose the problems. Perhaps the patient requires full mouth reconstruction to restore the mouth to optimum functioning. The dentist reviews with the patient the ideal plan as well as acceptable alternatives based on the patient's wants and financial limitations. Once the patient accepts the treatment plan and the method of payment, the plan is ready to be implemented.

The dentist selects the appropriate person to perform the necessary services from a staff of specialists and designs a realistic timetable to coordinate who will do what first, second, and so on, until treatment has been completed.

When treatment has been completed, the patient is placed on a 6-month recall and returns to have an evaluation of the care that was rendered. Any modifications or adjustments are done at this time. The patient is then placed on a maintenance plan and returns periodically for a routine examination. This becomes an ongoing process for the patient and the dentist. The difference between the planning steps for an individual patient and the planning steps for a community is that dealing with more than one individual at a time requires more complex steps. The box on p. 226 compares the provision of dental care for a private patient with that for a community.

Planning dental care for the community

Usually a planner is contacted because a problem has been identified within the community, for example, a high incidence of nursing bottle caries among young children. The planner, like the den-

---

A COMPARISON OF THE PROVISION OF DENTAL CARE FOR A PRIVATE PATIENT AND FOR A COMMUNITY

Private patient

1. The dentist conducts a dental and medical history and a clinical examination of the patient.
2. The dentist diagnoses the oral health of the patient.
3. The dentist develops a treatment plan based on the diagnosis, the priorities, the patient's attitude, and the method of payment for the services.
4. The dentist obtains patient consent for treatment.
5. The dentist selects the appropriate labor to provide the care: dentist, specialist, laboratory technician, dental hygienist, dental assistant.
6. The dentist selects the appropriate dental service for the patient: preventive services, restorative services, endodontic services, and so on.
7. The dentist evaluates the treatment rendered to the patient: clinical examination, radiographs, patient oral hygiene, patient satisfaction.

Community

1. The planner conducts a survey of the community's structure and dental status.
2. The planner analyzes the survey data of the community.
3. The planner develops a program plan based on the analysis of the survey data, the priorities and alternatives, the community's attitudes, and the resources available.
4. The planner obtains community approval of the plan.
5. The planner selects the appropriate labor to implement the program: dentist, dental hygienist, dental assistant, dental technician, nutritionist, health educator, schoolteacher, social worker, health aides, public health nurses.
6. The planner selects the appropriate activities for the community: community water fluoridation, school-based fluoride rinse programs, comprehensive dental services, oral cancer screening and referral programs.
7. The planner evaluates the community program: comparison of baseline survey with subsequent survey, attainment of goals and objective, cost-effectiveness of activities, appropriateness of activities, community satisfaction.

Modified from Young W, Striffler D: *The dentist, his practice, and the community,* Philadelphia, 1969, WB Saunders Co.

---

tist, begins by conducting a needs assessment of these children and their families. Included in the needs assessment will be the population's health problems and beliefs, ethnic makeup, diet, education and socioeconomic status, number of children with nursing bottle caries, and the severity of the disease.[8] Again, this information will help the planner in determining an appropriate plan.

Once the information has been gathered and analyzed, the planner, along with the community, sets priorities for dealing with the problem. The planner may decide that the first priority is to treat all existing nursing bottle cases within the community, followed by reeducating the mothers and fathers of these children and those individuals who

recommended sweetening the contents of the children's bottles. The planner then sets a reasonable goal to reduce the incidence of nursing bottle caries within that community within a specified time period and proposes methods or objectives to accomplish the goal.

Next, the planner identifies what resources are available to the community. Who will provide the treatment, how will the care be financed, and where will the care be provided? If too many constraints exist (for example, no transportation available to bring the children to the dental office or a lack of funds necessary to provide the treatment), then the planner has to consider alternative strategies to accomplish the intended goal. The planner might identify and recruit volunteer dentists or dental students to treat the children at no cost to the community.

Once the decision is made and approved by the community, it is ready for implementation. An implementation timetable is developed to provide a schedule for putting the plan into action.

After the children have been treated, a 6-month follow-up examination is instituted to evaluate the effectiveness of the plan. At that time, the planner addresses questions such as the following: How many children identified as having nursing bottle caries were treated? How many dropped out of treatment and why? How many developed new nursing bottle caries? The answers to these questions will help the planner to modify and adjust the program according to the needs of the community.[6]

The steps taken by a dentist to plan a course of action for the patient are a simplified version of the steps taken by a planner to plan for a community. However, because of time, cost, or labor limitations, the planner may find it necessary to modify the plan by considering various options that will ultimately reach the same end.

Who are the individuals who do the planning? There are many kinds of planners; some have been professionally trained or educated, whereas others have received on-the-job experience within their organization. There are two perspectives about planning: planning by individuals within the system or organization and planning by those brought in from outside.[1] A planner hired from within the system is usually an individual whose work responsibility is to plan for the system on a full-time basis. The advantage of hiring from within is that the planner already has a true understanding of the issues and operation of the system, including the subtleties of that system. This knowledge enables the planner to begin making decisions more quickly regarding appropriate action. The disadvantage, however, is that the planner may already have acquired certain biases about the system that could influence his or her objectivity.

The planner brought in from outside is usually an individual who contracts to work for the company or agency on a consulting basis for a short period of time. The planner's job is to assist the organization in its planning by formulating a new proposal and/or making recommendations for changing an existing plan. The advantage of this type of planner is that she or he potentially brings to the organization a fresher outlook, less bias, and a greater sense of objectivity than someone from the inside. The drawback is that the planner requires more time to reach a level of understanding of the system sufficient to plan an appropriate course of action.

One of the most important concerns for any planner should be to take into consideration the human element. Statistics alone do not tell the whole story. For example, a planner who reviews the health labor statistics on a multiethnic community and who sees that, overall, sufficient numbers of practitioners work within the community may think that the community does not need any new practitioners. A closer examination of the practitioner and patient populations may reveal that the practitioners are primarily of a certain ethnic background and do not like treating patients of different ethnic backgrounds, of which there are a great number in the community. Thus there may be large subgroups of the population who do not have access to dental care, even though statistically there are enough dentists available in the community.[5] Although statistics can be most useful in analyzing data, a planner must be aware of their limitations.

PLANNING: A DEFINITION

E.C. Banfield presents a basic definition of the term *planning:* "A plan is a decision about a course of action." In other words, a plan is a systematic approach to defining the problem, setting priorities, developing specific goals and objectives, and determining alternative strategies and a method of implementation.

There are many types of health planning. Each varies according to the factors affecting the health system, such as the geography of a region, the sociocultural background of the population, economic considerations, and the political situation.

Some types of health planning, as outlined by Spiegel and associates,[7] include the following:

1. Problem-solving planning involves the identification and resolution of a problem. An example of problem solving was the appearance of dental fluorosis among residents of a

community in Colorado. This enamel disorder was identified through a scientific study of possible causative factors.

2. Program planning entails designing a course of action for a circumscribed health problem. School-based fluoride rinse programs are an example of designing a course of action for the problem of dental caries within a community setting.

3. Coordination of efforts and activities planning aims to increase the availability, efficiency, productivity, effectiveness, and other aspects of activities and programs. This often involves an adjustment process, such as a merger or a closing of services and facilities. An example of this is the closing of obstetric and pediatric wards in hospitals located in areas with a declining birth rate.

4. Planning for the allocation of resources involves selecting the best alternative to achieve a desired goal when the amount of resources is limited. Planners are called on to allocate the budget, the labor, and the facilities in a system so that it may meet existing needs and demands. An example of this is the decision by a state government with limited financial resources for the provision of dental services to cut services to medically indigent adults based on the cost-effectiveness of providing preventive dental care to a younger population.

5. Creation of a plan involves the development of a blueprint or proposal for action containing recommendations and supporting data. It is common for a commission or special task force to be created to prepare the plan. A state health plan that describes the health status and the distribution of health services for the population in that state is a good example of such planning.

6. Design of standard operating procedures requires planners to come forth with a set of standards of practice or criteria for operation and evaluation. This can be a result of legislation or can be created voluntarily by the parties concerned. Guidelines for evaluating the quality of dental care as part of a quality assurance program for an insurance company is one example.

This chapter describes various types of health planning but concentrates specifically on the program-planning process. This process of program planning uses a systematic approach, as seen in Figure 10-1, and should be used as a guide to solving a particular problem. The process can be compared with the ability of a jazz musician to take the notes of a standard musical scale and use them to create a unique melody. In a similar fashion a planner uses the program-planning steps to create a plan that is unique for the specific situation or system.

The process of planning is dynamic. Within a fluctuating and ever-changing system the process itself must remain fluid and flexible, responsive to the presentation of new factors and issues.

This chapter discusses the components of program planning and focuses on the various options available to the planner. Let us first discuss the initial step in the planning process: conducting a needs assessment.

CONDUCTING A NEEDS ASSESSMENT

There are several reasons why a planner should conduct a needs assessment. The primary reason is to define the problem and to identify its extent and severity. Second, it is used to obtain a profile of the community to ascertain the causes of the problem. This information will help in developing the appropriate goals and objectives in the problem solution.

Another important reason to conduct a needs assessment is to evaluate the effectiveness of the program. This is accomplished by obtaining baseline information and, over time, measuring the amount of progress achieved in solving the specific problem.

Suppose the planner designed a program to administer fluoride tablets to all school-aged children in a given community. To determine how effective a fluoride tablet program is in terms of reduction of dental caries the planner would first take a baseline needs assessment of the caries rate among the schoolchildren prior to implementing the fluoride tablet program. After the initial assessment,

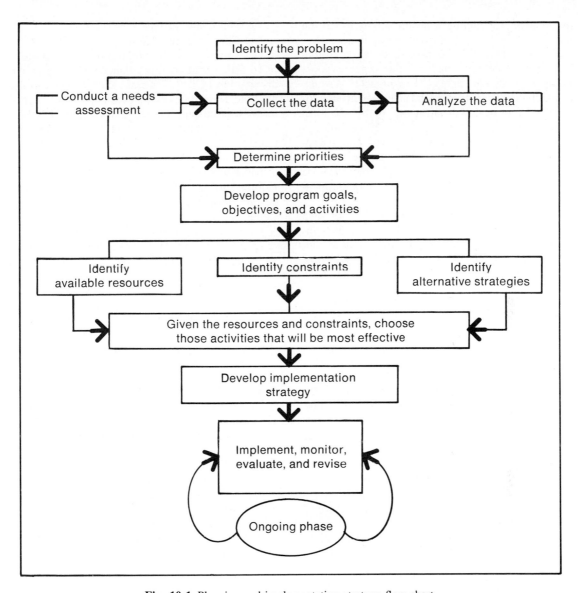

Fig. 10-1 Planning and implementation strategy flow chart.

the program is implemented. To measure the effectiveness of such a preventive regimen, the planner would then make periodic assessments of the schoolchildren at various time intervals and compare these results with the initial assessment.

Conducting a needs assessment for a community can be a very costly endeavor with respect to funds, labor, and time. If the funds are not readily available, the planner has several options.

One option is to coordinate with the research activities of other agencies interested in obtaining similar health information on the given population. For example, a neighborhood health center may be involved in conducting a health survey of all the residents living in a defined geographic area.

Another method is to investigate surveys that have been done in the past by other organizations. Frequently, dental surveys are conducted through research departments of dental schools, through local and state health departments, or by the local health systems agencies (HSAs). If no surveys have ever been done, the planner may either want to solicit the assistance of these agencies and organizations or inform them that a survey will be conducted. This will prevent overlap or duplication of activities.

Whether the planner conducts his or her own survey, combines efforts with others, or uses information from past surveys, it is important to consider what type of information is needed and how it should be obtained.

Data can be obtained by various techniques such as survey questionnaires or clinical examinations or more informally through personal communications. The technique the planner chooses is based on who is to be examined. Factors the planner should consider are the number of individuals involved, the extent and degree of severity of the problem, and the attitudes of the individuals to be surveyed. The greater the number of individuals to be examined, the more formal the survey. If the problem is clinical, as opposed to attitudinal, a more clinical examination might be recommended. If the planner wants to interview a small group of individuals on their attitudes and feelings about a particular issue, a personal communication might be more appropriate.

To gather general information on a population, a population profile should be obtained. Such a profile includes the following:

1. Number of individuals in the population
2. Geographic distribution of the population
3. Rate of growth
4. Population density and degree of urbanization
5. Ethnic backgrounds
6. Diet and nutritional levels
7. Standard of living, including types of housing
8. Amount and type of public services and utilities

9. Public and private school system
10. General health profile
11. Patterns and distribution of dental disease

To gather epidemiologic data on the patterns and distribution of dental disease the planner can use a clinical examination, review patients' dental records, or consult the National Health Survey for data on a population residing in a similar geographic region with similar characteristics.

In addition to assessing the incidence and the distribution of dental disease, the planner needs to inquire into the history and current status of dental programs in the community. Questions to ask should include the following:

1. What types of programs currently exist?
2. Are these programs oriented toward prevention, treatment, education, research, or a combination?
3. Who or what organization is responsible for the planning, implementation, and/or administration of the program(s)?
4. How successful have those responsible been?
5. What was the community's acceptance of such a program?

The planner must learn the way in which policies are developed and decisions are made within the community to better understand the community as a whole, especially if she or he is new to the community. The following areas need to be explored:

1. Who are the financial leaders (bankers, businesspeople) and who are the political leaders (mayor, city council, other public officials)?
2. Who sets the policies for the community?
3. What is the organizational structure of the community?
4. What are the community leaders' attitudes toward oral health and community dental programs?

After learning how the community operates, the planner needs to examine the types of resources that are available to the community to implement a program. These include the funds, the facilities, and the labor. The following questions might be asked:

1. Funds
   a. What is the source of funding at the state and local level for dental care?

b. Is third-party coverage available to the community through the workplace?

c. Is federal funding available through special eligibility programs?

d. Are private funds available through foundations or endowments?

2. Facilities

a. Where is the closest major medical center?

b. What specialty services does it provide?

c. What dental facilities exist and where are they located (in public schools, health centers, hospitals)?

d. How well are the facilities used by the population?

e. Are the facilities easily accessible to the population served?

f. Are the dental services provided appropriately, adequately, and efficiently?

g. Does the facility meet the required Occupational, Safety, and Health Administration (OSHA) standards for bloodborne pathogens?

h. Is the equipment adequate and running efficiently?

i. How many operatories are available?

j. How many dental laboratories are available?

3. Labor

a. How many active licensed dentists, hygienists, and assistants are available?

b. How many laboratory technicians are available?

c. How many dental and dental auxiliary schools are located nearby?

d. How many active community health aides are available?

e. How many public health nurses are available?

f. How many school nurses are available?

g. How many public health hygienists, voluntary health agencies, and nutritionists are available?

When planning a preventive dental program for a community or institution, it is important for the planner to determine where the population obtains water and the fluoride status of that water. In certain regions of the country, particularly in rural areas, many persons obtain their water from either individual wells or nearby rivers, lakes, or streams. The amount of fluoride in the water sources might indicate to the planner that a fluoride supplement program may not be necessary for that community. If individual wells are being used, the planner would need to get a report on the fluoride status of each well because wells may be receiving their water from different sources.

If a community is obtaining water from a central area, the planner needs the following information:

1. What type of drinking water is available to the community?

2. What is the fluoride content of the water?

3. Does the water contain optimum levels of fluoride?

4. What efforts, if any, have been made in the past to gain fluoridation?

5. What are the attitudes of the community, the dental profession, and decision makers toward fluoridation?

6. What are the laws with regard to fluoridation?

7. Is a referendum possible or required?

8. Are the school's water supplies fluoridated?

To prevent duplication of fluoride administration the planner also should inquire into the type of fluoride being administered to individuals in private offices, the schools, and the health centers.

1. Do local dentists or physicians prescribe fluoride supplements to their patients?

2. Do schools (preschool, parochial, public) have a fluoride tablet or rinse program?

3. Do the health centers or hospitals administer fluoride to their patients?

4. Do fluoride brush-in programs exist in the schools?

5. If so, how often do children brush with a fluoride toothpaste?

6. How successful have these programs been and how are they supported?

All the information presented in this section can easily be obtained through the various survey instruments discussed. If, however, a survey cannot be conducted, the necessary information on an institution or a community can also be obtained through other means. This approach will require the planner to investigate all available sources that might have data relevant to the population or the community. Such sources include the local, state, and federal agencies and private organizations.

In a small community one can find a tremendous amount of information on the community's residents by visiting the local health department. The local health department maintains statistics on the population's health status, morbidity and mortality, general health problems, and health service utilization. A trip to the chamber of commerce and town hall will provide useful information on the community profile, including population distribution, age breakdown, income, educational levels, school systems, and transportation.

In a larger community where health information may not be as readily accessible as in a small community, a good source for data is the HSA. The HSAs are federally mandated health planning agencies that develop specific plans to address the health problems of a designated region. They have data on health statistics of a population and health resources available in a given district. The state health department can also provide health-related information for all communities, cities, and towns within the state.

The federal government has large volumes of health statistics data from many of its agencies. The most familiar and widely used sources of data are the National Health Surveys and the U.S. Census Bureau. These sources provide longitudinal and comparative data regarding large population groups. Because of the magnitude of the data gathering for these surveys, they are usually conducted once every 10 years. Consideration of the publication date of such data and its relevancy and applicability to specific populations is important.

Other sources for obtaining such data are research studies and investigative reports. Many of these studies are funded by government agencies and are conducted by local organizations, research companies, or consulting groups. A considerable volume of data is usually generated from their reports. A computer literature search (MEDLINE) may be helpful. The National Library of Medicine provides these computer searches for a nominal fee. Most medical libraries affiliated with universities also provide this service.

Once the data are obtained, the information must be analyzed before it can be put into a plan

of action. Let us examine the data presented in the following case study and consider ways of using the information to develop an appropriate program.

Analysis of data: a case study
BACKGROUND

Tide Water is the fifth-largest city in Massachusetts and is situated in the southeastern section of the state on the shore of Deep Water Bay. Excellent water resources and deep-water shipping potential brought industrial growth to Tide Water, and it became the "spindle city of the world" as the cotton industry flourished. Native granite was used to construct multistory factories, some of which are still in use. This prosperity ended quickly when the cotton manufacturers moved to the South in the 1930s and 1940s. The problem of vacant mill space, in addition to the depression, made Tide Water's economic situation one of the worst in the country. Tide Water was able to make a strong recovery with a growing garment industry, which replaced the cotton mills and other manufacturers and provided a more diversified industrial base.

The following information is available about Tide Water:

POPULATION

1990 census: 96,988 persons
Ethnic and racial characteristics
1. Foreign born: 16%
2. Foreign stock: 48%
3. Race: White 99%
   Black 0.5%
   Other 0.5%
4. Density (persons per square mile): 2,946

AGE DISTRIBUTION

	Total male	Total female
Under 5 years	4,223	4,047
5 to 14 years	8,120	7,893
15 to 19 years	3,782	4,028
20 to 64 years	23,992	27,458
Over 64 years	4,902	8,453

EDUCATION*

Median number of school years completed: 8.8

*Figures reflect a large immigrant population, principally Portuguese.

Persons completing high school or more: 25.6%
Persons completing fewer than 5 grades: 13.3%

PERSONAL INCOME

Salary	Families
Less than $1,000	616
$1,000 to $2,999	2,341
$3,000 to $4,999	2,988
$5,000 to $6,999	3,922
$7,000 to $8,999	4,474
$9,000 to $11,999	5,761
$12,000 to $14,999	2,838
$15,000 to $24,999	2,079
$25,000 to $49,999	407
$50,000 or more	95
Total families	25,521
Median income	$8,000

TRANSPORTATION

Bus service: intracity and intercity
Taxi service: 3 companies, with a total of 65 radio-equipped cabs
Highways and streets
    4 major highways (2 N-S; 2 E-W)
    600 miles of streets, 99% paved

FLUORIDE STATUS

Tide Water has a community water supply that has been fluoridated since 1985.

HEALTH RESOURCES (LABOR)

140 physicians
43 dentists

FACILITIES

2 hospitals (725-bed capacity)
1 community health center (diagnosis, primary health dental care, education and prevention; sliding fee)
Mental health centers (many facilities, inpatient and outpatient clinics and residencies; free and sliding-scale fee)
AIDS, venereal disease, and tuberculosis programs (free)
Alcohol and drug programs (free)
15 nursing homes (1,150-bed capacity, representing all levels of care)

GOVERNMENT

City size: 33 square miles
Mayor (2-year term) and council (2-year term; 191 members) form of govenment
Democrats: 31,311

Republicans: 4,875
Independents: 10,204

EDUCATIONAL FACILITIES

20 day-care centers (50% free and/or sliding fee)

	Number	Enrollment
Public schools		
Elementary	32	10,007
Middle	1	982
Junior high school	2	1,852
Academic high school	1	1,948
Girls' vocational high school	1	214
Total	37	15,003
Catholic parochial schools		
Elementary	15	3,379
High schools	2	992

Other
    Regional/technical high school
County agricultural high school
Colleges
Community college: offers wide range of courses, many in health disciplines
Southeastern University: 4-year programs in most areas

It is important to first look into the socioeconomic structure of the community and determine the type of employment that exists. Tide Water has a large, industrial garment area. This leads to the following questions: is there a high percentage of industrial workers, and, if so, are they union employees? If this is the case, are they provided with a comprehensive health benefits package, including the provision of dental care? This information is important because it tells whether this population might be able to afford dental care through their jobs.

The population breakdown shows a large percentage of Portuguese living within the community. This indicates that possible cultural and language issues should be considered. In addition, the age distribution indicates that the highest proportion of people are between 20 and 60 years of age, or in the age bracket for the adult working population. There is a large population of school-aged children between the ages of 5 and 19 years living in the community. The age distribution of a community is important to consider because it tells where the target groups are and thus sets up certain priorities for planning. For example, if the majority of the population was of middle to older age, it would not be effective to design a program that would only affect a young population, such as the implementation of schoolwide fluoride rinse programs.

The educational status of a community provides two perspectives for planning. It first tells the educational level, in years of schooling obtained, by the majority of community members; second, it may indicate what the community's values are toward obtaining an education. Planning a health awareness program centered around an educational institution would be successful only if people are attending schools and value the information they receive there.

Knowing the median income of a community is very important to a health planner because it indicates the population's ability to purchase health services. If a segment of the population's income falls below poverty level, those individuals would be eligible for federal and state medical assistance programs (provided the individual state participates in such a program), thus making health services financially accessible to these individuals.

Health care must be geographically accessible as well as financially accessible if people are going to use it. A look into the community's public transportation system provides the planner with information regarding a population's ability to get to health care services. This is especially true for rural communities where roads are unpaved and public transportation is scarce.

Looking at the health care facilities in the communities tells the planner what type of services are being provided, the amount of services, and the cost of receiving those services.

The labor data give information as to the number of dentists providing care. (The federal government has developed certain labor-to-population ratios that indicate whether a population is considered to be residing in a medically underserved area.) However, just looking at the number of dentists in the community will not give the planner a true picture of whether the number of dentists within the community is sufficient to provide services to the population residing there.

Although the number of dentists in the community may be adequate, the planner must question whether the dentists are available to provide the care. How long does it take to get appointments? What are their hours (for example, do they work after 5 PM and/or on the weekends)? In addition to knowing the number of dentists, it is necessary to consider what types of services are being provided to whom, as well as for what cost.

Another consideration is the type of practice. Do the dentists accept third-party payments or Medicaid payments? Do they provide comprehensive services, including preventive care? Do they provide dental health education to their patients?

Knowing the fluoride status of a community is also essential for dental planning. In the case study community profile it states that water has been fluoridated since 1985. This indicates that those children born from 1985 on will receive maximum benefits from the fluoridated water. However, it is safe to say that those children born prior to 1985 may need additional attention with other fluoride measures.

In most cases the politics of the community will determine the direction the program will take. A conservative town government attempting to cut costs may be opposed to programs that provide prosthetic services to the medically indigent or elderly. Each local government's policies may vary in its methods of instituting new programs, allocating funds, hiring personnel, or setting priorities. In addition, the politics of the state government will also shape the overall direction taken by the communities within the state.

By looking at the educational system of a community the planner can determine the number of schools, the enrollment for each, and the distribution of children among the schools within the community. This information can assist the planner who is developing a school-based program for the community. The public and parochial schools are the ideal settings for dental programs. Moreover, as in countries like New Zealand, schools also serve as excellent vehicles for providing routine dental care.

The educational facilities should be designed appropriately to accommodate such programs. Teachers, parents, and school administrators should be in support of the programs, and, most important, the need must exist among the school-aged population to warrant such programs. In this particular community with the high percentage of Portuguese-American children the schools can be a good meeting place to use to open communication channels with the families and offer support services when needed.

If the planner is designing a dental treatment program for a specific population that is not receiving any care, there are methods developed by the Indian Health Service to convert the survey data into specific resource requirements for treating the population. The Indian Health Service (IHS) is a federal agency within the Public Health Service. It has been involved with extensive surveys on the oral health status of Native Americans. One method it has developed with the use of specific oral health surveys assesses the dental disease prevalence among the population and translates that data into time and cost estimates to treat the population. These surveys for disease prevalence include the decayed, missing, and filled (DMF) index, the Periodontal Index, and the Oral Hygiene Index—Simplified (OHI-S). In addition to determining the dental need, IHS also assesses treatment needs, which include prosthetic status, periodontal status, orthodontal status, oral pathology status, and restorative status.

By using a mathematical model, dental resource requirements can be computed and projected over a period of time. The data are then translated into time, labor, and facility requirements.

The basic measurement is time. Clinical dental services requirements and labor capability both can be expressed in time units. Various time requirement studies have been done by IHS to determine the amount of chair time that is necessary to complete a clinical service. This unit of time is called a service minute. For example:

Clinical service	Time required in service minutes[9]
Complete oral examination	10
Prophylaxis	17
Single surface amalgam	10

Labor and facility requirements

The number of dentists and dental auxiliaries, as well as of facilities and operatories necessary to treat the population, is determined by obtaining the total number of service minutes required for a given population. For example, a random sample of a population was examined and calculations showed that 70,000 service minutes would be required per year to treat approximately 60% of that population. Based on that figure the amount of staff required to provide approximately 70,000 service minutes would be one dentist and two dental assistants.[9] The number of operatories needed to accommodate this dental staff for maximum efficiency would be three.[9] The ratios (one dentist to two dental assistants to three operatories) have been derived from efficiency studies by the Indian Health Service.

This evaluation is highly statistical. Statistics can set parameters to the problem, but the values and attitudes of persons are equally important. The planner must take into consideration the sociocultural interests or the psychologic readiness of a people to want or use health services. If the community does not agree on which of the array of statistics represents the community's priorities, little will be done to translate the need identified in the data into effective programs.

DETERMINING PRIORITIES

"Priority determination is a method of imposing people's values and judgments of what is important onto the raw data."[7] The method can be used for different purposes such as for setting priorities among problems elicited through a needs assessment. It also can be used for ranking the solutions to the problem.

Given the community profile and analysis of dental survey data, how are priorities established? At this point, the community should be involved to assist in the establishment of these priorities. A health advisory committee or task force representing consumers, community leaders, and providers should be established to assist in the development of policies and priorities. Planning with community representation will aid in the program's implementation and acceptance.

Few dental public health programs meet all of the dental needs of the population. With limited resources, it becomes necessary to establish priorities to allow the most efficient allocation of resources. If priorities are not determined, the program may not serve those individuals or groups who need the care most.

Certain factors should be considered in determining priorities. For example, a problem that affects a large number of people generally takes priority over a problem that affects a small number of people. However, if the problem is common colds affecting a large number of people competing with Lyme disease affecting few people, then the more serious problem should take priority.

If the health problem is dental disease, generally more than one population group is affected. The following are groups commonly associated with high-risk dental needs:

1. Preschool and school-aged children
2. Mentally and/or physically handicapped persons
3. Chronically ill and/or medically compromised persons
4. Elderly persons
5. Expectant mothers
6. Low-income minority groups (urban and rural)

If the community decides to address the problem of dental caries first, specific groups are more susceptible to dental caries, such as preschool and school-aged children and low-income minority groups. The planner then begins to develop plans geared to an identifiable population group.

Once the target group has been identified (based on the dental problem), the type of program should be established. To do this, the planner begins to set program goals and objectives.

DEVELOPMENT OF PROGRAM GOALS AND OBJECTIVES

Program goals are broad statements on the overall purpose of a program to meet a defined problem. An example of a program goal for a community that has an identifiable problem of dental caries among school-aged children would be "to improve the oral health of the school-aged children in community X."

Program objectives are more specific and describe in a measurable way the desired end result of program activities. The objectives should specify the following:

1. What: the nature of the situation or condition to be attained
2. Extent: the scope and magnitude of the situation or condition to be attained
3. Who: the particular group or portion of the environment in which attainment is desired

4. Where: the geographic areas of the program
5. When: the time "at" or "by" which the desired situation or condition is intended to exist

An objective might state, "By the year 2005, more than 90% of the population aged 6 to 17 years in community X will not have lost any teeth as a result of caries, and at least 40% will be caries-free." This is known as an outcome objective and provides a means by which to measure quantitatively the outcome of the specific objective. This approach helps the evaluator and the community know both where the program is and where it hopes to be with respect to a given health problem. It also aids in establishing a realistic timetable for reducing or preventing principal health problems.

Second, objectives are the specific avenues by which goals are met. Process objectives state a specific process by which a public health problem can be reduced and prevented. For example, by 1995 community X will have a public fluoride program to guarantee access to fluoride exposure via the following:

1. Fluoridation of the public water supply to the optimum level
2. Appropriately monitored fluoridation of school water supplies in areas where community fluoridation is impossible or impractical
3. Initiation of the most cost-effective topical and/or systemic fluoride supplement programs available to all schools if both (1) and (2) are impossible
4. Provision of topical fluoride application for persons with rampant caries and use of pit and fissure sealants where indicated[4]

Once the problem has been identified and program goals and objectives have been established describing a solution to or a reduction of the problem, the next step is to state how to bring about the desired results. This area of program planning is referred to as program activities, and it describes how the objectives will be accomplished.

Activities include three components: (1) what is going to be done, (2) who will be doing it, and (3) when it will be done.

Activity 1: Beginning January 1, 1995, two dental hygienists will be hired to administer a self-applied fluoride rinse program within the public school systems.

ple

ing these program activities, care-
fully consider the type of resources available, as
well as the program constraints.

Resource identification

Selection of resources for an activity, such as per-sonnel, equipment and supplies, facilities, and fi-nancial resources, must be determined by consid-eration of what would be most effective, adequate,efficient, and appropriate for the tasks to be ac-complished. Some criteria that are commonly used to determine what resources should be used follow:

1. Appropriateness: the most suitable resources to get the job done
2. Adequacy: the extent or degree to which the resources would complete the job
3. Effectiveness: how capable the resources are at completing the job
4. Efficiency: the dollar cost and amount of time expended to complete the job

As discussed previously in the chapter, obtain-ing the community profile provides the planner with valuable information on available resources.

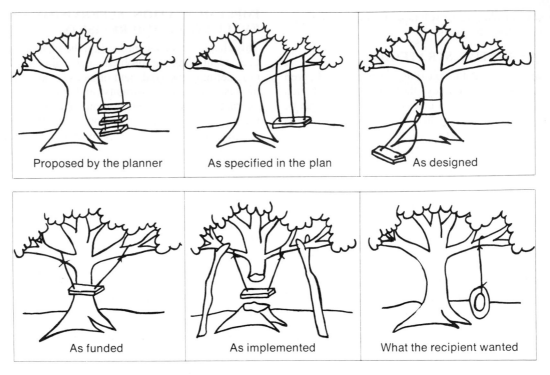

Fig. 10-3 A perspective on planning.

2. What: the activities required to achieve the objective
3. Who: individuals responsible for each activity
4. When: chronological sequence of activities
5. How: materials, media, methods, and techniques to be used
6. How much: a cost estimate of materials and time

To develop an implementation strategy, planners must know what specific activity they want to do. The most effective method is to work backward to identify the events that must occur prior to initiating the activity. The National Heart, Lung, and Blood Institute[10] has developed the *Handbook for Improving High Blood Pressure Control in the Community,* which provides examples of implementation strategies that can be applied to any type of health program. The box at the bottom of p. 239 lists rules for implementation strategy development. By review-

ing these rules, the details of operating a program will become clear to those responsible for instituting the program.

Monitoring, evaluating, and revising the program

Once it has been implemented, the program requires continuous surveillance of all activities. The program's success is determined by monitoring how well the program is meeting its stated objectives, how well individuals are doing their jobs, how well equipment functions, and how appropriate and adequate facilities are. Before problems arise in any of these areas, adjustments must be made to fine-tune the program.

Evaluation, both informal and formal, is a necessary and important aspect of the program. Evaluation allows us to (1) measure the progress of each activity, (2) measure the effectiveness of each activity, (3) identify problems in carrying out the activities, (4) plan revision and modification, and (5) justify the dollar costs of administering the program and, if necessary, justify seeking additional funds.

Each objective should be examined periodically to determine how well it is meeting the program goals. The objective should be stated in measurable terms so that a comparison can be made of what the objective intended to accomplish and what the objective actually accomplished.

Evaluation should also address the quality of what is being done. For example, if one of the activities was placing pit and fissure sealants on specific teeth of school-aged children, an evaluator would want to assess how well that sealant was placed, the appropriateness of the tooth chosen, and the time involved in placing the sealant on the tooth.

The attitudes of the recipients of the program should be examined to determine whether the program was acceptable to them. There are many programs that are considered successful by those who run the program; however, the people who have been the recipients of the service may have wanted something very different. Figure 10-3 illustrates this point and gives us a perspective on planning by showing the concept of the planner, the actual plan, the design, the constraints involved, the alternative strategy, and, finally, what in fact the recipient wanted in the first place.

SUMMARY

Merely hanging up a shingle is no longer all that is necessary for a health care provider to deliver health services to a given community. Consumers of health care are more involved than ever before in learning about the types of health care they should be receiving and are actively questioning the choices available to them. We as health professionals need to be responsive to consumers.

We must be prepared to meet the challenges of the 1990s through the development of good planning skills. These skills can then be used to achieve such goals as the following:

1. The construction of well-planned and accessible health facilities
2. The selection of appropriate, well-qualified, and sensitive health personnel
3. The provision of appropriate and effective health services
4. The time and the funds to provide the needed care

5. The active participation of representatives of those communities, organizations, and/or individuals who will be the recipients of the health care given

Only through fully understanding the needs of the community, the organization, and the individual can we begin to coordinate our planning efforts to develop acceptable, appropriate, and effective health care programs today and for the future.

REFERENCES

1. Blum HL: *Note on comprehensive planning for health,* Berkeley, Calif, 1968, Comprehensive Health Planning Unit, School of Public Health, University of California.
2. Bruhn J: Planning for social change, *Am J Public Health* 63:7, 1972.
3. Dubos R: *So human an animal,* New York, 1968, Charles Scribner's Sons.
4. *Model standards for community preventive health services,* a report to the U.S. Congress for the Secretary of Health, Education and Welfare, August 1979.
5. *Provision of dental care in the community, University of Michigan, School of Public Health, Ann Arbor, 1973,* Proceedings from the third annual course in dental public health, Waldenwoods Conference Center, Hartland, Mich, May 22-26, 1966.
6. Schulbert H and others: *Program evaluation in the health fields,* New York, 1969, Human Sciences.
7. Spiegel A and others: *Basic health planning methods,* Germantown, Md, 1978, Aspen Systems.
8. Striffler D: *Surveying a community and developing a working policy: the administration of local dental programs, University of Michigan, School of Public Health,* Proceedings from fifth workshop on dental public health, Ann Arbor, 1963.
9. U.S. Department of Health, Education and Welfare, Public Health Service: *Dental program efficiency criteria and standards for the Indian Health Service,* 1974.
10. U.S. Department of Health, Education, and Welfare, Public Health Services, National Institutes of Health, National Heart, Lung and Blood Institute: *Handbook for improving high blood pressure control in the community,* DHEW Pub No 78-1086. Washington, DC, 1977, US Government Printing Office.
11. Young W, Striffler D: *The dentist, his practice, and the community,* Philadelphia, 1969, WB Saunders Co.

SECTION FIVE

Research and Evaluation in Dental Care

Dentistry is referred to both as an art and as a science. The art of dentistry relates to skill in the less tangible aspects of dental care: judgments and esthetics, the proper contouring of restorations, the gentle touch in the manipulation of a curette, the chairside approach to the patient, and the development of patient motivation toward oral hygiene.

The science of dental care involves knowledge acquired through research and evaluation and requires the use of tools such as biostatistics to assist in the development of new information. Biostatistics enables the analysis of data in a systematic fashion and thus the processing of data that can be used to improve the state of dental health of individual patients and the community. Chapter 11 introduces some fundamental concepts in biostatistics to permit the student to evaluate programs and the research literature.

Chapter 12 further develops the concept of program evaluation that was introduced previously. Chapter 10 described the process of program development and touched on the evaluation of programs; Chapter 12 analyzes the process of evaluation and gives the student tools with which to improve a program.

Chapter 13 provides a substantive overview of research activities in dentistry, as well as useful guidelines for carrying out a research study. Clinical and social science research is emphasized, and a clear point-by-point method is provided for each type. A brief discussion on how to read the research literature is also included.

11 Introduction to Biostatistics

Familiarity with biostatistics or the mathematics of collection, organization, and interpretation of numeric data having to do with living organisms is essential for today's health care professional. Many people, however, are statistic shy. The goal of this chapter is to make clear the basics of biostatistics and to make the reader more comfortable with their usage.*

Dental health professionals have a variety of uses for data: in designing a health care program or facility, in evaluating the effectiveness of an ongoing program, in determining the needs of a specific population, and in evaluating the scientific accuracy of a journal article, to name just a few. These data are helpful only to the extent that they may be ordered and interpreted. Therefore what has been established is a system of managing data by using various techniques. Two statistical techniques are generally accepted: descriptive statistical technique enables an individual to describe and summarize a set of data numerically; inferential statistical technique provides a basis for making a generalization about the probable results of a large group when only a select portion of the group has been observed. Inferential statistics are used to generalize results to a larger population of interest, whereas descriptive statistics attempt only to generalize the group actually studied.

Before elaborating on terms relating to descriptive and inferential techniques, it is necessary to identify what is meant by the terms *population* and *sample*.

A population is any entire group of items (objects, materials, people, and so on) that possess at least one basic defined characteristic in common. Examples of populations might be all dentists, all U.S. citizens, all periodontally involved teeth, all individuals in a given school, or all patients treated at a particular private office. It is often impossible to collect information from an entire population because of the size of the population or because of such limitations as finances, time, or distance between population members. In cases where it is impossible to collect data on the entire population, complete and reliable information can be collected from a representative portion of the population called a *sample*. By observing and measuring a sample, it is possible to obtain information and make statements about the total population.

Statistics is a science that describes data for the purpose of making inferences about the population from which the data are obtained. When we collect a specific piece of information—data—from each member of a population, we obtain a characteristic of the population called a *parameter*. Similarly, when we collect a piece of information from each member of a sample, we obtain a characteristic of the sample called a *statistic*. Because most studies are conducted by using samples, statistics are most commonly used. Using statistics (characteristics of a sample), we try to infer what the parameters (characteristics of a population) will be.

SAMPLING

Samples, by definition, cannot have exactly the same characteristics as a population. However, a sample truly representative of the population can be obtained by using probability sampling methods and by taking a sufficiently large sample.

A *random sample* is defined as one in which every element in the population has an equal and independent chance of being selected. The following example illustrates two random sampling procedures: assume a population of 5,000 seniors in the predental program at 50 universities. Each senior class has 100 predental students divided into five equal sections of 20 students each. The ob-

---

*A complete treatment of biostatistics is not possible in this text. The interested reader is referred to the standard tests in the bibliography of this chapter that cover this material in detail.

jective is to determine the grade point average (GPA) of each predental student by selecting a representative sample of 1,000 students (that is, a sampling ratio of one fifth, or 20%). A simple random sample to select the 1,000 students would be completed in the following manner: a list of 5,000 students needs to be compiled and numbered 1 through 5,000. A numbered tag is prepared for each student and from the 5,000 well-mixed tags, 1,000 are drawn by a lottery. After each selection, the tag is replaced and another tag is drawn. This is the most basic random sample approach.

A similar procedure may be applied for selecting a random sample by using a table of random numbers, which can be found in most statistics textbooks. For this example, it would be necessary to use four columns of digits in the tables so that each student, one through 5,000, would have an equal probability of being selected. Selection would begin by blindly identifying a number on the table that corresponds to a member of the total population (one through 5,000). The selection process continues by taking numbers horizontally or vertically until the desired sample size is reached. Repeated numbers are omitted when encountered during sample selection in both procedures.

Random sampling is the procedure of choice whenever possible. It prevents the possibility of selection bias on the part of the researcher. What if GPA is related to school? A simple random sample may not ensure representation of the entire population of predental students. It may be necessary to select individuals according to certain strata or subgroups to diminish the chance of sample fluctuation. This method of selection is called *stratified sampling*. It is accomplished by randomly selecting a proportionate number of subjects from each subgroup for the sample. In the preceding example the subgroup would be the university attended. Therefore to produce a stratified random sample, one would (1) prepare a list of students at each of the 50 universities and (2) draw at random one fifth of the students at each university. Because the sampling ratio is used in each stratum, there is a proportional allocation by school. This eliminates the possibility of sampling bias that could result by selecting at random and giving no consideration to school.

Another type of sampling is the systematic sam-

ple. A systematic sample is not a true random sample because everyone may not have an independent chance of being selected. This type of sample is usually obtained by drawing a number and then selecting every *n*th individual, for example, having a list of names and deciding to test every even-numbered person on the list. All odd-numbered names are systematically excluded.

Two types of samples that may introduce serious bias in estimating population parameters are (1) the judgment sample and (2) the convenience sample. In a judgment sample someone with knowledge of the population may select a sample in arbitrary ways to represent the population. In a convenience sample a group is chosen because it happens to be convenient and may represent the population; for example, one classroom within a school is selected because the teacher gives permission to work with the pupils, or the patients at a particular private office are used because the dentist allows access to the patient list. Results relating to that particular classroom or that particular dentist's office may be valid, but when generalized to include the larger population of school classrooms or dentists' offices, their reliability is questionable.

Once a sample has been selected, raw data are collected and consideration must then be given to data analysis. Data analysis requires the application of statistical tests to data for the purpose of organizing, describing, and summarizing findings. Among the steps that may be applied in data analysis are the following:

1. Organizing data from lowest to highest
2. Constructing a frequency distribution
3. Grouping and regrouping data, based on relevant information
4. Tabulating scores
5. Constructing tables and graphs for efficient communication of obtained results

DESCRIPTIVE DATA DISPLAY
Frequency distributions

Often, to better explain data that has been collected, the data are grouped according to the variable they measure and ordered into an array. An array is simply a group of scores arranged from lowest to highest score. It can be organized into a frequency distribution by tabulating the frequency with which each score occurs. Three types of frequency distributions may be employed: ungrouped, grouped, and cumulative. The following example illustrates the descriptive displays of data.

A group of 33 dental students has taken Part I of the National Boards examinations. Their exam scores have been recorded. The dean of the dental school wishes to summarize these scores at the next school faculty meeting. Here are a few of the ways that the information could be presented.

First, an ungrouped frequency distribution table of the National Board scores is presented in Table 11-1. The variable of interest is the exam score, which is shown in the first column of the table. The exam scores for the group are listed in descending order. The next column of the table contains the frequency with which each score occurs in the data set. Next, the frequency of occurrence is expressed as a relative frequency, that is, as a

Table 11-1 Frequency distribution table for national board scores (NB1)

| | National Boards 1 | | | |
| | | | Cumulative | Cumulative |
NB1	Frequency	Percent	frequency	percent
56	1	3.0	1	3.0
57	1	3.0	2	6.1
63	1	3.0	3	9.1
65	2	6.1	5	15.2
66	1	3.0	6	18.2
68	2	6.1	8	24.2
69	2	6.1	10	30.3
70	1	3.0	11	33.3
71	1	3.0	12	36.4
72	2	6.1	14	42.4
74	1	3.0	15	45.5
75	1	3.0	16	48.5
76	2	6.1	18	54.5
77	3	9.1	21	63.6
78	2	6.1	23	69.7
79	1	3.0	24	72.7
80	1	3.0	25	75.8
81	3	9.1	28	84.8
82	1	3.0	29	87.9
83	1	3.0	30	90.9
84	1	3.0	31	93.9
88	1	3.0	32	97.0
89	1	3.0	33	100.0

percent of the total number of scores represented in the table. For example, three students scored 77 on the exam. This represents 9.1% of the group of 33 students.

Second, the data can be displayed as a cumulative frequency distribution. Table 11-1 shows the cumulative frequency and cumulative percent for the National Board scores. These descriptive measures express the frequency of occurrence of scores up to and including any given value in the data set. For example, 25 students (75.8% of the group) scored 80 or below on this exam.

Instead of displaying each individual value in a data set, the frequency distribution for a variable can group values of the variable into consecutive intervals. Then, the number of observations belonging to an interval are counted.

A grouped frequency distribution for the National Board scores is illustrated in Table 11-2. Note that although the data are condensed in a useful fashion, some information is lost. The frequency of occurrence of an individual data point cannot be obtained from a grouped frequency distribution. For example, seven students scored between 74 and 77, but the number of students who scored 75 is not shown here.

Graphing techniques

Graphing represents another alternative in displaying descriptive data pictorially and allowing rapid assimilation of findings by the reader. A general rule for constructing graphs along the X and Y axes is that the vertical Y axis usually represents the frequency of scores occurring along the scale

Table 11-2 Grouped frequency distribution of National Board scores

Scores	Number of students	Percent
56-61	2	6
62-65	3	9
66-69	5	15
70-73	4	12
74-77	7	21
78-81	7	21
82-85	3	9
86-89	2	6

of measurement, whereas the X axis represents the scale that measures the variable of most interest.

A bar graph is a two-dimensional pictorial display of data that is discrete in nature.

A histogram is a graphic representation formed directly from a frequency distribution. It is a display in which the horizontal (abscissa) and vertical (ordinate) axes of a graph are formed according to the scale values and the frequencies of the distribution, respectively. A histogram consists of a set of rectangles whose base is on the horizontal axis and which extends in height along the vertical axis proportional to the frequency. If the points are widespread, a double bar (//) or a double curved line ($\approx$) is used to indicate breaks in the graph. Graphically, a histogram is similar to a bar graph except that rectangles touch one another in a histogram (Fig. 11-1).

When the concern is to depict the continuous nature of the data, a line graph called a *frequency polygon* is used. To construct it one would place a point at the center of each rectangle found in a histogram and connect each point with a straight line. Polygons are used the most frequently of all graphing techniques, and often polygons are superimposed on a line graph to display pictorially two or more distributions in one figure (Fig. 11-2).

When material is presented in tabular form, the table should be able to stand alone; that is, correctly presented material in tabular form should be understandable even if the written discussion of the data is not read. Following are suggestions for the display of data in graphic or tabular form:*

1. The contents of a table as a whole and the items in each separate column should be clearly and fully defined. The unit of measurement must be included.
2. If the table includes rates, the basis upon which they are measured must be clearly stated—death rate percent, per thousand, per million, as the case may be
3. Whenever possible, the frequency distribu-

---

*Hill AB: *Principles of medical statistics,* ed 7, London, 1961, Lancet.

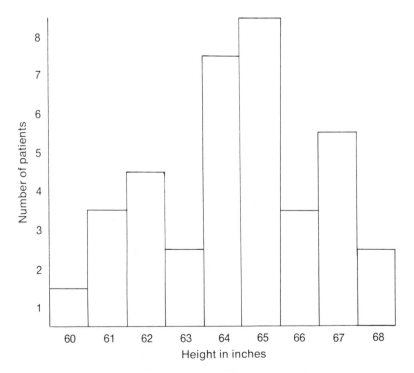

Fig. 11-1 Histogram of patient height.

tions should be given in full. These are basic data from which conclusions are being drawn, and their presentation allows the reader to check the validity of the author's arguments.

4. Rates or proportions should not be given alone without any information as to the numbers of observations upon which they are based. By giving only rates of observations and omitting the actual number of observations or frequency distributions, we are excluding the basic data.

5. Where percentages are used, it must be clearly indicated that these are not absolute numbers. Rather than combine too many types of figures in one table, it is often best to divide the material into two or three small tables.

6. Full particulars of any exclusion of observations from a collected series must be given. The reasons for and the criteria of exclusions must be clearly defined.

Figures (graphs) are used for a different purpose than tables. Figures are the presentation of material in a simplified manner to clearly illustrate a particular set of data. A major concern in the presentation of both figures and tables is readability. Tables and figures must be clearly understood and clearly labeled so that the reader is aided by the information rather than confused. The student is again directed to standard biostatistic texts for a formal discussion on summarizing data in graphic and tabular form. Also, standard writing style manuals generally contain discussions on the formal display of tables and graphs.

Measures of central tendency

The display of data in graphic or tabular form may be tedious, time-consuming, and unwieldy when every piece of data is not necessary. Sometimes a summary that can describe the total collection of data with just one number is preferable. Three measures in common use describe the central tendency of a distribution of scores: the mode, the mean, and the median.

The *mode* is that value that occurs with the

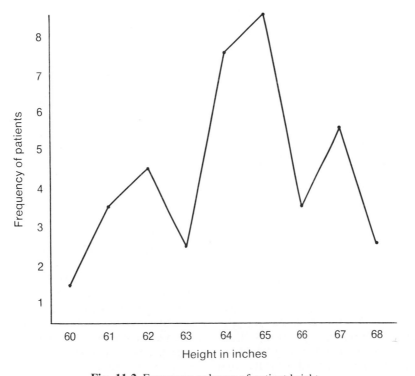

Fig. 11-2 Frequency polygon of patient height.

greatest frequency. It is possible for a distribution to have more than one mode when two or more values have equally large frequencies. For example, the distribution of scores in Table 11-1 has two modes, 77 and 81. Both occur with the equally high frequency of three. The primary value of the mode lies in its ease of computation and in its convenience as a quick indicator of the central value in a distribution. Beyond this, its statistical uses are extremely limited.

The measure of central tendency, called the *mean,* is the same as the arithmetic average that one learns to calculate in the elementary grades. It is computed by adding a list of scores and then dividing by the number of scores. The symbol for mean is a capital letter X with a bar above it $(\overline{X})$. The mean is by far the most common measure of central tendency used to describe a set of data because it fluctuates least from sample to sample and is sensitive to any change in any score in the distribution. The presence of a few extremely high or extremely low scores can change the value of the mean considerably.

The *median* is that point that divides the distribution of scores into two equal parts, that is, the point at which 50% of the scores lie above it and 50% lie below it. For example, given the scores 1, 3, 5, 6, 8, 9, and 10, the median is 6, because two equal-sized parts (1, 3, 5; 8, 9, 10) are above and below 6. The median is not affected by extreme scores in a given direction and is more stable than the mode.

An area in which the median is most often used and clearly illustrates its advantage over the mean or the mode is salary or dollar values. For illustrative purposes, suppose seven dental hygienists and two dentists work in a productive private office. Their salaries are as follows:

$75,000	$28,500	$22,300
$72,000	$26,000	$22,300
$29,000	$25,000	$22,300

The owner of the office declares that the average member's salary is $35,522—the mean. The business manager declares in a later report that the average salary is $22,300—the mode. Neither person has intentionally reported false results. Both have used a measure of central tendency. However, the statistical tool reported was the one best suited to the reporter's objective rather than the one that best described the data, in this case, the median. In this illustration the median is $26,000. This value gives a much clearer picture of where the salaries lie for the individual in the middle of the salary range. The mode in this example was extremely low compared with the majority of salaries, and the mean was influenced by two extremely high salaries.

Variability

Measures of central tendency indicate the typical performance for a group. However, this is not enough information to describe a distribution of scores. How widely scores are dispersed around that central point must also be known. Suppose Dr. A has a class of dental hygienists whose mean intelligence quotient (IQ) is 110. Some students in this class have IQs of 80 to 90 and others have IQs of 130 to 140. Dr. B's class of hygienists also has a mean IQ of 110, but the lowest is 100 and the highest is 124. The two hygiene classes have the same mean; however, we can see that the abilities of one class are definitely different from those of the other class because we know something about the spread of scores around the average.

Three terms are commonly associated with variability: range, variance, and standard deviation. The *range* is the difference between the high score and the low score in a distribution. In Table 11-1 the range is 33 (89 to 56). Often, ranges are stated as lowest and highest score, that is, the range is 56 to 89. The range has the advantage of being easy to calculate. However, it is unstable and affected by one extremely high or extremely low score. Also, only two scores are considered, and these happen to be the extreme scores of the distribution. Standard deviation and variance have much more utility than the range.

The *variance* is a measure of the average deviation or spread of scores around the mean. The variance, as is the standard deviation, is based on each score in the distribution. It is possible to have zero variance. However, it is impossible to have negative variance. Zero variance would occur when all scores in a distribution are equal, for instance, when everyone gets 100% as a test score, or when everyone in a group has the same weight or height. The following steps show how the variance is calculated:

1. Obtain the mean of the distribution.
2. Subtract the mean from each score (deviation scores).
3. Square each deviation score.
4. Add these squared deviation scores.
5. Divide the sum by the number of cases added.

The standard deviation of a set of scores is simply the positive square root of the variance. Table 11-3 illustrates the calculation of variance and standard deviation for the IQ scores of 10 students.

The variance and the standard deviation are relatively easy to interpret. The greater the dispersion of scores from the mean of the distribution, the greater the standard deviation and the variance. A large standard deviation indicates a wide dispersion around the mean. Consider the following statistics:

A. $\overline{X} = 60$ $s = 4$
B. $\overline{X} = 60$ $s = 9$
C. $\overline{X} = 60$ $s = 21$

Group A is the most homogeneous group with a small standard deviation and therefore small dispersion around the mean. Group C is the most heterogeneous group, with $s = 21$, indicating a major spread of scores around the mean.

Normal curve

The normal curve is one of the most used frequency distributions in biostatistics. It is a bell-shaped curve that is symmetrical around the mean of the distribution. The normal curve may vary from rather narrow distributions that are pointy in the center to wide distributions whose center is flat. The mean of the distribution is the focal point from which all assumptions and statements may be made. The mean is used for two reasons: (1) most distributions do not have a zero point to be used as a starting point (what is zero intelligence?), and (2) the normal curve theoretically does not touch the baseline at any point because of the remote possibility of an extreme score in the distribution. Curves that meet the criteria for normality can be separated into areas under the curve. Refer to Figure 11-3 for an example of this separation.

The total area bounded by the curve is 1, or 100%. A curve that meets the criteria of normality has the mean equal to the median, which is equal to the mode. The total area is broken into segments of single units (1 standard deviation). As indicated in Figure 11-3, the portion of the area under the curve between the mean and one standard deviation is 34.13% of the total area. The same area is found 1 unit below the mean. Similarly, two units above and below the mean cut off an additional 13.59% of the area under the curve, and so on for 3 standard deviations. Area under

Table 11-3 Calculation of variance and standard deviation for sample of 10 students

IQ scores χ	Deviation from mean ($\chi - \overline{\chi}$)	(Deviation)^2 ($\chi - \overline{\chi}$)^2
109	-2	4
99	-12	144
123	12	144
116	5	25
131	20	400
98	-13	169
116	5	25
89	-22	484
128	17	289
101	-10	100
1,110 = Sum of IQs	0	1,784 = Sum of the deviation squared
111 = Mean IQ		

Variance (s^2) = 1784 ÷ 10 = 178.4
Standard deviation (s) = 13.36

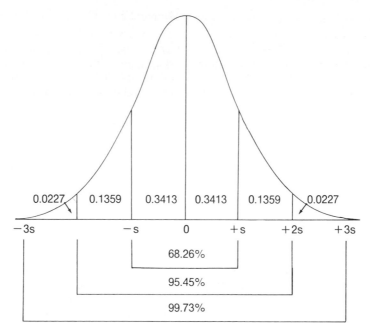

Fig. 11-3 The normal frequency curve.

the curve can best be understood by imagining a test that is administered to a large group of students. When the tests are scored, the distribution will probably take the form of a normal curve. In that case, 34.13% of the students who took the test would score between the mean and one standard deviation above the mean, another 13.59% would score between the first and second standard deviations above the mean, and 2.21% would score between the second and third standard deviations above the mean. Thinking of the area under the curve in terms of percent of persons makes it easier to interpret the distribution of the normal curve.

SIGNIFICANCE RELATED TO INFERENTIAL STATISTICS

With large populations, it is often impossible to study each member in the group because of time, cost, and so on. Instead, we select a sample from the population and from that sample attempt to generalize to the population as a whole. In using inferential statistical procedures (trying to infer about a group larger than our sample), we must deal with statistical probability—the mathematical

assumption that a certain situation will occur according to chance a specific portion of time. For example, if a coin is flipped an infinite number of times, by chance the coin will come up heads 50% of the time and tails 50% of the time.

The main thing to remember in inferential statistical procedures is that we are trying to generalize about a group larger than the one for which we actually have data. If we have a good sample, our generalization will be accurate; if our sample is poor, we will be hampered in our ability to generalize to the population. For example, suppose we are interested in determining the general status of a patient's oral health. We could examine each tooth of an individual and then make our judgment. However, if we had 1,000 persons to examine in a limited time we might look for an alternative method. Perhaps we would select four teeth, one from each quadrant, and then base our decision regarding the oral cavity on the results of examining those four teeth. In this case, we have taken a sample of 4 teeth from the population of 32 teeth. Our assessment of the oral cavity will be accurate if the teeth we have chosen are the best representatives of teeth in each quadrant. Needless to say, we should be certain to examine the same 4 teeth of each individual when making our assessment. A more detailed example may serve to clarify the use of inferential statistical procedures: a graduate student in public health wishes to implement a community-based education program for a group of urban mothers. He finds through the literature that an education program has been offered to a similar group of mothers using an entirely different approach. He is interested in testing how much the participants in his program learn as compared with the other program. Assume both groups started with the same knowledge level. The student tests the mothers and compares the mean result of his program with that obtained in the other program. He finds that his group tests higher, but he is not sure if it is such a difference that he can clearly say his program is better. There is a procedure available called *Student's* t-*test* that allows the graduate student to compare the mean results from his program with the mean results of the other program. The purpose of using Student's *t*-test is to determine the probability that the difference between the two means is real and not a result produced by a chance difference. What this public health student wishes to find is a statistically significant difference between the first and second means, that is, the mean produced by his program and the mean produced by the other program.

The distinction between statistically significant and practically significant results is important. For example, in the case just discussed, two programs are offered in health education and one is found to produce greater test scores among participants than the other, say 5 points greater. Based on test results, the program of choice is the one producing the greater score. Suppose this program, which produces a 5-point gain, also costs $100 more per participant to produce. In all likelihood a group of decision makers might decide that $100 per participant is too high a price to pay for the "moderate" gain; although the greater test scores were statistically significant and statistically better, the difference between program results was not practically significant. Pragmatic decisions play a much greater role in research than many scientists are willing to admit.

CORRELATION AND INFERENTIAL STATISTICS

The science of statistics has given us a large number of tests that can be applied to public health data. Only a few of these will be discussed in this section. Discussions will center on the chi-square test, the calculation of the coefficient of correlation, and Student's *t*-test. Each is best adapted to data of a certain type. An understanding of the tests will guide an individual toward the efficient collection of data that will meet the assumptions of the statistical procedures particularly well.

Chi-square test

The chi-square test is based on the comparison of the observed measurement of a given characteristic and the expected measurement if the sample differs in no way from what is expected by chance. The chi-square statistic (X^2) measures the discrepancy between observed and expected frequencies by adding together all values:

$$\frac{(\text{Observed number} - \text{expected number})^2}{\text{Expected number}}$$

The X^2 test is set up in such a way that the original number of cases entering into each sample becomes part of the calculation and affects interpretation of the answer. Therefore all observations play an equally important role, whether negative or positive. A zero observation is as important as a large positive or negative value.

Chi-square will equal zero if all comparisons between observed and expected values are zero. The accurate interpretation of X^2 depends on the computation of a figure called the *degrees of freedom*. This indicates the number of cells in a two-dimensional grid that can be filled independently without the totals for the problem being incorrect. It is calculated by subtracting 1 from the number of rows and 1 from the number of columns in the grid and then multiplying these figures together:

$$(r - 1) \times (c - 1) = df$$

After calculating the X^2 value and the degrees of freedom, the next step is to use a master table and find the numbers closest to the value computed for X^2 in the line of the table that represents the figure for degrees of freedom. Having located the number, one then follows to the head of the column and reads the probability of chance occurrence of such a value of X^2.

The following problem illustrates the procedure for calculating the X^2 value: suppose we are interested in whether vaccination, apart from whether it has only prophylactic effect, reduces the severity of any actual attack of smallpox. Chi-square could be used to determine whether vaccination has an effect.

First we must discuss several areas illustrated in Table 11-4. To perform X^2 analysis it must be possible to place each piece of information into only one cell. For instance, an individual who was never vaccinated could not be placed in both the abundant and the sparse categories. This would cause one person to be counted twice and invalidate our results. Next, expected frequencies must be determined before we are able to make comparisons with the observed frequencies. The formula for calculating expected frequency follows:

$$eij = \frac{(Tr \times Tc)}{N}$$

where e is the expected frequency of cell ij, Tr is the total for row r, Tc is the total for column c, and N is the total frequency. Table 11-5 provides an example showing the expected frequencies used in Table 11-4 and how they were calculated.

The master table value for X^2 with 2 degrees of freedom is 5.99 at the 5% confidence level. Because our calculated value was 230.17, we have determined that there is a statistically significant difference between what was expected by chance and what actually occurred. Therefore vaccination in this example had a significant effect.

With X^2, we deal with one variable but test its occurrence in a number of different situations.

Table 11-4 Calculation of chi-square

	Hemorrhagic or confluent	Abundant	Sparse	Row totals
Observed frequencies				
Vaccinated within 10 years of attack	10	150	240	400
Never vaccinated	60	30	10	100
TOTAL	70	180	250	500
Expected frequencies				
Vaccinated with 10 years of attack	56	144	200	400
Never vaccinated	14	36	50	100
TOTAL	70	180	250	500

$$\chi^2 = \frac{(10 - 56)^2}{56} + \frac{(150 - 144)^2}{144} + \frac{(240 - 200)^2}{200} + \frac{(60 - 14)^2}{14} + \frac{(30 - 36)^2}{36} + \frac{(10 - 50)^2}{50}$$

$\chi^2 = 230.17$
$df = (r - 1)(c - 1)$
$df = (2 - 1)(3 - 1)$
$ds = 2$

Table 11-5 Expected frequencies calculated for Table 11-4

	Confluent	Abundant	Sparse	Total
Vaccinated within 10 years of attack	$\frac{(400 \times 70)}{500} = 56$	$\frac{(400 \times 180)}{500} = 144$	$\frac{(400 \times 250)}{500} = 200$	400
Never vaccinated	$\frac{(100 \times 70)}{70} = 14$	$\frac{(100 \times 180)}{180} = 36$	$\frac{(100 \times 250)}{250} = 50$	100
TOTAL	70	180		250 = 500

This comparison of categorical-type information is the type of problem for which X^2 is best suited. In a sense, therefore, we are really dealing with two variables, although values for the second variable need not be related to the other in any recognizable pattern.

Correlation

Correlation analysis allows us to deal with another quite common type of problem in which there are two variables, each measuring some different characteristic. Each unit in the data we are testing consists of a pair of measurements, and our objective is to determine the strength of the relationship. One measurement in the unit is for the first variable, and one is for the second variable. Correlation is best applied when the number of pairs is very large; the larger the number, the more reliable the results. The relationship between pairs is easiest to grasp by using what is called a *scatter diagram* (Figs. 11-4 and 11-5).

In Figure 11-4 there appears to be no relationship between the two variables and no way to predict the value of Y from a value of X. In Figure 11-5, however, a relation becomes apparent, not perfect, but recognizable: as one variable changes, the second variable changes in the same direction.

The measure of the direction and strength of the relationship between two variables is summarized by the correlation coefficient. Figure 11-4 has a correlation coefficient of 0; Figure 11-5 has a correlation coefficient of $+0.87$. A correlation of $+1$ would mean that all the points in Figure 11-5 were located exactly on the ascending diagonal line. Values for X would thus increase as values for Y increased (although the ratio need not be $1:1$), and for every possible value of X it would be possible to predict exactly the corresponding value for Y. Inverse or negative correlation would imply a descending line, with values for X decreasing as values for Y increased. If the correlation coefficient were -1, then all points would be located exactly on this descending straight line. The plus or minus sign indicates the direction of the relationship, same or inverse, respectively, whereas the absolute value indicates the strength of the relationship. The closer the coefficient is to 1, the stronger the relationship. Confidence can seldom be given to a correlation coefficient built on less than a dozen pairs of observations unless the correlation is almost perfect, that is, where r approximates either $+1$ or -1. Often 30 cases are used as the recognized minimum number of pairs, and most researchers believe that using 100 pairs produces stability and confidence in the correlation coefficient.

Student's *t*-test

The t statistic is used to compare two means to determine the probability that the difference between means is greater than that expected by chance. Note that if more than two means are to be compared, then another statistical procedure such as analysis of variance (ANOVA) is indicated and not the t-test. Before proceeding, the student is cautioned against performing analyses or accepting results that have more than two means and proceed to calculate a large series of t-tests using different combinations of means, two at a time. This is blatantly incorrect statistical application, although it may be found in many published articles.

The theoretic distribution for testing statistical significance is Student's t distribution. The t distribution varies. Graphs for t distributions with different degrees of freedom are pictured in Figure

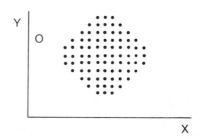

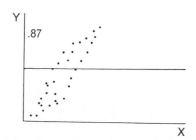

Fig. 11-4 Hypothetical scatter diagram showing correlation coefficients of 0.

Fig. 11-5 Hypothetical scatter diagram showing correlation coefficients of $+0.87$.

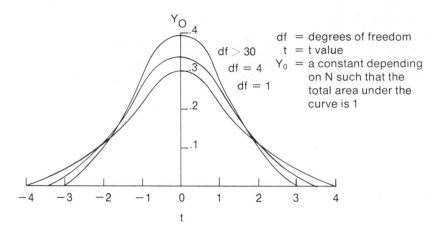

Fig. 11-6 Distribution of *t* for several different degrees of freedom.

11-6 in three examples. As the degrees of freedom approach 30, the curve begins to closely approximate the normal curve.

A calculated *t* value can be positive or negative. The following example helps to clarify the use of the *t*-test.

	Group *X*	**Group *Y***
Number of individuals	10	10
$\overline{X}$	14.8	8.8
Variance	22.84	25.96
Standard deviation	4.78	5.09

Based on this information, the *t*-test is the statistic of choice. Assume the level of significance is 0.05 because no level is specified and after calculation, $t = 2.101$ is produced. One more step remains before the determination can be made as to the degree of difference between means: calculation of the degrees of freedom. The number of degrees of freedom is equal to the number of independent scores that are used to estimate a parameter. For the *t*-test, the parameter estimated is the standard error. For each sample a standard error is estimated. Thus for most examples with two samples:

$$df = n_1 + n_2 - 2 = 18$$

The previous discussion has dealt primarily (with the exception of the X^2) with statistical tests called *parametric tests*. The user of these tests must accept the following two assumptions:

1. Normal distribution. Scores are equally distributed (systematically) around the mean.
There are equal numbers of low and high scores, and most scores are found within 3 standard deviations of the group mean.

2. Continuous equal interval measures. A score must be a whole number or a fractional part, that is, 1, 2, 3, 6.9, or 7.1. This is not a situation where the only possible scores are whole numbers.

One final type of statistical test is nonparametric. This test is used in situations where the data clearly does not fit the two assumptions just indicated. These tests have minimal assumptions specific to each test, but generally these assumptions are less rigorous than those for parametric tests. Again, the student is directed to standard statistical texts for an expanded discussion of these and other statistical topics.

BIBLIOGRAPHY

Boyer EM: *Basic statistical concepts and techniques applied in dental health,* Des Moines, 1975, University of Iowa.

Darby ML, Bowen DM: *Research methods for oral health professionals: an introduction,* St. Louis, 1980, Mosby–Year Book.

Dunning JM: *Principles of dental public health,* ed 2, Cambridge, 1975, Harvard University Press.

Emory CW: *Business research methods,* ed 3, Homewood, Ill, 1985, Richard D Irwin.

Hill AB: *Principles of medical statistics,* ed 7, New York, 1961, Oxford University Press.

Richards LE, LaCava JLJ: *Business statistics: why and when,* New York, 1983, McGraw-Hill.

Snedecor GW, Cochran WG: *Statistical methods,* ed 6, Ames, 1971, Iowa State University Press.

12 Program Evaluation in Health Care

PURPOSE OF PROGRAM EVALUATION

Program evaluation is concerned with finding out how well programs work by using social and behavioral science research techniques to assess information of importance to program administrators and public policy makers. The fundamental purpose of program evaluation is to provide information for decision making. Ultimately, evaluation is a judgment of merit or worth about a particular person, place, or thing.

IS EVALUATION RESEARCH?

The term *research* refers to systematic inquiry that leads one to discover or revise knowledge about a particular subject. So-called basic research is generally focused on discovering facts, relationships, behaviors, and underlying principles. Applied research often deals with the same phenomena, but the focus is usually less on the discovery of basic knowledge and more on the development of tools or the application of knowledge to develop solutions to actual problems. Evaluation is an example of applied research. Administrators, educators, policy makers, and others face questions (problems) about designing, implementing, continuing, and improving social, educational, health, and other programs. Evaluators assess or evaluate those programs to discover or revise knowledge about them and the problems they were designed to address so that informed judgments can be made, modifications can be implemented, and solutions can be achieved.

As researchers, program evaluators engage in scientific inquiry. They use tests, questionnaires, and other measurement devices. They collect and analyze data systematically by using common statistical procedures. Finally, they typically describe their findings in formal reports.[8]

An important difference between basic and evaluation research is the generality of their findings. Ideally, the basic scientist is searching for basic knowledge; the more basic or fundamental, the better. Fundamental facts and principles, such as Einstein's theory of relativity, have broad applicability. They generalize across wide areas of knowledge. Most applied scientists—and program evaluators, in particular—are usually dealing with specific problems in specific settings. Their findings or conclusions can seldom be generalized to "similar" problems.

To elaborate for a moment on this distinction between the basic science researcher and the evaluator, consider the role each individual might play in the testing of a fluoride rinse. In examining the value of fluoride rinse, the basic science researcher would probably be concerned with the effects of fluoride on teeth, the strength of the solution necessary to produce a reduction in caries, and whether the conclusions could be generalized across the population. The evaluator would be more concerned with determining whether the actual mouthrinse program, initiated to test the researcher's conclusion, was run correctly and followed the objectives it stated. The evaluator's concern for the fluoride rinse as such is only superficial. Once the evaluator can judge whether the program is an accurate test of the fluoride rinse, the secondary results might then relate to the positive or negative effects of fluoride rinse. In other words, the particular program's operation is of prime importance to the evaluator, and the effect of fluoride is important only in terms of its results as applied to a realistic, closely monitored program.

Determining the value of things is another difference between evaluation and basic research. Evaluation eventually comes down to making a decision about what should be done or which course of action is best. Basic researchers strive only to obtain accurate, truthful information. There is no requirement to attach assessments of merit to the discovered knowledge.[8] Theoretically at least, the basic scientist's task does not involve making value judgments. The evaluator may or may not make decisions based on value judgments, but the evaluation report almost always ends up in the hands of someone who does.

FOCUS OF EVALUATIONS

Evaluation studies ultimately focus on the goals, objectives, or intent of the program or activity being studied. At the simplest level we ask, does this program do what it was designed to do? There are, of course, many other facets to evaluation. One of the most useful frameworks for looking at the evaluation research task has been put forward by Donabedian.[4] He suggests that assessment or evaluation can profitably look at structure, process, and outcome.

Structure refers to the program setting and logistics (i.e., facilities, equipment, financing, human resources). *Process* refers to the actual ways or methods that are employed in the provision of program services (i.e., delivering health care, educating children). *Outcome* refers to the actual impacts, effects, and changes brought about as a result of the program being evaluated.

Donabedian rightly sees structure, process, and outcomes as inextricably linked: the interrelationships will be critical to the program's ability to meet its goals or fulfill its intent. Examining structure, process, and outcomes allows the evaluator to identify more clearly where problems and program liabilities lie and, hence, where corrections can be made if goals are to be met. Looking at goals, structure, process, and outcomes should be the primary focus for the evaluator. A second set of concerns also exists, however. These questions might be classified as "client" questions; that is, for whom and why is the evaluation research being conducted? This is not a trivial question. The researcher must understand, for example, whose decisions will determine the ultimate fate of a program and what their interests and concerns are. The evaluator must also know what kinds of decisions will be made.

To illustrate, let us say a dental school implements a new curriculum for its students. An evaluator who is brought in designs and carries out a carefully planned study to determine if the program has the resources it needs (structure), how

well the program is running (process), and how successful the graduates are (outcomes). Such an evaluation is appropriate if the client's interest is to determine if the curriculum is functioning properly and meeting its goals. The design would not be appropriate, however, if the client wanted to know if the graduates of the new curriculum were better trained professionals than those of the old. The evaluator must understand the client's focus.

Individuals interested in the results of evaluation may include program developers, program staff, program directors, policy makers (state or federal bureaucrats), program directors in other similar agencies, or epidemiologists.[12] Each group seeks different information about the same program. Program developers seek all kinds of information about ways to improve specific parts of the program that affect them directly. The director of the program is usually interested in knowing the overall effectiveness of the basic program, although he or she is generally more concerned with finding out what specific modifications will be needed to improve the organization and operation of the program. Financial issues are usually of concern to policy makers, who question whether a program should be continued as is, given more resources, or canceled. Staff from other programs are interested in whether the program can be generalized for possible adaptation or adoption. Epidemiologists may seek to compare the effect of different program principles and generalize about the factors responsible for success.

Clearly the evaluator faces a number of potentially competing interests. In responding to those interests the researcher must distinguish between different types of evaluation. As we have seen, Donabedian's framework allows us to focus on the critical features or components that make up a program. These factors must be taken into account if evaluation efforts are to be successful and truly useful. At the same time, Scriven[10] chooses to draw our attention to the fact that evaluation research may be one of two types. He uses the terms *formative* and *summative* to describe these types.

Formative evaluation

Formative evaluation refers to the internal evaluation of a program. It is an examination of the processes or activities of a program as they are taking place. It is usually carried out to aid in the development of a program in its early phases.

The following situation is one in which a formative evaluation is appropriate: a fluoride rinse program is initiated at a neighborhood health center in which paraprofessionals are trained to administer three types of fluoride rinses under a strict sequence of procedures. After 3 days of operation, the work of the paraprofessionals is observed to determine the extent to which the strict sequence of procedures is being adhered. The observation and determination of correct or incorrect procedure sequence provide an example of examining the activities of a program as they are occurring—formative evaluation. If the sequence is incorrect, formative evaluation allows the program to make remedial changes at that point and thereby improve performance. Obviously, such a strategy is much better than waiting until the program is completed and then announcing that there were procedural errors. Formation evaluation is used primarily by program developers and program staff members concerned with whether various components of a program are workable or whether changes should be made to improve program activities.

Summative evaluation

Summative evaluation, by contrast, judges the merit or worth of a program after it has been in operation. It is an attempt to determine whether a fully operational program is meeting the goals for which it was developed. Summative evaluation is aimed at program decision makers, who will decide whether to continue or terminate a program, and also at decision makers from other programs who might be considering adoption of the program.

Different evaluation designs are needed to carry out these two types of evaluation. Different types of measures and time schedules will also be required. Because most programs are ongoing, with changes often being made "on the fly," a discernible end point or completion date may not exist. In such cases the dichotomy between formative and summative evaluation may not be as precise as described here, and formative evaluation may continue to be important as the program develops and matures.

Most health programs can be divided into four phases of implementation, which should occur in sequence: (1) the pilot phase, whose development proceeds on a trial-and-error basis; (2) the controlled phase, in which a model of a particular program strategy is run under regulated conditions to judge its effectiveness; (3) the actualization phase, in which a model of the program strategy is subjected to realistic operating conditions; and (4) the operational phase, in which the program is an ongoing part of the structure. Often this ideal progression from phase 1 to phase 4 does not occur, and a program becomes lodged at one state of development. Each phase has different objectives to be met and thus different evaluation designs by which to best assess achievement of program objectives. Formative evaluation plays an important part in both the pilot and controlled phases of program implementation. Summative and formative evaluations are used during the actualization phase, whereas the final operational phase is evaluated using a summative evaluation design.[11]

SPECIFYING HEALTH PROGRAM OUTCOMES AND INPUTS

One generalization that can be made of health program evaluation is that it is primarily concerned with how well a program is meeting its goals, either at some formative stage (so that the information can be fed back into the program) or at the end. The first step in evaluation, then, is to discover what the program goals are and to then restate them as clear, specific objectives written in measurable terms.

This first step is often a formidable task. Many program directors and staff members develop only general goals expressed as vague abstractions. They find it difficult to translate them into concrete specifications of the changes in behavior, attitude, or knowledge that they hope to effect. In addition, programs often have multiple goals. Some are more important than others, some are more immediate (as opposed to long-range), some are easier to study, and some may be incompatible with others. Yet each program director and staff member must establish a sense of goal priorities if they, or external evaluators, are to assess the operation of their program. In many instances, directors and staff members are unable to clearly sort out goals, objectives, and priorities and find it useful to bring in outside evaluators or administrative consultants to assist in this process.

The frequency of ambiguous and unclear goal statements has led some observers to speculate about the underlying reasons for this state of affairs. One view is that it usually requires support from diverse groups and individuals to get a program accepted. Program goals have to be formulated in ways that satisfy the diversity of interests represented. Another speculation is that program planners lack experience with expressing their thoughts in measurable terms and concentrate mainly on the specifics of program operation. In one sense, ambiguous goal statements serve a useful function: they hide differences among diverse groups by allowing for a variety of interpretations. However, such differences between groups and staff or within the staff could be disruptive if the program is implemented. Once a program has been initiated, if there is lack of true consensus as to what the program is specifically attempting to achieve, progress is difficult. Each staff member may be pulling in a different direction and trying to implement a different interpretation of the goal. As an outside agent or more objective observer, the evaluation study director can make a substantial contribution to program planning and administration in formulating goals, clarifying priorities, and reconciling divergent viewpoints related to program direction.

Ultimately, of course, evaluation attempts to measure the outcomes of a particular program. If a program's goals cannot be operationalized (stated in a precise, measurable manner), it becomes nearly impossible to determine whether the desired outcomes of a program have been achieved. In other words, without clearly stated goals and objectives, evaluation becomes an imprecise tool of questionable usefulness.

One common difficulty in specifying desired objectives is that objectives are often long-range in nature, making it extremely difficult to measure success in meeting those objectives. In the interim, evaluation is conducted by relying on surrogate measures of attitudes, knowledge, skills, or behaviors that presumably are related to the ultimate objectives.

This problem is not unique to evaluation but is basic to program design as well. A program may be designed to produce certain intermediate changes on the assumption that they are necessary for the attainment of ultimate goals. In such cases, probably the best that evaluation can do, at least under the usual time constraints, is to discover whether intermediate goals are being met. It is up to more intensified research efforts to investigate the relation between these goals and desired final outcomes.

Measuring outcomes

To evaluate the effectiveness of health programs, specific measurement instruments must be set up for systematic collection of data on the attainment of each program objective and program goal. These procedures follow accepted principles of biostatistical and research design, which are discussed in Chapters 11 and 13.

Establishment of an effective health program evaluation requires specific description and measurement of each objective of a program. Depending on the nature of the program and the evaluation effort, some data will be collected as a part of the day-to-day operations of the program. Examples might include patient visits, staff turnover, program revenue, and supply costs. In most cases, data collection instruments addressing specific objectives will also be necessary. Examples of factors to be measured by such instruments might include patient satisfaction, employee morale, sealant wear, and the mastery of skills (such as toothbrushing). Usually, multiple instruments are required. If a program has several objectives, use of a simple summary instrument is likely to be superficial and misleading. If measurement instruments that are truly relevant to program intents are available, they should be used, thus moving the evaluation process several steps ahead. Time is saved, and the program and evaluation benefit from tested and validated instruments. Use of the same measurement instruments makes it easier to compare the relative effectiveness of one program with many other programs and adds significantly to the overall body of research knowledge. However, if existing instruments are not relevant to the program objectives, new measures that are constructed for the specific needs of the program must be developed.

Instrument reliability and validity

Measurement instruments used to assess program objectives and materials must be valid and reliable. A valid measurement instrument is one that provides a score that accurately describes the characteristics it is intended to measure. A reliable instrument consistently or repeatedly produces the same score. Validity and reliability are important because no test or other measurement instrument is perfect. Each time a test is administered, a range of scores results. We know that statistically each score contains a small amount of error because of testing and measurement procedures. If the procedure is repeated 10 times for 10 separate components of a health program, one can see how the amount of error can build, thus reducing the ability of the evaluation to assess program effectiveness accurately. The greater the reliability and validity, the more accurate the information collected during the evaluation process.

A simple example of a test that might be reliable but not valid would be the dental hygiene board examination administered to first-year dental students. Results of that test might prove to be highly reliable and consistent, yet not valid. One might guess that if first-year dental students took the dental hygiene board examination a number of times, their individual scores would not fluctuate much higher or lower than the scores they received at the first administration. Thus the test would be considered highly reliable. It repeatedly produced the same or nearly the same score. This test would not be considered valid because it measured material totally foreign to the first-year dental student. The test is designed to measure skills of graduate dental hygienists, not first-year dental students. Thus the test is reliable but not valid.

As a second example, let us assume a course is offered in which four tests are administered during the course of the semester. No one test was found to be perfectly reliable, thus error as a result of testing would result with each administration. Assume student A received the following scores:

	Score	Reliability	Testing error	Range
Test 1	80	0.80	5	75 to 85
Test 2	70	0.63	8	62 to 78
Test 3	80	0.55	12	68 to 92
Test 4	90	0.92	2	88 to 92
AVERAGE	80			73 to 87

In this example, student A obtained an average of 80 and probably would receive a course grade of B− or B. Yet, because of normal error associated with the unreliability of the four tests, that student's true performance may be between 73 and 87. These scores indicate that student A's course grade could actually be between C− and B+, a substantial difference for most students. The more reliable the test, the smaller the error. Compare the reliability scores with the test error. The test with high reliability (0.92) has the smallest error (2), whereas the test with low reliability (0.55) has the greatest amount of error.

Difficulties in obtaining necessary information

After considering what measurement instruments to use and when to measure outcomes, a final concern must be how to measure. In this area two problems are particularly important: bias and sampling. The possibility of bias is great if one evaluates her or his own work. Bias may be avoided by using objective measures rather than subjective measures and also by using several people rather than a single person to measure outcomes. Sampling is used in evaluating a health program when it is not possible or practical to obtain information from every person involved in an activity or when it is not possible to assess every activity that a program initiates.

Sample size depends on the activity to be studied. The student is advised to consult a standard research design text for a more formal discussion of bias and sampling problems related to evaluation and research.

Constant intrusions into the program to collect data can be a source of friction with program staff. The evaluation is a service to the program, not vice versa; therefore evaluation activities should be limited to only those found essential to furthering program effectiveness. One thoughtfully constructed test or questionnaire is often better than three imperfectly conceived ones. When the evaluation is clear about what is needed and why, measures can be constructed and data collected with a minimum of disruption.

Programs may intend to bring about changes not only in people but also in agencies, larger social systems, or the public at large. Measures have to be relevant to such changes. Cost-benefit analysis is another measurement technique. Cost-benefit analysis is not a suitable substitute for usual methods of evaluation but a logical extension of it. Evaluation defines the program's benefits; cost-benefit analysis adds consideration of the value of the benefits. Costs of the program are compared with benefits as a way of judging whether the program is a worthwhile investment.

How does one decide which program activities to measure? Difficulties arise when theory and knowledge are inadequate to define the factors that affect success. In most program areas the general rule of thumb is that each stated objective of the program should be measured. A clearly stated objective indicates what achievement is sought, and thus such an objective will aid in the identification of what procedures to use for measuring program outcomes.

Table 12-1 indicates six general factors where evaluation of health programs may begin. Below each general factor are listed specific areas in which various program members would find evaluation information of interest. This list is not intended to be all-inclusive, but it should provide a few ideas to an individual who is not sure where to begin.

To conclude this section on measurement instruments the following outline identifies three factors to consider in instrument selection: importance, statistical adequacy, and feasibility.[9]

1. Importance

   Is the information that is gained by administering the instrument the measure that is needed to assess health status or health program effectiveness? Does the program require this information to perform its function?

2. Statistical adequacy

   a. Validity: Does the instrument accurately assess what you are trying to measure?

   b. Reliability: Will repeated application of the computational method for the measure yield similar results? How reliable are the data used to calculate the results?

   c. Sensitivity: Can the instrument adequately distinguish among levels of performance?

3. Feasibility

   a. Clarity of measure: How precise is the measure? Is the wording understandable? Are its limitations explained?

   b. Data availability and cost: Does the program have the information needed to assess the objective? Are the instruments appropriate for their specific use within the program?

   c. Compatibility: Can data collected for this program be compared with similar data on a statewide or national basis? Can they be compared with similar data from different types of programs?

   d. Ease of use and interpretation: Can collection and interpretation of data for implementation of the measure be done without specialized or statistical knowledge?

STUDY DESIGNS APPROPRIATE FOR SPECIFIC PROGRAMS

In planning an evaluation study one is immediately struck with the fact that there are a multitude of possible study designs from which to choose.[7] Choosing the best design is one of the most critical tasks the evaluator faces. In the broadest sense, evaluation research designs are divided into two groups: experimental and nonexperimental. Experimental design has long been considered the ideal for evaluation. The design requires that people, objects, and other factors be randomly assigned either to the program or to a control group. A control group is a group of individuals in an experiment whose selection and experiences are identical in every way possible to the program participants except that they are not part of the program. The control group may receive a pseudoprogram (the social science equivalent of the laboratory placebo), the standard program (the traditional rather than the innovative program), or no program at all. Relevant measurements are taken before and after the program. If the program recipients show greater positive change than the controls, the outcome can clearly be attributed to the program. Experimental design is the study design all researchers choose when given a choice.[2]

Toothbrushing studies are a perfect example of the true experimental design model. For illustration purposes the study shown in Table 12-2 is designed to demonstrate the effectiveness of a fluo-

Table 12-1 Component factors of health system characteristics

Availability	Accessibility	Cost	Quality	Continuity	Acceptability
Supply of services: Existing service capacity Used capacity Supply of resources: Personnel Equipment Facilities Financial resources	Ability to obtain services in terms of the following factors: Economic Out of pocket cost Health insurance coverage and benefits Opportunity cost to patient/client, family and others Temporal Travel time Waiting time Locational Architectural Cultural Organizational Informational Use of services by specified population subgroups	Service cost Costs incurred by providers Costs incurred by financing mechanisms Sources of payment for services	Structure Competence and qualifications of resources Existence and extent of review and assurance mechanisms Minimal volume of specialized services Process Accuracy of services Appropriateness of services Documentation of treatment Outcome Health status Behavior Environment	Coordination of settings among health system components and to/from other nonhealth systems Regular source of care Degree of interruptions or delays in service plan given a logical sequence of services Patient transfer Medical and health information transfer Follow-up	Consumer satisfactions with Availability Accessibility Cost Continuity Courtesy and consideration Provider satisfaction

Modified from Hadley SA, Gillespie JF Jr: Operational measures: indicators of health system performance, *Am J Health Plan* 3:44, 1978.

ride toothpaste for the reduction of new carious lesions. The study is of 3-year duration and of longitudinal design. Both experimental and control groups brush daily under supervision. The study is double-blind; all experimental materials are color coded, and look and taste are identical. All participants use the same brand and model of brush, with the type of paste (that is, fluoride paste and nonfluoride paste) being the one variable examined in the study. Results of the study show a significant reduction in the numbers of new lesions, thus allowing the researcher to assume the reduction was a result of the one differing variable (i.e., fluoride versus nonfluoride).

One major problem arises when one tries to implement experimental procedures in health programs. It is nearly impossible to implement the design in the busy day-to-day activities of the pro-

Table 12-2 Longitudinal results of 3-year fluoride toothpaste study

	Randomly assigned groups	
	Experimental (fluoride paste)	Control (nonfluoride paste)
Baseline examination (DMFS) (prior to beginning testing of paste)	97.4	97.5
After 1 year	91.5	95.0
After 2 years	86.3	93.4
After 3 years	80.0	90.3
Difference	17.4	7.2

DMFS, decayed, missing, filled surfaces.

gram. One must question how random services can be tested on people who come to drop-in, multiservice, or neighborhood health centers. In addition, there is resistance from the program staff and difficulty resulting from the very nature of the recipient groups and from outside events that "contaminate" the controls placed on the study. These contaminations reduce the validity of the evaluation.

Two types of validity affect the ability to implement evaluation research designs according to strict experimental requirements: internal validity and external validity. These kinds of validity are different from the term used earlier relating to measurement instruments. A program has internal validity if its outcomes are a result of the approach or techniques being tested rather than a result of other causes that have nothing to do with the program being implemented. Internal validity determines whether the results can be accepted based on the evaluation design of the program.[2]

A program has external validity if the results obtained would be generalizable everywhere to similar programs or approaches. External validity affects one's ability to credit the evaluation results with generality based on the procedures used.[2]

The process of conducting an experimental evaluation design by its nature exercises some degree of control over the program, thus contributing to internal validity, while producing some limitations in external validity. A catch-22 situation is produced. As the circumstances of a program are controlled, the chances increase that what happens in the program will be exactly what the evaluator hopes to find (internal validity). However, the more conditions are controlled, the less chance there is that the program will continue to work when the controls are removed (external validity).

The constant struggle between external and internal validity is an important one; external validity is of little value without some reasonable degree of internal validity to provide confidence in the conclusions. There is no advantage in being able to generalize results that are based on invalid or inconsistent program activities. The two sets of validity demands must strike a balance. There should be enough internal validity so that an experiment can be conclusive and yet sufficiently realistic to be generalized. In program evaluation, internal validity becomes the major concern because most programs attempt only superficially to generalize results beyond their program.

Perhaps "the source" in the area of research design is Donald T. Campbell. Campbell[1] suggests that experimental design is possible in most health programs with careful planning and administrative backing, and control groups can be used in somewhat turbulent programs.

In reality, it is often impossible to fully apply rules relating to internal validity. To evaluate programs in such situations the evaluator must choose some approach other than experimental. If circumstances eliminate experimental design situations, Campbell and Stanley[2] have developed quasiexperimental designs that are often suitable. Campbell[1] offers three types useful in evaluation: interrupted time series, control series, and regression discontinuity designs. Although the results do not provide the certainty and the potential for generalization of experimental designs, they guard against most of the important threats to valid interpretation. Again, for the interested student, a standard research methods text is suggested for more comprehensive discussion of research design. It should also be noted that evaluation is concerned with making decisions about specific programs. Therefore internal validity is often more important than external validity to the evaluator.

CONSTRAINTS ON USING THE RESULTS OF EVALUATION

Once the evaluation is completed, the logical expectation is that the results will be used to make rational decisions about future programming. All too often, however, the results are ignored. With all the money, time, effort, skills, and irritation that went into the acquisition of information, why does it generally have so little impact? One reason may be that evaluation results do not match the informational needs of decision makers.

Individuals responsible for conducting evaluations should have a better understanding of decision processes and of informational requirements relevant to decision making. An allied issue is that of timing. Evaluation results should be ready in time to be considered, not after the decisions on future programming have been reached. Moreover, the evaluation results may not be relevant to the level of the decision maker who receives them. For example, overall assessments of program merit may be most useful to directors in other agencies who want to know whether a new program strategy works and under what conditions. Such people may never receive the report or may receive it in a nearly unreadable form.

Another constraint on the use of results may be a lack of clear direction for future programming. Results may be ambiguous and implications unclear. They have to be translated into terms that make sense for pending decisions and that delineate alternatives that are indicated. There seems to be a large void between the findings of program evaluation and the planning of future programs. Someone is needed to translate the evaluation results into explicit recommendations for future programs.

In practice, evaluation is sometimes undertaken for dubious reasons. Evaluation may be used by program decision makers to delay a decision, to justify a decision already made, to pass the responsibility of future decisions to others, to vindicate a program in the eyes of its observers, or to satisfy funding conditions of government or foundation agencies.[11] These noninformational reasons for evaluation are not rare, and individuals conducting evaluation should be forewarned if they learn that one of these is the underlying purpose of evaluation. It is as important to spend enough time in-

vestigating who wants to know what, and why, as it is to carry out the evaluation activities. Evaluations for political ends or where there is no commitment to using the data for decision making might well be eliminated rather than waste the talents of the individuals involved.[5]

External evaluators (persons called in who are not part of the program) are often reluctant to draw conclusions from their data. However, judgments and recommendations for action have to be made somewhere. Unless the evaluator plays a leading role in the process, it may not get done.

A further constraint on use of results is that organizations are comfortable with the status quo. When presented with negative results, their prestige, ideology, and even resources are threatened. They frequently react by rejecting the results.

Campbell[1] suggests that one way out of this dilemma is for reformers to change their stance. Instead of committing themselves to new programs as though they were proven solutions, they would do better to commit themselves to seeking solutions to the problem. Then they could run a series of experimental programs until genuine solutions were found.

The prevalence of negative findings in a wide range of program fields is not something to bemoan or cover up, even when it provokes political controversy or organizational resistance. Rather, the evidence that so many programs are having little constructive effect represents a fundamental critique of current approaches to social programming. This is a matter to which society will, in time, have to respond.

SUMMARY

Evaluation involves research into the operation and accomplishments of programs that are usually, but not exclusively, designed to impact on social problems. By their very nature, evaluation efforts are linked more or less directly to a set of values that provide the criteria for judging relative success.

In looking at programs the evaluator must recognize that program structure, process, and outcomes are all interrelated, and that these are functionally related to the program's goals and objectives. Performing a good evaluation involves formulating (or clarifying) objectives, specifying the criteria to be used in measuring success, determining and explaining the degree of observed success, and (usually) recommending modifications in program activity to improve performance.[6]

Evaluations are undertaken not simply to reveal success or failure. If that were the case, most evaluations of programs would reveal lack of total success in attaining goals and objectives. Good evaluation does more than demonstrate degree of attainment. It also identifies problems and points out how a structural problem, for example, links with and affects process and outcome variables. Identified problems may also relate to ill-conceived, ill-defined, or simply misdirected goals. Ideally, good evaluations identify opportunities and ways to correct programs and improve program efficiency. The evaluation of programs assumes that (1) programs have been planned to expend funds to enable materials to be developed and activities to be performed and that (2) the activities are intended to cause the achievement of program goals.

A program may not achieve its goals for the following reasons[3]:

1. Resources were not used as planned.
2. The assumptions linking resources to activities were invalid.
3. Activities were not performed as planned.
4. The assumptions linking activities to objectives were invalid.
5. The assumptions linking objectives to the program goals were invalid.

A sixth reason, which is technically included in this list but often overlooked and thus deserving of special mention, is that the behavior of the program staff and/or the client population may consciously or unconsciously undermine program performance. In other words, the best-designed program in the world cannot succeed if the providers and clients do not like it and are openly or tacitly unwilling to cooperate.

If evaluation can identify the problems, subsequent program planning should proceed more effectively than it could in the absence of evaluation. Thus a successful evaluation in the hands of a thoughtful administrator can improve the planning and management of programs, thereby increasing program effectiveness.

REFERENCES

1. Campbell DT: *Reform as experiments in evaluating action programs,* Boston, 1972, Allyn & Bacon.
2. Campbell DT, Stanley JC: *Experimental and quasi-experimental design for research,* Chicago, 1966, Rand McNally.
3. Deniston OL, Rosenstock IM, Getting VA: Evaluation of program effectiveness, *Public Health Rep* 83:323, 1968.
4. Donabedian A: The quality of care: how can it be assessed? *JAMA* 260:1743, 1988.
5. Elinson J: *Effectiveness of social action programs in health and welfare, assessing the effectiveness of child health services.* Report of the fifty-sixth Ross Conference on Pediatric Research, Columbus, Ohio, 1967.
6. Glossary of administrative terms in public health, *Am J Public Health* 50:225, 1960.
7. Isaac S, Michael WB: *Handbook in research and evaluation,* San Diego, Calif, 1981, Edits.
8. Popham JW: *Educational evaluation,* Englewood Cliffs, NJ, 1975, Prentice Hall.
9. Schulberg HC, Sheldon A, and Baker F: *Program evaluation in the health fields,* New York, 1969, Behavioral Publications.
10. Scriven M: *The methodology of evaluation.* In Tyler RN, Gagne RM, Scriven M, editors: *Perspectives of curriculum evaluation,* AERA monograph series on curriculum evaluation, No 1. Chicago, 1967, Rand McNally.
11. Suchman EA: *Action for what? A critique of evaluation research. In* O'Toole R, editor: *The organization, management, and tactics of social research,* Cambridge, Mass, 1970, Schenkman.
12. Weiss CH: *Evaluating action programs: readings in social action and education,* Boston, 1972, Allyn & Bacon.

BIBLIOGRAPHY

Anderson SB and others: *Encyclopedia of educational evaluation,* San Francisco, 1976, Jossey Bass.
Baker EL: *Formative evaluation.* In Popham JW: *Evaluation in education: current applications,* Berkeley, Calif, 1974, McCutchan.
Bloom BS, Hastings ST, Madaus GF: *Handbook on formative and summative evaluation of student learning,* New York, 1971, McGraw-Hill.
Cook TD, Campbell DT: *Quasi-experimental design and analysis issues for field settings,* Boston, 1979, Houghton Mifflin.
Donabedian A: The seven pillars of quality, *Arch Pathol Lab Med* 114:1115, 1990.
FitzGibbon CT, Morris LL: *How to design a program evaluation,* Beverly Hills, Calif, 1978, Sage.
FitzGibbon CT, Morris LL: *How to present an evaluation report,* Beverly Hills, Calif, 1978, Sage.
Guba EG: *Development, diffusion and evaluation.* In Eidell TE, Kitchell JM, editors: *Knowledge production and utilization in educational administration,* Eugene, 1968, Center for the Advanced Study of Educational Administration, University of Oregon.
Guba EG: Failure of educational evaluation, *Educ Tech* 9:29, 1969.
Polit DF, Hungler BP: *Nursing research: principles and methods,* ed 2, Philadelphia, 1983, JB Lippincott.
Rosenstock IM: Evaluating health programs, *Public Health Rep* 85:835, 1970.

Rosenstock IM, Welch W, Getting VA: Evaluation of program efficiency, *Public Health Rep* 83:603, 1968.

Rossi PH, Freeman HE: *Evaluation: a systematic approach,* Newbury Park, Calif, 1989, Sage.

Stufflebeam DL and others: *Educational evaluation and decision making,* Itasca, Ill, 1971, FE Peacock.

Suchman EA: *Evaluation research: principles and practice in public service and action programs,* New York, 1967, Russell Sage Foundation.

Tuchman BW: *Conducting educational research,* ed 2, New York, 1978, Harcourt Brace Jovanovich.

Wholey JS and others: *Federal evaluation policy,* Washington, DC, 1970, Urban Institute.

Worthen BR: Toward a taxonomy of evaluation designs, *Educ Tech* 8:3, 1968.

13 Research in Community Dental Health

If it can be said that biomedical research falls into one of two categories—basic (laboratory) research or applied (clinical) research—there is no doubt that research in community dentistry is predominantly applied research. The research invariably involves people who are not only the experimental subjects but also often the immediate as well as the long-range beneficiaries. Not until a new material or technique has been tested on a human population is a researcher able to say with some degree of certainty, "This method really works," or "This method clearly does not work." It is unfortunate that a procedure or a material sometimes slips into the standard armamentarium of the clinician or educator without having been tested adequately in controlled research. A case in point is the assumption that a rubber cup prophylaxis *must* precede the application of topical fluoride. The clinician has always believed that this is indeed the case, but is it so? Clinical research is only beginning to apply rigid criteria to research regarding this and other firmly held, and often arbitrary, assumptions.

This chapter deals with several aspects of research in community dentistry:

1. Various types of research commonly carried out in this field
2. Role of the federal government in supporting such research
3. Ethical issues related to research involving human subjects
4. Techniques for designing research studies and writing protocols (for example, a typical clinical trial and a questionnaire survey)
5. Methods for reading and critically evaluating the published dental research literature

In a detailed discussion of research methodology, one cannot avoid the troublesome subjects of epidemiology and biostatistics; these disciplines are basic tools of the clinical investigator. However, there is serious danger of an introductory discussion of research becoming submerged in epidemiologic and statistical jargon. In the interest of making this chapter readable to the widest possible audience, we do not deal explicitly with these topics, and jargon is kept to a minimum. For detailed discussions of biostatistics and epidemiology, the reader is referred to Chapters 11 and 7, respectively.

TYPES OF RESEARCH IN COMMUNITY DENTISTRY

Community dentistry research falls into three different areas: (1) clinical trials and tests of techniques and of therapeutic agents, (2) research in educational techniques and the behavioral sciences, and (3) research related to the administration and evaluation of community dental programs.

Investigators and their funding agencies are increasingly aware of the importance of cost in relation to effectiveness. This awareness has permeated all aspects of community dental care research and has become, to a great extent, the yardstick by which research outcome is measured. No longer is it sufficient to say that a therapeutic agent works or that it prevents some proportion of oral disease. The critical question becomes, how much does it cost to prevent this oral disease, and are there other techniques that can accomplish as much at a lower cost?

Table 13-1 shows several different methods for preventing dental caries that are commonly used in publicly supported programs. The efficacy of all these approaches is well demonstrated in the research literature. However, from the point of view of community dentistry, one must ask the question, what are the relative costs of these methods? This question is especially important in view of the substantial decline in dental caries prevalence among U.S. schoolchildren, which is obviously beneficial in terms of overall oral health but which

Table 13-1 Efficacy and practicality of various community-based preventive procedures

Procedure	Median annual cost/person ($)[16]	Average caries reduction (%)	Caries reduction (surfaces/year)*	Cost of saving each surface ($)
Fluoridation Fluoride	0.26	30[24]	0.28	0.93
Supplements Fluoride	2.26	30[18]	0.28	8.07
Mouthrinses School	1.3	30[21]	0.28	4.64
Fluoridation	4.26	30[18]	0.28	15.21
Sealants	23.73	80[25]	0.74	32.07

* Based on estimated average 1-year caries increment of 0.92 surfaces for 11- to 15-year-old children in United States in 1986-87.[7]

has the annoying characteristic of making the prevention of additional dental caries relatively more costly. *Clinical* effectiveness of the various techniques, except for sealants, is comparable, but the *cost*-effectiveness (cost of preventing one carious tooth surface) covers a wide range, from the very high cost-effectiveness of water fluoridation to the very low cost-effectiveness of sealants.[16]

Clinical trials of techniques and therapeutic agents

Clinical trials of techniques and therapeutic agents usually follow as the practical applications of laboratory (in vitro and animal) research, epidemiologic observation, or both. A case in point is the clinical use of fluorides for the prevention of dental caries. Although the student is referred to other sources for a definitive history of fluorides,[13] the subject is summarized briefly here.

In the early 1900s the observation was made that populations in certain parts of the United States, for example, eastern Colorado, displayed teeth with severe staining and mottling. Concurrently, it was observed that this disfigurement invariably was accompanied by relatively low dental caries prevalence. It was not until the 1930s that the observational techniques of epidemiology and the analytical techniques of chemistry were able to establish the connection between mottling of the teeth and fluoride content in the drinking water. The inferential step from the mottling-fluoride observation and the mottling–low caries observation is obvious. In the late 1930s and early 1940s, clinical researchers begin asking two questions: (1) if the presence of fluoride in drinking water reduces dental caries and causes mottling of the teeth,

might there be some optimum concentration of fluoride in the drinking water that would minimize mottling and maximize the anticaries effect?[10,12] and (2) if fluoride in drinking water inhibits dental caries, might not a prepared fluoride solution applied topically to the teeth have a similar effect?[4,8,20]

The first question was answered by careful evaluation of the amount of mottling and the level of dental caries in communities having varying concentrations of fluoride in the drinking water.[11] The optimum amount was found to be approximately 1 part per million of fluoride ion. In the mid-1940s this epidemiologic conclusion led directly to the controlled addition of fluoride compounds to the drinking water in several communities in the United States and Canada.[1] These clinical "community dentistry" research projects have demonstrated conclusively over the past 4 decades that drinking water fluoridated at the proper concentration can prevent a large proportion of dental caries in a population. In the earlier clinical trials, when water was virtually the only source of fluoride in the diet, children in fluoridated communities had up to 65% less caries than children in comparable fluoride-deficient communities. More recently, as fluoride has become more ubiquitous in the diet and in fluoride-containing preventive agents, the relative effectiveness of water fluoridation has dropped to about 30%.

The second question led directly to laboratory research measuring the effect of topical fluoride applications on incidence of dental caries in laboratory animals.[3] Those studies were quite successful, and application of topical fluorides to the teeth of human subjects was first attempted in the early

1940s.[4,8,20] Ultimately the technique gained wide acceptance within the profession and today is used almost universally in private dental offices and in community programs, not only professionally applied but self-applied as well.[22] In addition to solutions and gels, fluoride-containing dentifrices and mouthrinses are in this same category of topical fluorides.

Before beginning a clinical trial of some therapeutic agent (for example, a toothpaste with a new form of fluoride or a mouthrinse containing a chemical that could inhibit plaque formation—in short, any drug that has not previously been used in that manner in human populations), the investigator may need to consider certain federal regulations. For instance, a license to use the new drug in a human population may frequently be required from the federal Food and Drug Administration. Further information regarding this license, called an IND (investigative exemption for a new drug), can be secured from the Food and Drug Administration, 5600 Fishers Lane, Rockville, MD 20852. Also, the research study probably needs to be approved by the Institutional Review Board for Studies Involving Human Subjects (IRB) of the institution where the investigator is employed or is a student. These issues are discussed in more detail later in this chapter under Ethics of Dental Research. Finally, the drug or chemical compound may be protected by a patent as, for instance, are some of the formulations incorporated in therapeutic toothpastes.

Having conceived a worthwhile clinical study based on favorable research in laboratory studies or on well-established epidemiologic observations, and having dealt with the federal and institutional guidelines previously described, the investigator is ready to design and implement a research study. The design of a clinical trial is dealt with in more detail later under Research Design.

Educational and behavioral research

Educational and behavioral research is frequently carried out by undergraduate dental students and dental hygiene students. Both types of research have the advantage of not usually requiring large numbers of study subjects, and often the study can be completed in a relatively short period of time.

Typically the study deals with applying some behavioral or educational technique to the oral hygiene practices of an individual or a group.

Experimental subjects can be approached on several different levels involving changes in knowledge, attitudes, or behavior. Much traditional dental health education and accompanying research has been based on changing the level of knowledge regarding oral health and disease in a population. Research evidence firmly establishes that, although increases in levels of knowledge may be easy to accomplish, this approach is probably of little value in terms of improving oral health.[15] Most persons, when asked what they *should* do to maintain good oral health, verbally respond with the correct answers, although intraoral evidence may show that this knowledge is not being put into practice. If persons are not able to link their knowledge of oral health to their own personal oral health needs, their behavior will not change.[15] Ultimately, permanent changes in behavior are essential for improving oral health. These issues and their resolution are discussed in more detail in Chapter 9.

Administrative and evaluative research

Administrative and evaluative research typically deals with the way in which a program (for example, a school-based clinical dental program) operates and how it can be improved, or with how some innovation (for instance, use of pit and fissure sealants) has been accepted in the professional community. Administrative and evaluative research involvement in evaluation of programs is discussed in detail in Chapter 12.

The questionnaire survey. An important tool of administrative and evaluative research is the questionnaire survey. Carefully designed questionnaires can be extremely effective for securing information from a population under study. The questionnaire itself, referred to as the *survey instrument,* requires a great deal of thought and careful planning. Not only is the content itself important, but equally significant are the structure and appearance of the questionnaire. A method for designing and carrying out a questionnaire survey is discussed in detail under Research Design.

Government role in community dentistry research

For the past few years the federal government has played an increasingly important role in dental research. A great deal of this research falls within the scope of community dentistry. With an operating budget of almost $130 million (1990), the National Institute of Dental Research is able to exert an enormous amount of influence on the dental research community. Although many individual researchers may object to this influence, there is no doubt that the effect over the past few years has been largely positive. This influence has been of three types: (1) defining research priorities, (2) conducting intramural research, and (3) funding extramural research.

Defining research priorities. Areas of potentially fruitful research are identified and published primarily through the mechanism of sponsoring conferences of recognized experts in some particular field. These research areas subsequently tend to become areas for which funding is available. A good example of this is the recent publication of the National Institute of Dental Research, *Broadening the Scope—Long-Range Research Plan for the Nineties,*[6] which grew out of a series of meetings of prominent researchers from throughout the United States in late 1989.

Intramural research. Some agencies (particularly the National Institute of Dental Research, located in Bethesda, Maryland) carry out a great deal of intramural research with staffs of highly competent researchers.

Extramural research. The bulk of dental research is conducted by means of extramural funding mechanisms. A contractual arrangement is made between the federal agency and some institution competent to carry out the research in question. Funding of extramural research is of two basic types: grants and contracts.

A *grant* is awarded either to an institution or to an individual for the purpose of attaining some research goal that has been defined by the individual or the institution. Although the general area of research may previously have been suggested by the federal agency, the research design is developed by the grantee. By contrast, *contract* research evolves from a research protocol that has been designed and stipulated in detail by the federal agency.

Most government research in dentistry is sponsored by the Department of Health and Human Services through the National Institute of Dental Research of the National Institutes of Health. The approval and funding processes, regardless of the agency involved, are generally the same. Initially the agency issues an announcement to appropriate institutions. These announcements are of two types: requests for proposal and requests for applications.

The *request for proposal* (RFP) is a device used when contract research is anticipated. The RFP is a detailed definition of the goals and parameters of the research project. Institutions that are interested and feel competent to carry out the research are invited to submit detailed proposals in which they describe exactly how they would meet the terms of the proposal (the scope of work). Responses to RFPs must meet all the conditions of the RFP, and any deviation from the defined protocol must be submitted as an alternative proposal.

The *request for applications* (RFA) suggests a general area where the federal government places a high research priority. Applicants are invited to submit grant applications (as opposed to contract proposals) that are addressed to this general area or priority. In the resulting grant application, researchers define their own research goals and develop their own protocol.

In either case, whether for a grant or a contract, the proposal is submitted to review by a group of experts who are peers of the principal investigator. For proposals that meet the standards of excellence defined by the peer group, there is a final negotiation process and ultimate funding of the project, assuming funds are available.

ETHICS OF DENTAL RESEARCH

To the extent that proposed research involves human subjects, an elaborate system of safeguards has evolved out of concern for the welfare of human beings and the protection of the rights of persons who could be victims of inappropriate or poorly conceived research.

The Nuremberg Code of Ethics for Medical Research grew out of the deliberations of the Nuremberg War Crimes Tribunal and the revelations regarding biomedical research that was carried out by the Nazis during World War II. The principles established were reinforced by the Declaration of Helsinki, which was adopted by the World Medical Association in 1966.[17]

In the early 1950s the Department of Health, Education, and Welfare (now called the Department of Health and Human Services) became involved in establishing guidelines for the design and conduct of research involving human subjects at the federal level. For any institution using Department of Health, Education, and Welfare funds, these guidelines became mandatory in 1974.[17]

The formal mechanism for monitoring research that uses humans as experimental subjects is the Institutional Review Board for Studies Involving Human Subjects, established according to federal regulations at all institutions conducting research paid for by federal funds.

Minimally the institution must have a committee consisting of five members including both males and females. It should represent a variety of professions, include at least one nonscientist, and include at least one person who is not associated with the institution.[12] The IRB must review all research involving humans, whether or not it is to be supported with federal funds. No project involving humans is to be approved unless evidence is presented that the rights of the human subjects have been adequately protected. In the case of federally funded projects the institution must submit a form that indicates that the appropriate review has been carried out.

Concept of informed consent

For a person to be involved legitimately as an experimental subject in a research project, she or he must have given free and informed consent to the researcher. Although this discussion is directed to informed consent in relation to research studies, the same principles prevail in regard to consent for receiving clinical treatment.[2,23]

Informed consent (over and above that informed consent required for regular clinical care) is required whenever a person will receive some treatment or be involved in some technique of physical or psychologic manipulation that is regarded as

experimental in nature. Informed consent may not be required if the individual is not directly involved in the research, for instance, if patient records, radiographs, or previously extracted teeth are used in a situation where the patient is not directly identified. However, if the records or radiographs were collected for the purposes of the research, informed consent would be required. Assume, for instance, a patient is scheduled for extractions for orthodontic reasons. If prior to the extractions some experimental treatment is to be carried out on the teeth scheduled for extraction, even if it will be absolutely harmless, consent is required for the procedure. In general, if a patient or experimental subject is manipulated in any way for experimental purposes, even though the manipulation is minimal and the risk or inconvenience is inconsequential, consent is still required.

The following case studies illustrate what may often be the thin line between requiring and not requiring informed consent for participation in experimental research. The issue of informed consent prior to routine treatment or therapy is not considered here.

Case study 1

A clinician wishes to determine which of two commonly used methods for educating patients in plaque control, A or B, is more effective. To help answer this question, clinical records of 100 patients previously exposed to each of the two methods were examined. Routinely, a plaque measure has been recorded on a patient's chart prior to exposure to the educational program and then at regular intervals after this exposure. These data were collected for each of the patients in the two groups, as well as other data such as age, sex, educational level, and socioeconomic background. All these data became a part of the patient's regular record. The data are tabulated according to the identified variables, and the clinician determines that method A produces better results than method B.

Informed consent is not required for this study for the following reasons:

1. Only existing patient records were used.
2. The patients, within the context of the research, became experimental subjects but were not manipulated in any way beyond the normal treatment procedure.
3. The patients' confidentiality (their right to

privacy) was not invaded by the research because no data were used that could serve to identify them.

Case study 2

A research protocol is conceived precisely the same as that described in Case study 1, except that it is conceived before the fact of the regular care and that the research subjects are placed randomly in two groups, one group to receive program A and the other to receive program B. In all other respects, the project is exactly the same.

Informed consent is required for this project for the following reasons:

1. It is decided a priori that the patients would be part of a research project.
2. The patients are manipulated to the extent that they are each placed arbitrarily and randomly in one of the two experimental groups.
3. Even though the outcome is the same, and even though there is no invasion of the patients' privacy, the prior intention of the activity is to collect research data and the patients are being manipulated to that extent.

Several elements are necessary in a properly designed informed consent document:[9]

1. A fair explanation of the procedures to be followed and their purposes, including identification of any procedures that are experimental,
2. A description of any attendant discomforts and risks reasonably to be expected,
3. A description of any benefits reasonably to be expected,
4. A disclosure of any appropriate alternative procedures that might be advantageous for the subject,
5. A statement describing the confidentiality of records,
6. For research involving more than minimal risk, an explanation as to whether compensation and medical treatment are available if physical injury occurs and, if so, what they consist of and where further information may be obtained,
7. An explanation of whom to contact for answers to pertinent questions about the research and research subjects' rights and whom to contact in the event of a research-related injury to the subject,
8. A statement that the person is free to withdraw consent and to discontinue participation in the project or activity at any time without prejudice to the subject.

The box on p. 274 is an example of a consent form used in a research project. The necessary elements described previously are clearly evident.

The use of placebos

A *placebo* is an agent that is known to have no physiologic effect on the patient, although it can have an extremely beneficial effect on a patient whose problem is basically psychologic rather than organic. One of the important elements of research design is to compare an experimental drug or technique with some other drug or technique, the efficacy of which is known with a great degree of accuracy. It is quite understandable, therefore, that the most common comparison in biomedical research has been to the placebo, the physiologic efficacy of which is known to be zero. Typically a study population is divided randomly in half, with one group taking the experimental drug and the other group taking a placebo that looks, smells, and tastes like the experimental drug. The degree to which the experimental drug group is different from the placebo drug group in its outcome is a measure of the efficacy of the experimental drug.

With the growing armamentarium of effective drugs—for example, fluorides for the prevention of dental caries—it is considered unethical to design a study in which half of the study population is denied a preventive treatment of known efficacy.[5] However, in a situation where a drug or technique of known efficacy is available (this is commonly the case), the dilemma is dealt with easily by the use of an active control, rather than a placebo control. Practically speaking, this presents no problem because the clinical value of the experimental drug or technique ultimately must be measured against previously accepted alternatives.

RESEARCH DESIGN

This section considers the design of two types of research common in community dentistry: the clin-

EFFECT OF PRENATAL FLUORIDE SUPPLEMENTS
IN PREVENTING DENTAL CARIES

Consent form

Dear _____:

The Center for Community Dental Health at the Maine Medical Center, the Eastman Dental Center in Rochester, New York, and the National Institute of Dental Research (National Institutes of Health) are cooperating in conducting a study to determine the value of using fluorides during pregnancy in preventing tooth decay in the baby teeth of offspring. As an expectant mother, you are being asked to consider participating in this study.

If you participate, you will be asked to consume a daily tablet, beginning during the fourth month of your pregnancy and continuing until the birth of your baby. For the study to yield valid data, half of the women will consume a tablet containing one milligram of fluoride and the other half will consume a tablet that will look and taste the same, but will not contain fluoride. This is called a "blind" study, and it is the only way that we can measure a difference in effect between consuming, and not consuming, fluoride during pregnancy. Assignment to group will be random, so you will have a 50/50 chance of being in the fluoride group. At the completion of the study, 5 years from now, all subjects will be told which group they were in.

After your child is born, you will be given (free of charge) fluoride for him or her to take until the age of 5. The fluorides will be in the form of drops during the first 2 years and chewable tablets after that. If your child is receiving a vitamin supplement from his or her physician or pediatrician, it should not contain fluoride because this prescribed dosage is adequate. All children will receive fluoride, regardless of which group the mother was in.

At the age of 3, your child will receive a dental examination (without radiographs) and at the age of 5 another dental examination, including a single radiograph on each side of the mouth. If any dental problems are found, you will be notified immediately. In any case, your family dentist will be given the exam results, if he or she so requests. There is no charge for the dental examinations. You, as the parent, would be responsible for seeking any dental care that might be necessary.

Risks

There are no known risks involved in this study. The amount of fluoride you consume during pregnancy will be approximately the same amount you would consume if you lived in a community with fluoridated water. If you should move to a fluoridated community while either you or your child is taking daily fluoride supplements, you should discontinue the supplements, as the drinking water will contain the amount of fluoride needed for prevention of tooth decay. Regarding the dietary fluoride supplement for your child, this procedure is used routinely and probably would have been recommended by your pediatrician when your baby was born.

The dental examinations are routine and as recommended by most dentists, although you should take your child to your family dentist for regular checkups, in addition to participation to this study.

ical trial and the questionnaire survey. Typical examples are presented, together with accompanying discussions.

The clinical trial

Probably the most frequently conducted form of research in community dentistry is the clinical trial. Reasons for carrying out clinical trials and the essential antecedents to such research have been discussed earlier in this chapter. The clinical trial can be quite elaborate, involving several thousand research subjects and extending over a period of 2 or 3 years or more. The major clinical trial used to test the Salk polio vaccine, for instance,

---

EFFECT OF PRENATAL FLUORIDE SUPPLEMENTS
IN PREVENTING DENTAL CARIES—cont'd

Benefits

Your child will derive the benefit of daily fluoride supplements (at no cost to you) and two dental examinations. Additionally, if you are in the fluoride group, there is a possibility of even greater prevention of tooth decay. If this study should show a benefit from prenatal fluorides, children everywhere will have the opportunity to have fewer cavities.

If you have any questions regarding this study you may call Ms. Vaughan at (*phone number*) or Dr. Leverett at (*phone number*) (call collect, if long distance). Also, you are encouraged to discuss the study with your family dentist, obstetrician, or pediatrician.

Of course, this study is entirely voluntary, and if you elect not to participate, or withdraw before completion of the study, you will not jeopardize the status of your child or of you as patients in any of the participating institutions.

Whenever possible, the father of the child should be aware of the nature of this project and give his consent to your participation. If this is not possible, please so indicate on the line marked "Father's Signature."

☐ I *DO* consent to participate in the prenatal fluoride study. Also, I have discussed the study with my obstetrician, who has no objection to my participation.

_____   _____
Signature   Date

_____   _____
Print name   Your date of birth

_____   _____
Street   Expected date of birth of child

_____
City/ town

_____
Phone number

_____   _____
Father's signature   Name of obstetrician or prenatal clinic

☐ I *DO NOT* consent to participate in the prenatal fluoride study.

_____   _____
Signature   Date

_____
Print name

---

involved more than 400,000 children.[14] A typical clinical trial intended to test the efficacy of some caries-preventive agent, for example, a fluoride mouthrinse, would begin with several hundred children in the caries-prone age range of 11 to 13 years and continue for 2 to 3 years. This population size and time frame are made necessary by the fact that differences in dental caries increment manifest themselves slowly and in relatively small numbers. However, a clinical trial that is intended to measure what is anticipated to be a large difference occurring in a short time could require much smaller numbers and a considerably shorter period of time.

EFFECT OF PRENATAL FLUORIDE SUPPLEMENTS
IN PREVENTING DENTAL CARIES

Background

There has been interest for many years in the use of prenatal dietary fluoride supplements. Because calcification of primary teeth begins in utero, it has been suggested that the ingestion of fluoride supplements by women during pregnancy could result in increased protection for these teeth in the offspring, enhancing the benefit derived from the use of supplements postnatally, as commonly prescribed. Although there is a reasonable amount of clinical evidence to support this practice, virtually all of the published studies of prenatal fluoride supplementation have major shortcomings in design or execution that compromise their value.

The insufficiency of clinical evidence was noted by the U.S. Food and Drug Administration in 1966. As a result, the FDA banned the marketing of fluoride products by manufacturers that made claims of caries prevention in the offspring of women who used the supplements during pregnancy. While questioning the efficacy of prenatal fluoride supplements, the FDA did not challenge the safety of the procedure because the amount of fluoride prescribed was approximately equivalent to the quantity consumed daily by persons residing in areas with optimally fluoridated drinking water.

Although the FDA action is still in effect, additional studies have since been conducted that have demonstrated the placental transfer of fluorides in humans, and clinical studies have also offered further support for the efficacy of prenatal fluoride supplementation in preventing dental caries. However, prenatal studies are still few compared with those that form the basis of the better-established caries-preventive procedures, such as water fluoridation or postnatal fluoride supplements, and most of the prenatal studies that exist are deficient in some important respect.

Thus it cannot be concluded from currently available data that prenatal fluoride supplementation should be recommended for the prevention of dental caries. Acceptance and promotion of any preventive procedure should be based upon scientifically sound and conclusive clinical data, and the available data are neither. However, the positive trend in the data clearly offers suggestive evidence that the procedure might benefit primary teeth. Hence, further research to determine efficacy is indicated.

Objective

The objective of this study is to determine whether children whose mothers regularly ingested fluoride supplements during pregnancy have a lower incidence of dental decay than children whose mothers did not ingest fluoride supplements during pregnancy.

Population

The population of this study will be women who are in the first 3 months of pregnancy and who reside in a community with a low level of fluoride in the drinking water (0.3 ppm or less) within York and Cumberland Counties, Maine.

---

*See consent form in the previous box.

The box on pp. 276 and 277 exemplifies the large-scale clinical trial. A typical brief protocol for a study that was presented for approval to the Institutional Review Board of the Eastman Dental Center is shown. This protocol, which should be considered as a summary protocol, is brief and concise, although it contains all of the elements of good study design and protocol writing. A typical grant application or contract proposal submitted to a federal agency for funding would be considerably more detailed. The consent form attached to this protocol has been described and evaluated earlier.

EFFECT OF PRENATAL FLUORIDE SUPPLEMENTS
IN PREVENTING DENTAL CARIES—cont'd

Method

After having the study explained to them, women who are interested will be asked to sign a consent form (see sample attached)* and will be assigned randomly to one of two study groups. Subjects in group 1 will consume one tablet containing 1 milligram of fluoride as sodium fluoride each day during their pregnancies, beginning during the fourth month. Subjects in group 2 will consume a tablet identical in appearance and flavor but containing no fluoride, beginning during the fourth month and continuing the remainder of their pregnancies.

Assignment to the two groups will be entirely random and "blind" (neither the study personnel nor the study subjects will know which group is which).

Upon completion of the term of pregnancy, all offspring, regardless of group assignment of their mothers, will receive daily fluoride supplements. Initially, the supplements will be in the form of drops and will be replaced by chewable tablets at approximately 2 years of age. These supplements will continue until each of the children reaches 5 years of age.

At 3 years of age each child will receive a thorough dental examination, without radiographs. At 5 years of age, each child will receive a second dental examination, including a single radiograph on each side of the mouth. The results of all dental examinations will be made available to family dentists, upon request.

Risk

There is no known risk to the procedures described. The amount of fluoride consumed by the mothers-to-be is approximately the same amount that would be consumed by a person residing in a community with a fluoridated public water supply. The use of dietary fluoride supplements of this type is widespread. For example, in southern Maine the Center for Community Dental Health, the Portland Health Department, and the State Office of Dental Health have been instrumental in establishing several community programs for using dietary fluoride supplements which have been in operation for up to 7 years.

Benefit

A certain benefit of this program is that all children participating will have provided to them dietary fluoride supplements for the first 5 years of their lives, which should result in less decay than in children not using fluoride supplements. Additionally, all children will receive two thorough dental examinations during that time. There also is a possibility that the children whose mothers consumed fluoride supplements during their pregnancies will have even less dental decay.

Obviously, there is also a substantial potential benefit to society at large, should the procedure prove to be efficacious.

The questionnaire survey

Typically, the incentive to conduct a questionnaire survey begins with the identification of a population containing individuals who possess what the researcher thinks may be useful information. The problem, of course, is to facilitate the willingness of the individuals to share this information in a useful and measurable manner. This section will describe a technique for developing and carrying out a questionnaire survey.

Let us suppose, for the sake of illustration, that we are concerned with the relative efficacy of undergraduate dental curricula in private and state-supported schools, and we decide that one method for beginning to address this issue is to conduct a questionnaire survey.

Selection of study population. For a study of this type we would select equal numbers of dentists who have graduated from the two types of dental schools. The number of subjects selected would depend on the number and complexity of questions asked in the survey and on the proportion that we expect to respond. The decision regarding sample size can best be handled by a statistician and will not be dealt with in this discussion. However, let us say that we decide to select as the study population 200 to 300 subjects from each of the two types of dental schools. Further, we should select subjects who are as much alike as possible, except for the variable under study (source of funding for school). Other differences, which are called *confounding* or *intervening variables,* could be minimized by selecting subjects from among graduates of American dental schools during a given 1-year or 2-year period, say, 1986 and 1987. By contacting appropriate dental schools, we could secure lists of names and addresses of graduates during those 2 years. If this procedure results in more subjects than are required for the study, some technique for randomly selecting from among the potential population would be instituted to end up with the desired population of 400 to 600 graduates.

Defining the goal of the study. The goal of the study would be to determine whether there are any measurable differences between the two study groups.

Hypotheses. The null hypotheses for this study would be that, when looking at dental graduates from the two types of schools, there are no differences in terms of (1) the structure and outcome of dental practice, (2) the performance of these persons as students in dental school, (3) involvement in professional activities outside the dental office, and (4) other similar measures that we may care to identify. At this point, we will focus on hypothesis 1, using it as an example of a way in which the questionnaire can be developed.

Core area objectives. In dealing with one of the hypotheses, we should make a statement from which measurable questionnaire items can be developed, for instance, "Graduates of private and publicly funded schools who enter private practice will not differ with regard to the ultimate structure and outcome of their dental practices."

Subgoals. The example of a core area objective refers to both structure and outcome of dental practice; therefore a more specific subgoal is required. Obviously, a rather specific statement is ultimately required and, if the core area objective is sufficiently specific, the statement of the subgoal may not be necessary. In terms of the example the subgoal might be "Graduates of private and publicly funded schools who enter private practice will not differ with regard to the form of their dental practices."

At this point we have a statement that is sufficiently specific and that represents a small enough chunk of our study goal that we can begin to make a quantifiable statement that, when converted to actual questionnaire items, will solicit the information we seek.

Subgoal statement. Graduates of private and publicly funded schools who enter private practice will not differ with regard to the form of dental practice. Specifically, they will be the same as follows:

1. Have the same proportion of general practitioners
2. Have the same distribution of specialty practices
3. Be as likely to enter solo or group practice
4. Have similar patterns of use of auxiliaries
5. Delegate clinical responsibilities to auxiliaries in the same manner
6. Have the same patterns of referral for specialty care
7. Have the same number of operatories
8. Have similar configurations of dental equipment

You may wish to add other statements of the same type.

Items. By a very careful process of refining, we have reached the point where we have defined quite specifically the quantifiable information that we wish to secure. Our next task is to write the actual questions, or *items,* that the respondent will be asked to answer. However, before taking this step, it would be worthwhile to explore the various formats used for questions.

The *dichotomous-response* type of question is

characterized by "yes/no," "true/false," or "present/absent" responses:

Do you have a recall system? Yes/No

Are you in general practice? Yes/No

This type of question is desirable in a questionnaire because it is very easy to answer accurately and the response is easy to analyze.

A *multiple-choice* question is necessary in a situation in which there is a list of possible responses:

Do you have any of the following equipment in your office?

Panoramic x-ray   Copying machine
Ultrasonic cleaner   Computer

When *quantifiable* items are involved, questions may lend themselves to a specific number as a response:

With how many other dentists do you practice? _____

How many operatories do you have? _____

How many continuing education courses did you take during the last year? _____

Occasionally it may be necessary to ask a question that requires a *written* response:

List all dental organizations of which you are an active member.

However, this type of question is best avoided because it is difficult to tabulate the completed data. You should, in a case such as this, provide a list, albeit a long one, of potential options and thereby convert the question to a multiple-choice type of question.

Sometimes, particularly if one is attempting to elicit feelings rather than facts, a question that resembles a multiple-choice question may be asked:

How successful have you been in maintaining low turnover of office personnel?
Very successful
Moderately successful
Neither successful nor unsuccessful
Moderately unsuccessful
Very unsuccessful

We are specifically soliciting one of five responses arranged in this format. However, the same responses can be arranged horizontally as follows:

/	/	/	/	/
Very successful	Moderately successful	Neither successful nor unsuccessful	Moderately unsuccessful	Very unsuccessful

In this case a respondent may make a mark anywhere along the scale, either at one of the five points or somewhere between. This type of scale is somewhat more difficult to score and should be avoided in most cases.

Occasionally, a combination of a dichotomous response and some other form may be indicated.

Do you have a recall system? Yes/No
If No, please skip to the next question.
If Yes, when is the appointment scheduled?
☐ At the time of the visit
☐ By mail, near time of recall
☐ By phone, near time of recall
☐ Patient reminded to call for appointment

With your recall system, what percent of patients respond affirmatively? _____

Some questions fall conveniently into a *matrix format*:

Which of the following clinical responsibilities do you delegate and to which auxiliaries?

	Hygienist	Assistant
1. Prophylaxis		
2. Fluoride treatments		
3. Taking radiographs		
4. Impressions for study models		

Now, returning to the example, here are some questionnaire items that are intended to derive specific quantifiable information suggested by the subgoal statements.

1. Are you a general practitioner? Yes ☐ No ☐
   If no, which specialty do you practice?
   ☐ Orthodontics
   ☐ Periodontics
   ☐ Pediatric dentistry
   ☐ Other (specify) _____

2. With how many other dentists do you practice?
3. How many operatories do you have in your office?

	Fully equipped including x-ray	Partially equipped (list equipment)
For dentist(s)		
For dental hygienist (2)		
Other (specify)		

Demographic and baseline data. Assuming that the questionnaire responses are anonymous (which is absolutely imperative for maintaining a high response rate), we will want to include questions that establish certain characteristics about the respondent: (1) year of birth, (2) year of graduation from dental school, (3) name of dental school, and (4) other useful data.

Data collection and evaluation. This topic is extremely important to the successful conduct of a questionnaire survey, but it is beyond the scope of this discussion. Because the method of collecting, tabulating, and analyzing data is dependent on the type of computer facilities available, the advice of persons at a local computer facility should be sought prior to establishing the final design of the survey instrument.

Pretesting. After the final design of the survey has been established, it should be tested on a small number of persons who are not in the selected study population but who have similar backgrounds. A final item on the pretest survey should solicit comments and criticisms (relating to the questionnaire itself) from the respondent. In this way errors and ambiguities can be corrected and the length of the questionnaire altered if it is too time-consuming.

Maximizing response to the questionnaire. No questionnaire survey can be successful if a significant proportion of the population does not respond. Here are a few suggestions for improving the rate of response:

1. Use a cover letter that is signed or cosigned by a person who represents authority and prestige to the study population, for example, a dean of a dental school, a president of a dental society, or a noted authority in the area under investigation. This letter should be brief but should emphasize the importance of the study and describe direct and indirect benefits to the respondent.
2. Have an esthetically pleasing questionnaire.
3. Provide a self-addressed, stamped envelope.
4. Provide some sort of follow-up reminder for nonrespondents.

If the questionnaire is truly anonymous, follow-up is not possible. However, there are ways to short-circuit the anonymity in this type of questionnaire. One method, not to be recommended, is to code the return envelope to identify the respondent. In this case the cover letter would contain a promise not to link the envelope with the questionnaire. A better method is to include a self-addressed postcard on which the respondent's name is printed. She or he is instructed to return the postcard several days after returning the questionnaire. In that way the dentist can be identified as a respondent, although still maintaining the anonymity of the response.

When the flow of responses has diminished to an average of about 1% per day (usually after approximately 2 weeks), a postcard reminder can be sent to nonrespondents. This usually will generate an increase in the rate of response. When the flow again returns to about 1%, a mailing identical to the first mailing should be sent to each nonrespondent, with the word "reminder" written at the top of the cover letter. Further follow-up will probably be unproductive, and the investigator should be satisfied with a response rate in excess of 60%. Certain demographic characteristics of nonrespondents— for example, year of birth, dental school, year of graduation, and specialty practice— can be secured from the latest edition of the *American Dental Association Directory,* and this information can be useful in determining to what extent the respondents differ from nonrespondents.

READING THE RESEARCH LITERATURE

In 1990 more than 25,000 articles were published in the dental periodical literature.[19] A substantial proportion of these articles report original dental research. A list of some of the more important journals publishing original research in community dentistry is given at the end of this chapter.

One would be foolish to believe that all journals maintain the same standards of quality or that all published dental research is of equal value and quality. Following are a few general guidelines that the student can use to identify the better and more reliable published dental research.

Date of publication. Of course there are a few "classic" articles in the literature, articles that probably will always represent preeminent contributions to the body of knowledge. The general rule, however, is that research tends to become dated and a contribution that was valid and useful a few years ago may be obsolete or even misleading when interpreted within the context of the current "state of the art." One should give greater credence to more recently published research.

Reputation of the journal. The more respected, or *refereed,* journals accept articles for publication only after they have been reviewed and critiqued by eminent researchers in the field. This *peer review* process tends to reject inadequate research and provide useful criticism of basically sound research.

Reputation of the author(s). Evaluation on this point may be beyond most casual readers who are not familiar with the important people in the field. However, a review of the Author Section of the *Index to Dental Literature* can give some idea of the publishing frequency of the authors and the subject areas in which they publish most often. The sequence of authors' names can be important. When a well-known researcher's name is not first in authorship, it may mean that he or she did not contribute substantially to the research.

Source of financial support. Usually the source of financial support, whether a government or commercial grant, is acknowledged with the published research. One should be somewhat cautious in accepting favorable findings reported in research sponsored by a commercial source that has a vested interest in the results.

Corroborations from other sources. Although the findings of a single study on a particular subject, even though quite dramatic, need to be accepted with caution, repeated corroboration from other sources substantially increases the reliability of the original report.

Quality of literature review. A careful researcher is thoroughly familiar with other research done in the area under investigation, which is reflected in the quality and completeness (not to be confused with the quantity) of his or her literature review. This is, of course, another area in which the less-informed reader will have difficulty making a sound judgment. However, one could seek the advice of a colleague or teacher. As a general rule of thumb, government-supported research published in refereed journals will have a high-quality literature review with the introduction.

Characteristics of study design. Characterizing the differences between good research and bad research in just a few words is impossible. However, there are a few characteristics of the protocol that should be noted.

1. Is the study design adequately described? Although it need not be long, the description should be complete enough that another investigator could replicate the study.
2. Is the sample size adequate? Samples may be both too small or too large. If a sample is too small, modest differences between groups may not reach the level of statistical significance and thus important findings may be overlooked. If sample size is too large, very small differences may reach levels of statistical significance. In the latter situation it is not unusual for investigators to report that a difference was "statistically significant," while ignoring the fact that the difference was so small that it was not "clinically significant."
3. Was the data analysis adequate? Were appropriate statistical tests used? Were any statistical tests used?
4. Are the conclusions based solidly on the data? Does the author avoid generalizing beyond the limitations of the study?

Style of writing. This criterion is probably (and unfortunately) the least reliable of those listed. It is painfully true that some of our finest researchers are terrible writers, and the converse is probably also true—that some of our worst researchers are good writers. Nonetheless, good research that is well written should be considered better than excellent research that is poorly written because it is communicated better to the scientific world.

JOURNALS PUBLISHING ORIGINAL RESEARCH IN COMMUNITY DENTISTRY

Journal of Public Health Dentistry
Journal of the American Dental Association
American Journal of Public Health
Journal of Dental Research
Public Health Reports
Journal of Dental Education
Community Dental Health
Community Dentistry and Oral Epidemiology
Clinical Preventive Dentistry
Caries Research

REFERENCES

1. Ast DB, Fitzgerald B: Effectiveness of water fluoridation, *J Am Dent Assoc* 65:581, 1962.
2. Barber B: The ethics of experimentation with human subjects, *Sci Am* 234:25, 1976.
3. Bibby BG: Use of fluorine in the prevention of dental caries; I, rationale and approach, *J Am Dent Assoc* 31:228, 1944.
4. Bibby, BG: The use of fluorine in the prevention of dental caries; II, effect of sodium fluoride application, *J Am Dent Assoc* 31:317, 1944.
5. Bok S: The ethics of giving placebos, *Sci Am* 231:17, 1974.
6. *Broadening the scope—long-range research plan for the nineties,* 1990, National Institute of Dental Research, US Department of Health and Human Services, Public Health Service, National Institutes of Health.
7. Brunelle JA: Dental caries in United States children 1986-87, NIH Pub No 89-2247 Washington, DC, 1989, US Department of Health and Human Services.
8. Cheyne VD: Human dental caries and topically applied fluorine: a preliminary report, *J Am Dent Assoc* 29:804, 1942.
9. Code of Federal Regulations 45 CFR 46, revised as of March 8, 1983, Washington, DC, 1983, US Government Printing Office.
10. Dean HT: Endemic fluorosis and its relation to dental caries, *Public Health Rep* 53:1443, 1938.
11. Dean HT, Arnold FA Jr, Elvove E: Domestic water and dental caries; V, additional studies of the relation of fluoride domestic waters to dental caries experience in 4,425 white children, aged 12 to 14 years, of 13 cities in 4 states, *Public Health Rep* 57:1155, 1942.
12. Dean HT, Elvove E: Studies on the minimal threshold of the dental sign of chronic endemic fluorosis (mottled enamel), *Public Health Rep* 50:1719, 1935.
13. Dunning JM: *Principles of dental public health,* ed 4, Cambridge, 1986, Harvard University Press.
14. Francis T and others: An evaluation of the 1954 poliomyelitis vaccine trials, *Am J Public Health* 45(5, part 2):XIV-63, 1955.
15. Frazier PJ: A new look at dental health education in community programs, *Dent Hygiene* 52:176, 1978.
16. Garcia AI: Caries incidence and costs of prevention programs, *J Public Health Dent* 49:259, 1989.
17. Horowitz HS: Ethical considerations of study participants in dental caries clinical trials, *Community Dent Oral Epidemiol 4:43, 1976.*
18. Horowitz HS: Effectiveness of school water fluoridation and dietary fluoride supplements in school-aged children, *J Public Health Dent* 49:290, 1989.
19. *Index to dental literature, 1990,* Chicago, 1991, American Dental Association.
20. Knutson JW, Armstrong WD: Effect of topically applied sodium fluoride on dental caries experience, *Public Health Rep* 58:1701, 1943.
21. Leverett DH: Effectiveness of mouthrinsing with fluoride solutions in preventing coronal and root caries, *J Public Health Dent* 49:310, 1989.
22. Miller AJ, Brunelle JA: A summary of the NIDR community caries prevention demonstration program, *J Am Dent Assoc* 107:265, 1983.
23. Morganstein WM: Informed consent—the doctrine evolves, *J Am Dent Assoc* 93:637, 1976.
24. Newbrun E: Effectiveness of water fluoridation, *J Public Health Dent* 49:279, 1989.
25. Weintraub JA: Effectiveness of pit and fissure sealants, *J Public Health Dent* 49:317, 1989.

SECTION SIX

Management and Ethics in Dental Care

Dental students and dental auxiliary students have ahead of them 40 or 45 years of dental practice. For some, it will be a "private practice"; for others, a career in education, public health, group practice, or community health. Yet all practitioners of dentistry are faced with certain inevitable challenges—how to lead a happy, successful life—being one of tantamount importance.

As dental practice changes, as evidenced in Chapter 2 of this book, the skills of the practitioner must also change. Gone are the days of the solo practitioner working alone in the little office over the corner drugstore; here today is the team practice. Management of personnel may be the key to a successful practice, whether in a dental office providing care or in a health department administering government programs. As Dr. Moosbruker states in Chapter 14, "Effective management of job functions, communications, decision making, problem solving, finances, and interpersonal relations improves productivity and saves money."

Dental professionals are faced with ethical decisions throughout their practicing lives. Issues such as breach of confidentiality, iatrogenic disease, paternalistic behavior toward patients, as well as paternalistic public health laws are common. Chapter 15 discusses ethical principles in health care and the responsibility professionals have toward society. Several ethical dilemmas and a decision-making model are presented.

Chapter 16 provides clear and succinct information about the legal rights of practice and ways to eliminate or reduce them. Risk management depends on a careful understanding of how the legal system works in the regulation of health professional practice.

14 Team Management in Dental Practice

The practice of dentistry has changed dramatically during the past decade. The field of community dental health is now concerned with the efficient delivery of dental care as well as traditional concerns for preventive dentistry and dental health education. This chapter deals with the team approach to dental care and the skills and philosophy necessary to manage a modern dental practice. As the number of people who must interact on a regular basis increases, the need for management increases. Households require management; one's social life requires management; indeed, any situation in which a number of people are involved in complex processes requires management.

Although the dentist has traditionally been the team leader, it is likely that as dentistry moves through the 1990s other dental health professionals will also emerge as team leaders. Independently practicing dental hygienists, for instance, must acquire the skills of management if they are to be efficient practitioners. Whether one is the manager or the managed, the fundamental principles enumerated in this chapter will be of importance. Effective management of job functions, communications, decision making, problem solving, finances, and interpersonal relations improves productivity and saves money.

The most useful way of thinking of a group of people whose activities must be managed is as a team. This chapter focuses on the various processes that a successful team leader must be able to manage and some of the methods through which a team leader can accomplish the task.

It begins with a brief working definition of a team. A discussion of two alternate theories of management follows, together with the principles derived from these theories. Next, the major interpersonal and group processes that the team leader must be able to manage are described: communication, problem solving, and decision making. Because an understanding of the dynamics of func-

tioning groups is also extremely helpful in managing a team, there is a discussion of what to observe in an ongoing group process. Additional team management issues that are discussed include team roles and role negotiations, the supervisory function, conflict management, and team development.

WHAT IS A TEAM AND WHY DO YOU NEED ONE?

The definition of a *team* used here is "a group of interdependent individuals, usually with different roles and functions, whose combined efforts toward a mutually shared goal are required for the successful completion of a task."

A number of problems commonly occur when team functioning is attempted. The following nine items cover the major reasons for these problems and will be the focus of this chapter:

1. Absence of clear and shared goals and philosophy
2. Lack of a specified decision-making mechanism
3. Use of a decision-making mechanism that attributes more to educational background and professional status than to having the most relevant information
4. Lack of clarity about responsibilities of each team member
5. Closed or only partially open communication channels
6. Absence of a time and method for problem identification, analysis, and solution
7. Insufficient planning time or an inadequate planning process
8. Lack of a mechanism for resolving team conflicts
9. Inadequate selection procedures for team members

Unresolved team problems can be extremely costly. Friction among team members can be felt by patients and may result in inadequate care of patients, loss of patients, and high personnel turnover. Team rapport is needed to keep the dentist in touch with patients. In a busy practice, auxiliaries serve as a communication bridge. Continuity of care may depend on their relationship with the patient and their ability to bring the dentist into the relationship to share the ongoing conversation and learn the patient's concerns.

The need is even greater and the bridging task more sensitive if the patient is culturally different from the dental team because of ethnic, social class, or physical ability differences for example. Minority groups often receive less or different dental care from the majority population, and the type of care may be the result of provider behavior.[7] Differently-abled patients also represent an underserved population, even though there is evidence that exposing dental students to as little as 3 days of practice providing care for these patients results in more positive attitudes toward them, more felt competence in treating them, and more awareness of the need for dentists to provide such care.[6]

A question for any dental team's consideration is the extent to which the patient is regarded as a member of the team for discussion of and decisions about his or her own treatment. Jong[1] claims this is an ethical principle and calls it *autonomy,* or respect for the patient's rights. What is meant here is more than a brief description of the situation by the doctor and a rapid and uninformed decision by the patient. Ideally at least one meeting would take place with the dentist, auxiliaries, patient, and hygienist, if appropriate, concerning the specific problems of the patient, with the patient *not* sitting in the dental chair.

Including the patient in the team to this extent probably results in better rapport, more cooperation with the treatment plan, and perhaps even earlier payment of bills. However, taking the additional time for the team to talk with the patient may also result in decreased earnings or in higher fees to compensate.

THEORIES OF MANAGEMENT

Underlying assumptions, values, and beliefs are guiding factors in our behavior but are often not identified as such. The manner in which someone goes about managing or participating on a team is also determined in large measure by her or his un-

derlying beliefs about people: what motivates them, what they need, how they function. McGregor described two very different theories of management, outlining the underlying assumptions about people on which they are based and the principles of organization that logically follow.[3] The theories are designated simply X and Y. Theory X's assumptions about average people are the following:

1. They are lazy, preferring to work as little as possible.
2. They dislike responsibility or are incapable of handling it.
3. They prefer to be dependent on others, to be led.
4. They are incapable of self-control and therefore must be controlled by others.
5. They cannot find satisfaction of important needs in work and must, therefore, seek basic satisfaction outside the work setting.

These assumptions lead to an organizational structure that has a very clear chain of command, in which the top of the hierarchy both directs and controls the bottom. For example, each level directs the actions of the level below it by making assignments, coordinating activities, and perhaps explaining procedures. There is usually little communication up the line, with the result that the person directing does not know the effects of his or her directives. For example, beginning the day at 8:15 AM rather than 8:30 AM may mean an auxiliary has to catch an hourly bus that arrives at 7:30 AM rather than at 8:30 AM. The dentist may then wonder why the auxiliary is so tired at 4:30 PM but never asks about it.

A second outcome of accepting Theory X's assumptions about people is that one builds an organization with narrow task specialization. The assignments are made so that each individual has a small and narrowly defined task that she or he will do well. The result is that personnel cannot substitute for each other, even though the tasks are within the scope of their competence. More important, they often do not understand each other's jobs, so that needless conflicts can arise because of lack of knowledge and awareness. The best example of task specialization is the assembly line, but it has parallels in the dental office. For example, one auxiliary always sterilizes the instruments or takes the radiographs, and no one else but the dentist knows how to operate the equipment. If the knowledgeable individual is sick or very busy, a slowdown occurs.

The assumptions that Theory Y makes about people are quite different. They include the following:

1. They prefer to be active rather than passive.
2. They are capable of assuming responsibility and find satisfaction in doing so.
3. They prefer being independent, finding greater satisfaction in not having to look to others for direction.
4. They are capable of finding basic satisfaction and self-fulfillment in their work.
5. They are capable of self-control, not needing control from outside.

Acceptance of these assumptions about people leads to the formation of an organization with minimum hierarchy. If people find greater satisfaction in assuming responsibility and in being independent and are capable of self-control, then greater productivity and satisfaction will result from fewer people being in superior-subordinate relationships. The integrative force in the organization is mutual confidence rather than authority. There is shared responsibility in a Theory Y organization through wide participation in decisions rather than centralized decision making. The basic unit of organization is the small group rather than the individual. People plan task performance and assign jobs according to qualifications and interest. The role of the supervisor is as an agent for maintaining intragroup and intergroup communication rather than as an agent of higher authority.

It is also true, however, that the theories in operation are probably never absolute, nor would they be completely effective if they were. The individual worker and supervisor lend their own personalities to the functioning of any organization. It is possible for employees, for example, to be so conditioned to Theory X principles that they believe its assumptions about themselves and act accordingly, thus undermining Theory Y organization. Other employees may believe Theory Y assumptions about themselves, demanding more and more freedom, yet perform in a manner that causes management to treat them on the basis of Theory X principles.

COMMUNICATION

Because communications are necessary for any team's functioning, the ways or processes through which they are achieved have a large impact on efficiency, energy expended, quality of care provided, and satisfaction level of the team. Time is a major requirement for effective communication processes; that is, the team members need a set period of time, preferably daily, during which they can all share information, identify problems and issues, and give and receive feedback on their interactions. This can occur in the form of a *debriefing* session at the end of the day or at a specified time each day. The issues identified and worked through in this daily session can range from the discovery of a series of patients returning with sensitivities to the auxiliaries' feelings that they are being ordered around and not appreciated by the team leader. Fifteen minutes set aside at the end of the day for debriefing could improve the effectiveness of most dental teams.

The manner in which a team discussion is led can determine the amount of information that is actually shared. For example, compare "I did not see anything worth discussing occur today, did you?" with "What did you observe about the way I handled Jimmy's fears this morning?" If you are the team leader, there are several rules of thumb for getting group members to participate in a discussion:

1. Do not state your opinion first.
2. Ask an open-ended question that requires some thought, not one that can be answered by "yes" or "no."
3. Wait for a response, even if it seems like an interminably long time.
4. Do not do a lot of the talking yourself; make your point once and then stop to give the others a chance.

Team members can be most facilitative of each other's growth and development on the job if they ask for and give each other feedback on their daily functions. "What did you observe about the way I handled Jimmy's fears?" is a direct request for feedback. The kind of feedback designated here has two components: an objective observation of behavior and a subjective reaction to the observations. An auxiliary might respond that he or she had seen the dentist try to convince Jimmy to "take it like a man" and not to be a "crybaby." Then the auxiliary would describe her or his feeling reaction. It might be something like "I felt very close to you because that is just the way my father used to talk to my little brother" or "I felt very sorry for Jimmy and wanted to tell him I understood his being frightened, that everybody was afraid sometimes." These are both specific feeling reactions to the dentist's behavior that avoid the global noninformative value judgment of "I thought it was good (or bad)." After either of the first two reactions, the dentist might ask, "Can any of you think of another way to deal with Jimmy?" The pros and cons of the alternatives can then be discussed along with supporting data. For example, one of the auxiliaries may have seen Jimmy interact with his father or mother and could report the technique the parent uses and the results, or the auxiliary may have tried something that was successful.

The discussion thus far may suggest that only children have significant enough problems during dental care procedures to warrant a team discussion. Such is clearly not the case. Fear of going to the dentist is widespread. It is the subject of many jokes and stories and the bane of most dental professionals' existences in that it is the major cause of the reactions they receive on announcing, "I am a dentist" or "I work in a dental office." It is possible that careful discussions of patient management, with team members giving feedback to one another on their styles and skill development, could eventually change the image of dentistry.

A major issue in the communication between any two people or groups of people is the degree of openness that is considered acceptable. A particularly appropriate example for a dental office is telling someone that his or her breath has an odor. Generally, people do not trust one another's intentions sufficiently. If I think you are telling me I have bad breath because you have my best interests at heart and do not want me to offend patients, I will accept the feedback. If, by contrast, I think that you wish me ill, do not like me, or talk about me behind my back, then I will be offended by your feedback. Trust is an element that must be carefully fostered and protected in any group. Its development requires the freedom to check out one's perceptions, to ask questions about motivation, and to share feelings, which are all part of

being open. The conditions of trust and openness are interactive: trust is built through openness, and openness develops in a trusting environment. The team's task, then, is to strive constantly for more trust and openness, pushing the boundaries as far as they will go at any moment by being willing to take a risk.

Effective feedback tends to increase the trust level in the group. Feedback is more likely to be heard by and be useful to the person receiving it if it is as follows:

1. Descriptive: tells what you saw and heard
2. Specific: not global, but concrete and detailed
3. Objective: nonjudgmental, not "good" or "bad" or "right" or "wrong"
4. Well timed: close to the event, unless time is needed for calming down
5. Contracted for: the person says she or he wants to hear the feedback
6. Owned: "This is my feedback and nobody else's; I cannot speak for anybody else"
7. Involves a personal risk: givers put themselves on the line by sharing their personal reactions and feelings; judgmental feedback puts the receiver on the line
8. Checked out: the giver makes sure the receiver understands what the giver means to say

Communication is difficult. There are more misunderstood or half-understood messages than there are complete understandings. The difficulty occurs because people assume that they have understood and that communication is easy. If you doubt this point, try checking out all the communications you receive in a day. Not only are you likely to discover that your first perception of the message was at least partially inaccurate, because you either missed part or read in too much, but you will probably also be regarded as dim-witted for even suggesting that simple communications could go awry. The difficulty can be described in terms of a filter system, such that each of us screens in and out those messages to which we are especially attuned. The content heard and understood versus that screened out is determined by our own life experiences, knowledge, attitudes, values, and psychological makeup. For example, if I am a very religious person and you are sending messages about your negative attitudes toward religion, I may not hear those messages, especially if I like you and if it is also important to me to have my friends believe the way I do. "Hearing" in this sense could mean either not picking up the sound waves, not processing them mentally, or adding extenuating factors to the processing. The filters, then, are our perceptual system, which includes more than just sensory receptors. It includes mental processing of the information received.

PROBLEM SOLVING

If it is true that a good communication process requires an amount of time set aside for that purpose alone, then it is doubly true of problem solving. Many individuals have at least a moderate degree of difficulty in admitting that they even have a problem, particularly one that cannot be blamed on nature or other circumstances beyond their control, for example, an interpersonal problem. There seems to be an underlying belief that to have problems is to be weak or wrong. It would benefit us greatly if we could change that belief to one that held that the failure to acknowledge problems is wrong, but that the process of working to solve problems is strong and right. Accepting that any group of people working together has problems is the basic ingredient of an effective problem-solving process. Once that is achieved, there are many ways of finding solutions.

A second difficulty that groups often face in problem solving is approaching solutions before the problem has been clearly defined. It is important to begin with a statement of the problem with which everyone can agree to ensure that the whole team is really working on the same problem. Often the problem is stated as a solution, for example, "to synchronize our timing." It is not clear from this statement what the real problem is, and further analysis is prevented by a premature goal statement. The problem might be that "each member of the team has a lot of lag time." Such a statement allows for an analysis of the problem to ascertain who has lag time, when, how do they feel about it, whether money is being lost because of it, and what procedures could be changed with what cost. The analysis phase in problem solving includes data collection about the problem and determination of the ways in which it is a psycho-logical (feelings and needs), sociological (attitudes and norms), economic (dollars and cents), and/or political (power and influence) problem. For example, the question might be asked: "What negative feelings result for whom from this situation?" or "Whose feelings are operating to keep this problem in place and what, specifically, are those feelings?" For the economic analysis, "What does it cost (us, society, the organization) in dollars and cents to have this problem?" Costs of a solution cannot be determined until a solution approach is clearly defined.

In one particular situation a problem arose in the university dental clinic because intake procedures for all patients were standardized and initial diagnosis was performed by persons other than those carrying out the treatment procedures. This turned out to be primarily a psychological problem in that the long waiting time between diagnosis and treatment and the multiple contacts interfered with the patient's need to feel cared for and the frequent desire for immediate treatment. It thwarted the dental students' need to determine the treatment plan that they had to carry out. Occasionally, it became an economic problem, in that when the student decided or discovered that the plan was wrong, time and money were lost through an incorrect beginning. Had the team decided to try to change the clinic admission procedures, political factors would have had to be considered. As it was, they decided to allow an extra 15 minutes preplanning time for each new patient to check the diagnosis against the patient's actual needs.

A thorough analysis of the problem facilitates solution finding. As added preparation for the hard work of deciding on a solution agreeable to all, a brainstorming session can be used. The process is one wherein each person says what outcome situation he or she would like to see "in the best of all possible worlds." No contradictions, objections, or presentations of barriers are allowed. The group members just brainstorm their fantasies of an ideal solution. It is a helpful process because it builds solidarity within the group and promotes a creative solution. People are generally in more agreement about what they would like to see happen than about how to get there or about what is possible.

The next step in problem solving is the difficult

one of suggesting alternative solutions. Each proposal must be fully explored before a final decision is made. The suggestions are tested for desirability of the outcome, likelihood of the outcome, and feasibility in terms of the motivation and capability of those involved. Known and potential barriers must be analyzed, along with known and potential assets. When the solution approach is decided on, there remains the task of planning the steps of its implementation. A clear assignment of tasks, time frames, and checkpoints for evaluation needs to be built in. The major work is done, but the goal can be lost through inadequate planning and follow-through. The following model summarizes the steps that are likely to be necessary for an adequate problem-solving process (see box below).

The model, or part of it, is appropriate for any situation arising in a dental practice that requires more than mere fact-finding or improved communication between the people involved. For example, in a three-dentist group practice with a hygienist and several auxiliaries, patients have been raising objections to the practice of charging fees on the basis of time per visit, claiming that the dentists differ in their degree of speed and thoroughness. In a practice with one dentist one hygienist, one assistant, and one receptionist-bookkeeper, a certain group of patients is always breaking appointments. Either of these situations lends itself to use of the problem-solving process by the whole team.

LEADERSHIP AND DECISION MAKING

The decision-making mechanism adopted by team members is integrally related to the theory of management under which they are operating and to the leadership style of the team leader. At the far end of the Theory Y continuum, every member of the team would participate in every decision. The leader's style would be represented by the right-hand side of the diagram in Figure 14-1. At the extreme Theory X end of the continuum, the leader would make all the decisions alone, the style represented by the left-hand side of the diagram.[8] There are numerous positions along the continuum, both with respect to the leader's style as indicated in the diagram and with respect to the type of decision being made. Some decisions are more appropriately made by the team leader, either with or without first collecting data from the other team members, and other decisions are more appropriately made by the entire group.

Problems are most likely to occur when the team is not consciously aware of its decision-making process, operating instead in some haphazard fashion largely dependent on the mood of the leader. In that situation people do not know how they can have influence; unless the team is in perfect agreement or most members are extremely apathetic,

---

PROBLEM-SOLVING MODEL

Step 1. Define the problem.
Step 2. Collect data about the problem (all known information, plus a list of information that must be obtained).
Step 3. Problem analysis: in what sense is this a(n)
  a. Psychological problem?
  b. Sociological problem?
  c. Economic problem?
  d. Political problem?
Step 4. Redefine the problem, if necessary.
Step 5. Brainstorm fantasy solutions, "in the best of all possible worlds."
Step 6. Suggest and test alternate solutions.
Step 7. Decide on a solution approach.
Step 8. Plan implementation of the solution.
Step 9. Plan to evaluate the solution.

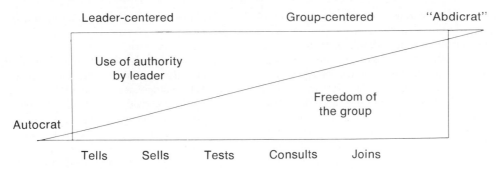

Fig. 14-1 Leadership continuum. (Reprinted by permission of *Harvard Business Review*. An excerpt from "How to choose a leadership pattern" by Tannenbaum RT and Schmidt WH, (March/April 1958). Copyright © 1958 by the President and Fellows of Harvard College; all rights reserved.)

dissatisfaction builds. A conscious awareness of how decisions are made opens the mechanism to review and possible change. One of the first decisions a team must face to operate logically is "How are we going to make decisions?"

Some criteria for determining how the decision should be made have been suggested by Vroom.[9]

1. The importance of the quality of the decision; for example, to what extent is there a "right" and a "wrong" decision?
2. The extent to which the leader possesses sufficient information or expertise to make a high-quality decision alone.
3. The extent to which the problem is structured; for example, is it known what information is needed and where it is located?
4. The extent to which acceptance or commitment on the part of subordinates is critical to effective implementation of the decision.
5. The prior probability that the leader's autocratic decision will receive acceptance by subordinates.
6. The extent to which subordinates are motivated to attain the group or team goals explicitly involved in the particular problem.
7. The extent to which subordinates are likely to be in conflict over preferred solutions.

The decision-making processes available include autocratic (decision making by the leader), consultative (decision making by the leader after sharing the problem and getting input from subordinates), and consensus (the group makes the decision).

In general, the decision is made in the manner that takes the least amount of time, providing certain rules are not violated. Some examples follow:

1. If a quality decision is required (one solution is more "right" than another) and either the leader does not possess enough information or the problem is unstructured, then the leader cannot make the decision alone. In the dental office the decision might be whether the amount of discomfort caused a patient by placement of a rubber dam is worth the advantage of a dry field. The dentist cannot make this decision alone because he or she does not know how much discomfort the patient experiences. In this case the dentist needs to consult both the patient and the auxiliary for the most complete information.
2. If the acceptance of the decision by subordinates is critical to effective implementation, and if it is not certain that an autocratic decision by the leader would receive acceptance, then the leader cannot make the decision alone. An example here would be whether sick days are actually time an employee can take off or for emergency use only. If employees do not agree with the leader's interpretation, they may continue to use their sick days as vacation time without the team leader's knowing.
3. If the employees do not share the team goals involved in the decision, then the group should not make the decision by itself or with the leader merely acting as a member. For example, salaried auxiliaries who do not share in the gross profits of the office ought

not to be allowed to decide the number of hours they will work.

4. If subordinates are likely to be in conflict over the appropriate decision, and if commitment is crucial for implementation, then group discussion is needed. For example, if the bookkeeper-receptionist and the dental assistant are both trained dental auxiliaries who were both hired for that role, and both strongly prefer assisting to bookkeeping, then the whole team needs to discuss and decide who will play what role when. An arbitrary decision by the dentist without hearing the feelings of those involved and having them hear each other's feeling would be likely to be rejected, with the result of poor desk work and continuing conflict.

PROCESS OBSERVATION

Managing the group processes of communication, problem solving, and decision making is greatly facilitated by an understanding of group dynamics. Observing an ongoing group (for example, a dental team's planning or debriefing session) is a good way to build that understanding. Some of the dimensions to be observed include the following:

Participation: Did everyone participate? Did some participate more than others? Did certain individuals participate only on certain issues? Was an effort made to draw people out? Did a few people dominate? Did some people appear to be excluded from the discussion?

Leadership: Was there a designated leader, or did one emerge? Was leadership shared? What leadership functions were exhibited, for example, initiating ideas, polling the group, summarizing?

Roles: Who proposed tasks, goals, or action? Who gave information? Who expressed feelings? Who clarified issues or interpreted ideas? Who attempted to reconcile disagreements? Who facilitated the participation of others? Who blocked the group's movement for personal or unstated reasons? Who distracted the group from its task?

Communication: Did people appear to feel free to talk? Did they listen to others? Was there any interrupting or cutting people off? Did

people take responsibility for their own statements by saying "I" and "me," rather than "they" or "one"?

Decision making: Were a lot of ideas suggested or only one? Was there thorough discussion before a decision was made? Was everyone's opinion considered in making the decision? Who influenced the decision? How?

Nonverbal: Who was looked at when speaking? Who was not? At whom did the speakers look? What postures were observable? What gestures? What facial expressions? What was the seating arrangement in the room? Did people move around at certain points in the discussion?

Climate: Was the group temperature cool and distant, warm and friendly, or hot and heavy? Was the tempo lively or slow? Was the emotional tone supportive, hostile, depressed, anxious, or resentful?

It is more difficult to observe an ongoing group process when one is involved in the content of the discussion. Providing an opportunity to observe without being involved greatly facilitates learning. The next skill level is to be able to participate in the discussion and still being aware of the process or dynamics of the group. The final skill is successful intervention into the process. *Successful* means helping the group accomplish its task to the greater satisfaction of its members. The same general rules for giving feedback to individuals apply, particularly the one about being nonjudgmental. The group's "process" is not a concrete fact; that is, there is no objective truth about what was really going on. The dynamics of the group are understood, or the group is "processed" by having each individual present express an opinion about what was happening and share feeling-level reactions. Examples of the latter are "I was bored," "I was angry at Dr. Williams for interrupting me twice," and "I was depressed about our inability to stay on the topic."

These same observation skills can be applied to the flow of the technical operation of the team and to interaction with the patient. An opportunity to observe another team's functioning may prove valuable. A word of caution, however: learning through observation requires a lot of concentration. The role itself can be somewhat trying, for example, standing quietly in a corner while others are active. There is a temptation to start a conversation with a fellow observer or to join the action in some way to avoid the tension of the observer role. What is needed is careful attention to overall flow and the details of what is occurring and an active attempt to form hypotheses, collect data to test them, and make connections to other experiences and knowledge bases.

ROLES AND ROLE NEGOTIATIONS

Team planning is particularly necessary in determining who is to do what. For example, what specific role functions are going to be performed by which member of the team? Because each individual needs to be aware not only of his or her own functions but also of the functions of each other member of the team, one-to-one planning does not contribute to as much team efficiency as a team discussion of roles.

The way in which people carry out their particular duties and functions is also an important aspect of their roles. For example, instruments can be put in a sterilizer quietly or noisily, gently or roughly, accompanied by singing or cursing. It is perfectly reasonable to have a personal reaction to the way others play out their roles. Sometimes there are even disagreements about the definition of a role. In these cases the process of role negotiation may be very appropriate.[2] Role negotiation consists of working out agreements among the members of the team regarding what activities each individual is to perform, such as what decisions they can make, what information they need to transmit to whom and how often, and who can legitimately tell them what to do and under what circumstances. The process has four steps.

The first step of a role negotiation process consists of each member of the team writing down for every other member a list of those things they would like to see the other person (1) do more or do better, (2) do less or stop doing, and (3) keep on doing the same way. These should be things that would enable the sender to do her or his job more effectively; for example, giving feedback on speed and quality of operations, sharing important information about the patient, explaining procedures to the patient, or disappearing for 5 to 10 minutes without notice.

In step two of the process each person makes a master list containing all the messages he or she received in each of the three categories. The lists are printed large enough to be posted and seen by the other team members.

In the third stage, members ask each other questions for clarification or additional information about the messages they have received. Defenses, rebuttals, and negotiations for changes are not allowed at this time. Nothing else is attempted until everyone fully understands all of his or her messages. The reasons for controlling the process at this point are to avoid misunderstandings and escalations of potential conflicts. Free expression of feelings at this point might lead to hostility, which would be hard to undo later.

Step four begins with persons marking on their own chart those behaviors that they are willing to, and feel that they can, change. Each person marks on the charts of others those behaviors that she or he most desires to have changed. Thus the most negotiable issues become clear. The rule of thumb for step four is that a quid pro quo provides the motivation for lasting change; that is, changes in behavior are negotiated: "I will make the coffee if you will stop complaining whenever I take a coffee break," or "I will stop yelling at you if you will keep the appointment book neater."

Whenever an agreement is reached between two or more persons, it is written down to give it the status of a formal contract. Participants to the agreement also discuss what incentives or sanctions they are willing to bring to bear on the agreement. The negotiating process continues until all agreements that participants are willing and able to make have been reached. Pressure is not exerted to go beyond what they think is possible. It is most helpful to have a behavioral science consultant available to guide the group through this process of role negotiation. The consultant could be useful in orienting the group toward constructive processes, adding the importance of an outside-the-group presence to the agreements, and reorienting potentially harmful conflicts.

THE SUPERVISORY FUNCTION

There are usually two goals of supervision: monitoring of performance and staff development. Achieving a balance between the two often presents difficulties. It is easy to fall into a pattern of only helping or only policing. The substantive issues in supervision can be described as quantitative and qualitative. For purposes of this discussion, quantitative relates to *how often* and *when* the supervisor checks; qualitative refers to the quality of the intervention or supervision, not quality standards for the operations themselves. If the team has afforded itself a time for communicating about problems and issues, supervision becomes much easier. The time can be used to discuss what checkpoints are most appropriate. Most people have a fairly good idea of their strengths and weaknesses and, when consulted, will probably have an opinion about what aspects of their work they would appreciate having checked. With this kind of an agreement, the whole process of supervision becomes a pleasant one.

The supervisors can now feel free to observe, but what happens when they think the quality of work is not sufficient? The answer depends on whether the supervisee agrees with the supervisor. If the supervisee thinks the work is not up to par, then the process is one of helping the employee to do it more effectively in the future. If he or she feels it is adequate or better, then a process of confrontation must occur before any help can be negotiated. Both are complicated interpersonal processes. The remainder of this section focuses first on confrontation and then on help.

Confrontation is a type of communication in which differences are acknowledged and dealt with. What is confronted is the fact that there is a disagreement or a difference of opinion. It is also possible that one of the parties has been unaware of the difference in perspective. Confrontations need not be full of anger and resentment. They can, instead, be motivated by caring for the other person and for the relationship. Angry feelings tend to build when confrontations are avoided beyond people's tolerance for frustration. The first couple of times someone slams a door, for example, it is easy enough to say, "You know it really jars me when you slam the door. I jump every time. Could you please close it more quietly?" When the frustration engendered by the slamming has built up for weeks or months, it is more likely that if you say anything, you will scream rather

than speak calmly, substituting anger for reasonableness.

Confronting differences of opinion and perspective to resolve them or to keep an open discussion going helps to maintain a good relationship. The energy required to start the discussion is an investment in the other person. It is unfortunate that the word *confrontation* has negative connotations because a confrontation can truly be an act of love and caring. Our cultural biases may tell us that differences imply inequality or other negatives, but *different* does not have to mean that one is better than the other or that one is right and the other is wrong. Differences openly confronted can provide energy and stimulation.

The helping part of supervision also requires a certain amount of skill. The tendency in offering help is to give advice or to take over the situation before fully understanding what the problem is and why the person needs help. To help a person do a better job in the future, it is necessary to understand that person's perception of the situation. One of the most useful things a helper can do is to ask open-ended questions.

For example, a dentist supervising a hygienist may notice some calculus remaining in a patient's mouth. It is possible that the hygienist is aware of what has been missed but decided that with this particular patient and at this time it was better to avoid trauma and pain. The hygienist may be planning to have the patient come in for another appointment when he or she can be more thorough. The dentist, in this situation, will not facilitate the hygienist's development without asking questions before evaluating. Appropriate questions might help the hygienist to evaluate whether she or he did, in fact, make the right decision.

The helping situation requires mutual trust, a recognition that helper and helpee are engaged in a joint exploration, and good listening on both sides, but particularly on the part of the helper. Disparaging or making light of the problem by the helper may cause the helpee to feel inferior or to lose trust. Defensiveness on the part of the helpee requires patience from the helper, not added pressure.

The helpee has a part in the process, too, such as giving the helper feedback on what is helpful, not trying to take the focus away from himself or herself, not just looking for sympathy, not responding in terms of "yes, but," and instead being ready to accept help and change behavior when it is appropriate and necessary.

Confrontation and helping are two components whenever there is a need felt by someone (supervisor, employee, patient) for an employee to do something differently.

CONFLICT UTILIZATION

"Conflict management" was a potential heading for this section. The word *utilization* was chosen because it highlights the positive effects of openly discussing different viewpoints. For example, open articulation of opinion forces one to think, thereby increasing understanding of one's own position. Further, a diversity of viewpoints leads to increased innovation and increased motivation and energy in the group or organization.

Walton's[10] model for third-party intervention in a two-party conflict situation includes many helpful ideas and will be the basis of much of what follows.[10] The discussion of a conflict is called a *confrontation*. The purposes of a confrontation can vary; the purpose might be to diagnose the conflict, to attempt to deescalate the conflict, to increase the authenticity in the relationship, or to increase commitment to improve the relationship. The phasing of the discussion moves from substantive issues to emotional issues and back, depending on the level of emotion and the degree to which substantive issues can be worked. The pair might begin by talking about policies and practices, resources, role conceptions, or role relationships. The process for these substantive issues is one of problem solving. When blocks become apparent (when, for example, there is no further progress being made), the third party suggests that the principals discuss their feelings toward each other. Underlying feelings may include any number of emotions, such as anger, fear, scorn, resentment, distrust, and rejection. Misperceptions about feelings often exist and are seldom discussed. Restructuring of perceptions and working through of feelings are likely to liberate energy for further work on substantive issues.

The model for confrontations suggests that a number of factors be in balance between the two parties, such as position or status in the organization, articulateness, ability to express feelings, and allies or supporters in the group or organization. Total situational power can be in balance, even if a "boss" and subordinates are confronting each other. For example, the subordinate may have a higher degree of verbal ability or the meeting may take place in his or her territory (office), or she or he may be paired with an ally during the meeting.

Motivation to work out the issues must be nearly equal between the two parties as well as their distance from and trust in the consultant. In other words, the third party must either be a neutral but respected figure to both or a close friend of both. A consultant who is close to one person and does not know the other may create an imbalance. Minimum requirements for the consultant's role are that both parties agree to the person's playing that role and feel they can trust him or her.

The actual functioning of the third party is similar to that of an orchestra conductor but is more subtle. Ideally, that person functions as an unobtrusive facilitator making suggestions to each of the principals but always encouraging them to talk directly to each other and not to the consultant. Interventions are concerned with getting the information out about the substantive matters, keeping both parties talking about the issues, or balancing the amount of talking being done so that each has equal time. The consultant may intervene to present her or his diagnosis of the conflict, to repeat what has been said as a way of clarifying the messages, or to give feedback to the principals. The consultant might also ask for feedback, particularly as to whether the clients are finding him or her helpful. Ending the meeting at an appropriate and agreed-on point is part of the third party's responsibility. It is almost always necessary to plan another meeting. Even if it appears that all these issues have been resolved, knowing that there is some checkpoint in the future will strengthen the new agreements. The discussion often will be a first step and is best understood that way; using conflict is an ongoing process.

A confrontation meeting might be used where two of the dentists in a group practice have some ongoing disagreements about use of office space, hours of covering the practice for each other, and fee schedules. In addition, there are some underlying feelings of distrust and resentment of unclear origin. Both dentists like, trust, and talk to the hygienist about their mutual difficulties. They feel that the hygienist understands their positions but is impartial. At some point, several hours of either the working day or after-hours time could be scheduled for the purpose of airing all the differences of opinion between the two with the help of the hygienist. He or she might watch, for example, to see that each has an equal amount of talking time, that one does not overpower the other, that they do not pile on issue after issue without attempting to solve any one of the problems, and that they do not engage in unsupported assertions or labeling of each other.

The example of the hygienist as consultant is used here purposefully because the third party should not be an authority figure but merely a facilitator. If the dentist plays this role between two employees, there is a danger that they will look to the boss for a solution, and the dentist will have to make it clear that he or she is there to help them work out their own problems, not to tell them what to do.

The confrontation meeting is appropriate whenever there is an ongoing conflict between two persons who are willing to talk about it and whenever a third neutral person is available to help them.

TEAM MEMBERSHIP GUIDELINES

The team leader cannot be held solely responsible for the team's success or failure because this responsibility is, by definition, shared. There are several requirements necessary to be an effective group member. Most important is a willingness to participate, to open up and share what is on your mind. Team members must also listen to each other, not just in a pro forma way, but actively for understanding. These first two guidelines have even more impact when there are disagreements among team members. The most effective way to deal with differences in perceptions, values, and opinions is to talk them through.

A spirit of cooperation is also very helpful. There is such a thing as "healthy competition," for example, that means trying to do something better than someone else in the interest of better overall team performance. When the attempt is to look good or make the other person look bad, however, it can become destructive competitiveness.

Another guideline is to attempt to solve problems rather than to establish blame. Helping one another and providing support toward doing a better job are effective team behaviors. Giving and being willing to accept feedback are important components of that process. Finally, inclusion of all team members is necessary for good team performance. Exclusiveness or scapegoating one or more members can decrease overall productivity.

TEAM DEVELOPMENT

It is possible to help a team move through a series of developmental stages to become a high-performing group in terms of task work and personal satisfaction. The team leader has a significant role to play in this process, but it is also possible to think of leadership as a function that members can perform too. There is general agreement in the small-group literature about the stages groups go through, although the names differ a bit.[5] Initially, group members need to be oriented to their task and to one another (role and role relationships). The leadership function here is to provide the right amount of structure, for example, holding regular meetings; encouraging team members to talk about their skills, interests, and perceptions; sharing information; and encouraging questions. Stage I is *orientation*.

Stage II is *conflict*, with one another and sometimes with the leader. It may look more like confusion over the tasks than outright conflict. People are concerned about their degree of influence and their place in the group. A team at this stage is not very productive. What is required is careful discussion of the differences of opinion and perception of the various team members about what they should be doing, how and why, and how they feel about other team members. The dilemma here is to match the group's tolerance for open discussion without pushing them beyond what they are willing to deal with. A norm needs to be established that expressing differences of opinion is all right. It is at this stage that the group needs to discuss its decision-making processes and engage in joint problem solving.

Stage III is *solidarity*. The group is celebrating having worked through some differences, and the leader may join them. There is in fact an attempt to co-opt the leader at this stage so that he or she will no longer be in charge. Usually, however, the leader is aware that the team could be a lot more productive with a little extra effort, and so is not willing to give up the role. This is also the stage at which teams become competitive with other teams, and an "us versus them" attitude may develop. The leadership functions needed to move beyond this stage include open communication about issues and feelings, requesting and giving both positive and constructive negative feedback, and delegation of challenging tasks.

The final stage is *productivity*. At this point the team is highly productive on tasks, and members are willing both to help and to challenge one another. There is a baseline of trust, warmth and openness that is not usually violated, even when task-related conflict arises. Members give feedback freely to each other and to the leader. Differences are accepted and openly discussed in the exploration of creative solutions to problems. The leadership functions needed include support of members to prevent burnout, providing challenging assignments, and knowing when to do each.

These stages are sometimes difficult to recognize because behaviors do not occur exclusively in their designated stages. It is also possible for a group to regress in response to an internal or external trauma or to changing membership.

When a new member joins a team, it might be appropriate to add some specific team-building exercises or processes to the usual team meeting. These might include all members sharing background information about themselves, sharing favorite activities or places to go on vacation, or sharing values like "the person I most admire" or "what I want most out of life." Values discussed might also be work related, such as "the most important thing to me about dentistry is . . ." or "the reason I chose dentistry as a field is. . . ." Exploring these questions in a group can often build or add to career commitment. If doubts about the choice are shared, that, too, builds support and understanding among team members and could suggest areas where people may need help in the future.

SUMMARY

This chapter has focused on the individual as a member of a team. Theories of management derived from social science literature formed the foundation for many of the guidelines presented. Whether we are talking about a private dental office, a community health center, or a major corporation, people function in similar ways. Successful team management requires the effective use of a number of ongoing interpersonal and group processes, such as communication, problem solving, decision making, role negotiation, supervision, and conflict utilization.

Whether one is the manager or the managed, it is important to practice personal skills of observation of interpersonal and group interaction, giving feedback, confrontation, and helping. A dental office is a small organization, yet few dentists or dental hygienists have had formal education in management. This chapter has provided some suggestions on how to manage and participate in an organization. It is hoped that this overview proves helpful for dentists, dental hygienists, and educators in furthering their understanding of the human aspects to team management.

REFERENCES

1. Jong AW: *Ethical issues in dental care.* In Jong AW: *Community dental health,* ed 2, St. Louis, 1988, Mosby–Year Book.
2. Harrison R: *Role negotiation: a tough minded approach to team development.* In Burke W, Hornstein HA, editors: *The social technology of organization development,* Fairfax, Va, 1972, NTL Learning Resources.
3. McGregor D: *The human side of enterprise,* New York, 1960, McGraw-Hill.
4. Moosbruker JB: *Using a stage theory model to understand and manage transitions in group dynamics.* In Reddy WB, Henderson C, editors: *Training theory and practice,* San Diego, 1986, University Associates.
5. Moosbruker JB: *Developing a productivity stage team: making groups at work work.* In Reddy WB, Jamison K, editors: *Team building blueprints for productivity and satisfaction,* Alexandria, Va, 1988, NTL Institute.
6. Moosbruker JB, Giddon DB: Effect of experience with aged, chronically ill, and handicapped patients on student attitudes, *J Dent Educ* p 278, Sept 1966.

7. Moosbruker JB, Jong AW: Racial similarities and differences in family dental care patterns, *Public Health Rep* 84:721, 1969.

8. Tannenbaum RT, Schmidt WH: How to choose a leadership pattern, *Harvard Business Rev* p 95, March/April 1958.

9. Vroom VH: A new look at managerial decision making, *Organizational Dynamics* p 66, Spring 1973.

10. Walton RE: Interpersonal peacemaking: confrontation and third party consultation, Reading, Mass, 1969, Addison-Wesley.

15 Ethical Issues in Dental Care

The practice of dentistry is governed by rules of conduct that are stated in law. In the United States these laws are generally assembled in the dental practice acts of each state, which specifically define the practice of dentistry and describe the duties that may be performed by dental auxiliaries. Federal laws may also apply to dentistry, as in the regulation of controlled substances or Occupational Safety and Health Administration (OSHA) regulations.

A more subtle regulation of conduct, however, lies in the ethics of a profession. Whereas laws are written and generally clearly defined, ethical rules of conduct are not always so clear. Laws are enforced by an arm of government, but ethical rules are generally only weakly enforced by professional societies such as the American Dental Association (ADA) and the American Dental Hygienists' Association (ADHA).

This chapter discusses some of the concepts of bioethics that form the foundation for the healing professions. Several case studies are presented and a framework for ethical decision making is developed.

PROFESSIONAL RESPONSIBILITY

Dentistry is treated by society as a learned profession, and therefore dental professionals have a responsibility to society. Contemporary professions arose during the Middle Ages and are represented by fields such as medicine, law, and the ministry. All professions have four common requirements: (1) a distinct body of knowledge generally requiring education beyond the usual level, (2) a component of service to society, (3) the right and responsibility to be self-governing, and (4) a code of ethics.

Society has conferred upon the professions a special status with unique rights and privileges. The professions, such as dentistry, determine their own standards for licensure and control the num-

bers of entering professionals, the length and conditions of education, the distribution of services, and to a great extent the cost of services. It is society's belief that professionals place the welfare of the patient above their own welfare, which helps support the independence of the professions in a regulated society. This covenant with society requires professionals to practice in an ethical manner, if society is to continue to accord these special privileges. Although the public at large is not aware of the details of the professional code of ethics of the ADA or the ADHA, it does expect that the professionals will behave in an ethical manner. In a recent Gallup Poll the public ranked the dental profession second with respect to ethical behavior among all professions.

Each of us establishes our own set of ethical standards. These standards may be higher or lower than those set by our respective professional groups. These standards are determined by our values and belief systems and are rarely at a conscious level. When we are confronted by an ethical question or dilemma, we may draw on our belief systems to find an answer. This chapter is designed to help dental professionals with those difficult questions.

ETHICAL PRINCIPLES

Ethics is the part of philosophy that deals with moral conduct and judgment. To provide a common basis for ethical reasoning, certain principles and terms are discussed in this chapter. There are several principles that health care professionals must be aware of in the practice of their profession. Knowing the names of these principles will not make us more ethical, but understanding the basis for certain behaviors may help us make more carefully reasoned decisions when confronted with ethical dilemmas. Although many ethical principles can be traced to early Greek physicians and philosophers, they also appear in many early Eastern philosophies. The major principles discussed in this chapter are to do no harm (nonmaleficence), to do good (beneficence), autonomy, justice, veracity or truthfulness, and confidentiality.

To do no harm or nonmaleficence is generally attributed to Hippocrates and is considered to be the foundation of social morality.[5] It is clear that although dental care professionals support this principle in theory they are at times guilty of transgressions. *Iatrogenic disease* is the name we give to doctor-induced illness, and all of us in the dental field have seen overhanging restorations cause periodontal disease or failure to sterilize instruments cause an infection. One example of a typical dilemma is whether a dental hygienist should use instruments that have not been adequately sterilized if the dentist employer tells the hygienist that sterilizing is not necessary. Because the dentist is ultimately responsible, is it the hygienist's concern? Each of us is responsible for our own actions. If we knowingly do harm to our patients, excusing our acts because someone else is legally responsible, we have still behaved in an unethical manner. The decision is not an easy one because refusing to use the instruments might cost the hygienist his or her job, but clearly there is a "right" answer in this case if we follow the ethical principle of "do no harm."

To do good, or beneficence, a concept also traced to Hippocrates, is required of all health care providers.[7] It should be the role of dentists and dental hygienists to benefit patients, as well as not to inflict harm. The expectation of the patient is that the care provider will initiate beneficial action and that there is an agreement between the doctor and the patient that some good will occur. It is not enough to say, "Well, it won't hurt the patient if I do this procedure." Will it help the patient? A dentist who feels pressured to produce more work to meet expenses might be tempted to recommend replacing a basically sound restoration in a patient who needs no work, using the argument that "it won't hurt the patient to have the filling replaced, and it will probably have to be done some time in the future anyway." The question is whether it will do the patient any good, and certainly, when examined closely, it would bring a number of "harms" to the patient: unnecessary anesthesia, po-

tential loss of some sound tooth structure, extra time in the chair, and, of course, paying for something that is unnecessary.

Autonomy is a principle that dictates that health care professionals respect the patients' right to make decisions concerning the treatment plan.[5] Patients should not be bystanders in their treatment but active participants. Informed consent, both a legal and an ethical concept, is an essential component of a patient's right to autonomy. This consent requires that the following four elements be present:

1. Disclosure of appropriate information, including risks and benefits involved in treatment, consequences of nontreatment, and alternative treatments, when applicable
2. Comprehension of the information by the patient
3. Voluntary consent
4. Competence to consent[5]

Dentists sometimes attempt to direct a patient toward a particular mode of treatment by stressing certain advantages and not mentioning disadvantages. The dentist may believe that it is in the "best interest" of the patient to have the treatment, but it is a breach of ethics to mislead or misinform patients. In addition, it may well become a legal problem. Dentists are often trained in a paternalistic setting and therefore practice in a paternalistic way after graduation from dental school. *Paternalism* is defined by the *Oxford English Dictionary* as the "principle of government as by a father," that is, a dictatorial "father knows best" attitude. Paternalism in health care can take the form of withholding information, restricting choices, or making the choice for the patient. Paternalism may also be expressed in laws that protect people from themselves as opposed to most laws, which protect people from other people. An example of a paternalistic law might be one requiring motorcyclists to wear crash helmets. This public health law is designed to protect those cyclists who might choose to ride without helmets. Another example is the law mandating fluoridation of community water supplies to protect people who might not avail themselves of self-administered fluoride drops or tablets. We may be able to justify paternalistic laws as being in the public's interest, but we should recognize that these laws limit the rights of a segment of the public because we judge that the laws are in their "best interest."

Justice is often described as fairness or equal treatment, giving to each her or his right or due. An oath often attributed to the Jewish physician Maimonides states, "Preserve the strength of my body and of my soul that they ever be ready to cheerfully help and support rich and poor, good and bad, enemy as well as friend. In the sufferer let me see only the human being."[7] In providing dental care it is difficult to distribute services to all who are in need, but it should be the concern of health care professionals to see that as even a distribution as possible occurs. Dentists can provide some free or discounted care in their offices to those who are truly needy, or they can provide financial support or donate some time to clinics for low-income patients. On a larger scale they can support local, state, or federal programs that seek to extend care to dentally needy clients; for example, dentists have not been vocal on extending dental services under the federal Medicare program for senior citizens. The Medicare program, established in 1965, provides relatively good medical and surgical coverage to citizens over age 65 but is relatively devoid of dental services.

Dentists often complain that they cannot treat Medicaid (a federal-state health care program for low-income people) patients because the fees are too low and the patients break too many appointments or that they cannot treat the mentally retarded because it takes too long. The question still must be answered: Who will treat the poor and needy in that only dental professionals can provide dental care?

Truthfulness or veracity is an ethical principle that one would expect to go unquestioned, yet many health care professionals practice in a less than truthful way.[5] Lying fails to show respect for persons and their autonomy, violates explicit agreements, and threatens relationships based on trust. As discussed previously, the dentist may feel that it would be better if the patient took a certain course of action and therefore manipulates the information that is given to the patient. Whatever the reason, the relationship will ultimately suffer and the dentist will be guilty of transgressing a major ethical principle.

Another example of the failure to be truthful re-

lates to the use of placebos. The following case study suggests a possible scenario.

Case study 1

A middle-aged patient who has been treated at Dr. Jones's office for a number of years complains of a pain in her upper molar area. When Dr. Jones reviews the patient record, he notices that Mrs. Carter has complained of pain numerous times over the past several years. In most cases the record indicates that nothing substantive was found. After a detailed clinical examination and radiographs, Dr. Jones can find nothing wrong. He tells Mrs. Carter that it may be a sinus problem but if the pain persists she should return next week. Mrs. Carter returns still complaining of the pain. She is a very noisy person and irritates most of the office staff. Because Dr. Jones can find nothing wrong, he decides to provide a "nontreatment" or placebo. He writes her a prescription for a sugar pill and tells her that it will reduce the pain and that he will adjust her bite because this is probably the problem. He pretends to reduce her occlusion, but merely runs the high-speed drill without touching any teeth. Mrs. Carter leaves "feeling better" and calls the next day to say that the pain has gone away. Dr. Jones tells his staff that she is just a faker and his nontreatment clearly shows she had no real problem.

The use of placebos can be argued against both scientifically and morally. Studies indicate that 30% to 40% of persons with pain of organic origin may show an analgesic response to a placebo. There is little evidence to suggest that pain relieved by a placebo is not real.[11] From an ethical point of view the use of placebos transgresses the principle of veracity. If Mrs. Carter were to learn of the deception she would obviously be upset, and the doctor-patient relationship, tenuous as it may be, will suffer.

Confidentiality is the last ethical principle that we will discuss in this chapter. It is a principle that can be traced to the Hippocratic oath[6] and exists today in the International Code of Medical Ethics, the principles of ethics of the ADA, ADHA, and the American Dental Assistants' Association. Patients have the right to expect that all communications and records pertaining to their care will be treated as confidential. It is very natural to want to gossip about a patient, particularly if it is someone famous or possibly a neighbor, but to do so would break a bond of trust between the dental professional and the patient. Dental students often discuss cases in school hallways or elevators without seeming to notice that others are within hearing distance. Confidentiality must be maintained at all times. Another case where confidentiality might be broken is when a dental hygienist uses another patient as an example, such as "Look, Connie, you really should do a better job with your flossing. My last patient has a terrible case of gingivitis, lots of bleeding, bad breath, and she may lose some of her teeth." At this point your patient might wonder, "Will she use me as an example with her next patient? I don't want everyone to know I have gingivitis." With the exception of required reportable diseases and extreme cases where disclosure is necessary to avert danger to others, confidentiality must be maintained.[6]

ETHICAL REASONING IN DECISION MAKING

The principles outlined in this chapter can be used as tools to solve our ethical dilemmas. Ethicists cannot give us answers, only insight into different ways of looking at issues, or words of caution about potential moral traps. Decision making on ethical issues is similar to any other decision making,[8] and the model provided by Harron and others[10] may be useful.

1. Analyzing: dividing a problem into its leading alternatives
2. Weighing: assessing the strengths and weaknesses of alternatives by balancing one against the other
3. Justifying: providing a compelling and sufficient moral reason that appeals to an established moral principle, such as to tell the truth
4. Choosing: selecting one or more of the alternatives for which some justification can be made
5. Evaluating: reexamining the choices and their justifications based on one's exposure to other similar moral cases

In the following case studies let us consider whether this model can assist in reaching the best decisions.

Case study 2

Ms. Johnson, a dental hygienist, has been working in a large group practice for 2 weeks and has been very happy in the new job. Her present patient, Susan Carter, *is a 17-year-old with no history of caries. Ms. Johnson has just completed a prophylaxis and had bitewing radiographs made. Dr. Smith enters the operatory, completes the clinical examination, and finds no caries or gingival problems. As he leaves the operatory he asks Ms. Johnson if she has done a topical fluoride treatment. Ms. Johnson responds that because the patient has never had any caries, is presently caries-free, and lives in a fluoridated community, she felt that a fluoride treatment was unnecessary. Dr. Smith states that it is office policy that all patients under age 21 routinely receive topical fluoride treatments. Ms. Johnson says that she knows the policy and that she had just applied fluoride to the patient's two younger siblings, also caries-free, but that the patient's mother had told her that they were having some difficult financial problems and could she please see to it that only necessary work was done. Mrs. Carter's bill already totals $265 for the examinations, prophylaxes, and bitewing radiographs for the three children and the fluoride treatments for Susan's two siblings. The fluoride treatment for Susan would add $30 more to the bill. Dr. Smith states that he is the dentist and he knows best. He further states that if Ms. Johnson wants to keep her job, she had better take a more positive attitude toward office policy.*

Ms. Johnson has a dilemma: should she "follow orders" and do the topical fluoride treatment that she believes is unnecessary, or should she follow her own conscience and not do the treatment?

Looking at the model for decision making, we begin by analyzing. What are the alternatives? (1) Do the fluoride treatment. (2) Refuse to do the treatment. (3) Tell Mrs. Carter that the treatment is probably not necessary for Susan but that it is office policy and it would be easier on her (Ms. Johnson) if Mrs. Carter would just tell the receptionist that she had to leave right away because she was already late and that she would make another appointment later for the fluoride. There are probably other alternatives. Try to think of a few.

Weighing the alternatives is the next step. What are the strengths and weaknesses of each alternative? Doing the treatment could be considered "doing harm" because if it lacks any benefit or has very little benefit to Susan, the $30 it costs Mrs. Carter is a form of harm. In this case Mrs. Carter has specifically asked that only important work be done, and Ms. Johnson would be breaking faith if she did the treatment when she believed it would not be beneficial. However, doing the treatment would put her back in the good graces of Dr. Smith, and Ms. Johnson likes her job. Alternative 2, refusing to do the treatment, could get her fired or at least cause problems with Dr. Smith. She might not get much support from others in the practice because this is not an absolutely clear professional decision, and there are *probably members of the profession who would support doing a topical fluoride treatment. Alternative 3 would seem to be the easiest because it would save Mrs. Carter the $30 without Ms. Johnson having to directly confront Dr. Smith. It might, however, cause Mrs. Carter to lose faith in the practice and possibly make her question the necessity of the fluoride treatments for her other two children and past fluoride treatments. It would also place Mrs. Carter in the position of having to tell a lie.*

Justifying requires that we find a compelling moral reason for each decision. Although there may be some reasons for "following office policy," (for example, it is generally helpful to have office policies so that patients are treated uniformly and employees will know what to do in most situations), there appears, in this case, to be no strong moral reason for alternative 1—doing the treatment. Alternative 2 could be justified on the basis of "doing no harm." Alternative 3 could also be justified on the basis of "doing no harm" and possibly "doing good" because Mrs. Carter would have some new information to aid her in making future decisions about topical fluoride treatments. The negative side of the alternative is that it encourages Mrs. Carter to lie to help Ms. Johnson and may cause Mrs. Carter to distrust Dr. Smith.

Choosing means selecting one of the alternatives and giving your justification or finding another alternative that you can justify.

Evaluating becomes easier as you face more and more ethical dilemmas because you will improve your decision-making powers and will have more experience to draw from. It is important to discuss your dilemmas with others and draw upon their experiences. You will find that you are not alone in these dilemmas and that many of your colleagues will have faced similar dilemmas in their professional lives. Making a decision is often difficult, but indecision itself is a decision and just "going along" with something may not lead to the outcome you really want. You must make the best decision that you can at the time, imperfect though it might be.

Case study 3

A young man comes to the office of a dentist and asks to have a tooth pulled because of a toothache. After taking a radiograph and conducting a clinical examination, the dentist determines that there is a small carious lesion in the lower first molar. A careful history of the type and intensity of the pain clearly supports the diagnosis of an early carious lesion on the occlusal surface penetrating the enamel but with only minimum penetra-

tion into the dentin. The dentist explains to the patient that the tooth can easily be restored with a silver or tooth-colored filling. The patient, however, wants the tooth extracted because he "had a tooth filled once and the drilling drove him crazy with pain." He insists that the dentist pull the tooth.

The dentist explains that the tooth is a very important one because it performs 60% of the chewing on that side of the mouth. If it is lost, the other teeth around it will shift and cause other problems. A bridge or partial denture might be needed, which would be costly and require several visits. The filling will take about a half an hour, and after the injection of a local anesthetic there should be no pain. The cost will be $55 for silver or $75 for a tooth-colored filling, within the same price range as an extraction. The patient is restless throughout the talk and persists in his desire for an extraction.

What should the dentist do? Does patient autonomy override the dentist's feelings about "good dentistry"? Can a patient dictate treatment, or should the professional make the decision?[3]

Use the decision-making process to reach a decision. In this case try to develop as many alternatives as possible. For instance, the dentist might convince the patient to have a temporary filling placed to sedate the tooth and allow the patient to make the decision when he is not in pain. There are often more alternatives than immediately come to mind. Discuss the case with your colleagues.

Case study 4

Dr. Lewis is a successful dentist in a suburb of a major metropolitan area. At age 45 he does not wish to treat acquired immunodeficiency syndrome (AIDS) patients. He chose dentistry and his office location because he wishes to treat only certain types of patients. He decides that because he cannot tell which patients have HIV infection he will instruct his receptionist not to take on any new patients that he considers to be in high-risk categories. Dr. Lewis is not very well informed about the disease, but he remembers that certain groups are considered "high risk." He lists Haitians, homosexuals, and IV drug users as the categories he wants his receptionist to turn away, as well as people who say they have AIDS or are HIV positive.

The receptionist is not very comfortable with these instructions and wonders how she'll determine if a person is in a high-risk group or how to ask about HIV disease. She discusses this with the dental hygienist and an associate who's recently joined the practice after completing a general practice residency. The staff agrees that it may not be possible even to determine if a patient is or is not infected. Furthermore, they concur that to have the practice selectively accept new pa-

tients is a violation of dental ethics and state and federal laws that prohibit discrimination based on the perception of disease. Instead, they decide that Dr. Lewis needs to realize that he may already be treating patients with AIDS and that he needs to continue following universal precautions and perhaps strengthen his office policies on infection control.

They decide to call an office meeting to discuss their concerns. Dr. Lewis reluctantly agrees that selecting out certain patients is not appropriate.

When the receptionist discussed this issue with other staff members, she began a process of decision making. She approached this process by first analyzing the problem to consider any alternatives that were available and weighing these alternatives, one against the other. The receptionist could have simply followed doctor's orders, made a list of questions to ask all new patients, and placed herself out of the process. Review the decision-making process and determine how else this case may have been resolved.

Sometimes outside influences can affect the decision. In this case, it is also important to view patient selection as a part of a dentist's code of professional conduct. Whereas the ADA code of professional conduct allows the dentist "reasonable discretion in selecting patients for their practice, dentists shall not refuse to accept patients into their practice or deny dental service to patients because of the patient's race, creed, color, sex, or national origin." The advisory opinion that follows this section states, "A decision not to provide treatment to an individual that has AIDS or is HIV seropositive, based solely on that fact, is unethical."

CODES OF ETHICS

As stated previously, a fundamental requirement for the status of profession is a formal code of ethics. All professional organizations have a published code to which members of the profession are expected to adhere. These codes have been developed over long periods of time; they reflect the customs and beliefs of current members of the profession and provide a historical link with the past. Some modern codes can trace their origins to statements made by Hippocrates or Hammurabi, long before the birth of Christ. Professional codes often state basic moral or ethical principles, such as not doing harm or injustice, but in essence these codes provide a pattern of behavior for how professionals should behave toward other professionals—a code of etiquette. In dentistry the code is the ADA's Principles of Ethics and Code of Professional Con-

duct.[1] This code contains five major sections.

1. Service to the public and quality of care
2. Education
3. Government of a profession
4. Research and development
5. Professional announcement

Sections 2, 3, and 4 each consist of one paragraph defining the principle. For example, section 3 starts: "Every profession owes society the responsibility to regulate itself. Such regulation is achieved largely through the influence of professional societies. All dentists, therefore, have the dual obligation of making themselves a part of a professional society and of observing its rules of ethics." In addition, section 4 has two brief paragraphs on inventions, patents, and copyrights. Sections 1 and 5 are much longer and consist of detailed codes of conduct related to each principle, such as statements on patient selection, patient records, community service, emergency service, consultation and referral, use of auxiliary personnel, and justifiable criticism. Some of these items of conduct relate to specific moral principles, such as "While dentists, in serving the public, may exercise reasonable discretion in selecting patients for their practices, dentists shall not refuse to accept patients into their practice or deny dental service to patients because of the patient's race, creed, color, sex, or national origin," which can be attributed to the principle of justice. Some statements relate laws to cultural norms of the profession, such as "Use of Auxiliaries." Dentists shall be obliged to protect the health of their patients by assigning to qualified auxiliaries only those duties that can be legally delegated. Dentists shall be further obliged to prescribe and supervise the work of all auxiliary personnel working under their direction and control. Other statements, however, are more closely related to cultural norms of the profession, which tend to restrict competition, such as the following:

Dentists who choose to announce specialization should use "specialist in" or "practice limited to" and shall limit their practice exclusively to the announced special area(s) of dental practice, provided at the time of announcement such dentists have met in each approved specialty for which they announce the existing educational requirements and standards set forth by the American Dental Association.

The statements that clearly relate to universal

moral or ethical principles are likely to remain in the code over time, whereas the more limited cultural norms are likely to change as society changes. A case in point relates to the statement restricting advertising that appeared in the code until 1979.

Case study 5

Ethics versus professional cultural norms. This case illustrates that professional codes of ethics do not necessarily espouse true ethical principles. Prior to 1977, professionals such as lawyers, physicians, dentists, and pharmacists were constrained from advertising by the code of ethics of their professional societies. The then-current 1962 ADA's Principles of Ethics and Code of Professional Conduct specifically stated: "The dentist has the obligation of advancing a reputation for fidelity, judgment, and skill solely through professional services to patients and to society. The use of advertising in any form to solicit patients is inconsistent with this obligation." State dental society bylaws very clearly spelled out the size and types of signs dentists could have outside their offices and the type of professional announcements dentists could send.

In the mid-1970s, as the consumer movement gathered strength, court cases encouraging competition appeared. In the 1975 *Goldfarb v Virginia State Bar* case, the court ruled that "learned" professions, including dentistry, were subject to the federal antitrust laws. Subsequently a 1976 ruling, *Virginia State Board of Pharmacy v Virginia Citizens Consumer Council,* permitted pharmacists to advertise prescription drug prices. Finally, in 1977, in the case of *Bates and O'Steen v State Bar of Arizona,* the U.S. Supreme Court ruled that the legal profession's restriction on advertising by its members was in restraint of trade. In January 1977 the Federal Trade Commission (FTC), a regulatory arm of the federal government, issued a complaint against the ADA and several of its constituent societies alleging violation of antitrust laws and section 5 of the FTC Act, which prohibits "unfair methods of competition in commerce and unfair or deceptive acts or practices in commerce." Some specific allegations were that restrictions on advertising resulted in the following:

1. Prices of dental services being stabilized or fixed
2. Competition among dentists in the provision of services being hindered, restrained, and frustrated

3. Consumers of dental services being deprived of information pertinent to the selection of a dentist and of the benefits of competition
4. Dentists being restrained in their ability to compete and make dental services readily and fully available to consumers
5. Development of innovative systems for the delivery of dental services being hindered and restrained[12]

In 1979 the ADA entered into a consent decree with the FTC to allow dentists to advertise. The ADA revised its Principles of Ethics and Code of Professional Conduct to read: "Although any dentist may advertise, no dentist shall advertise or solicit patients in any way that would be false or misleading in any material respect." Thus in 1979 the century-old restriction on advertising by professionals was ended. The courts did hold that professional associations could regulate advertising under their codes of ethics if they had a reasonable basis to believe that the advertising was false or misleading in a material respect.[2]

In the wake of the Supreme Court ruling and the FTC complaint, state dental practice acts were changed and restrictions on advertising were removed. An example is the 1981 amended Massachusetts Dental Practice Act, which states: "Unfair, misleading, deceptive and fraudulent advertising is prohibited. A dentist may advertise truthful and accurate information pertaining to dental services."[9]

Professional codes of ethics serve a useful purpose in that they assemble in a single document many of the cultural norms of a profession as well as promote some of the universally held principles of biomedical ethics. The professions must be careful, however, that they continue to remember that a professional is one who places the interests of the patient above his or her own.

Professions exist only at the pleasure of society; if professions fail to promote the good of society, they will cease to exist because society can regulate and thus limit the autonomy of professions at will.

CONCLUSION

Dental care professionals have an obligation to practice in an ethical manner. Based on our individual backgrounds, we have internalized values and standards by which we behave. Although this

ical, it has attempted to present some ethical principles that health care practitioners over the past centuries have held to be important and to provide a method for finding answers to ethical dilemmas. When we are faced with an ethical dilemma, a debate goes on in our heads. The more puzzling the question, the longer the debate. It is important that this debate occur. For example, a patient needs a three-unit bridge to replace a missing upper first molar tooth. The patient has dental insurance that will pay 50% of the cost of the bridge, but the insurance runs out next week because the patient has lost his job. The patient asks you to file for the bridge as if it were completed this week and then do the work, thus saving the patient $750. The patient states that he cannot afford to pay the entire fee and therefore could not have the work done unless the insurance paid half.

At first you are tempted to say yes. An inner debate begins: "It would mean a $1,800 case and I can certainly use the money." A second voice says, "It's unethical. It would mean lying on the insurance form." The first voice says, "The patient needs the bridge, so I would be doing a good service." You think again, "Am I going to turn into the kind of dentist I'm always complaining about, the kind I'd like to see thrown out of the profession?" A resounding *no* ends the debate.

You tell the patient that you cannot do what he asks, but you would be happy to do the bridge and could help him work out a plan to budget the costs over time. You also mention that, although the bridge should be done soon, a short delay until he gets dental coverage again would probably not be too harmful. You feel good about the decision and realize that the temptations are always there, but each time it seems to get a little easier to resist.

REFERENCES

1. American Dental Association Principles of Ethics and Code of Professional Conduct, *J Am Dent Assoc* 109:81, 1984.
2. *American Medical Association v Federal Trade Commission,* 636 F 2d 443 (2d Cir 1980).
3. Aronoff GM: Evaluation and treatment of chronic pain, 1991.
4. Beauchamp TL, Childress JF: *Principles of issues in bioethics,* Belmont, Calif, 1978, Wadsworth.
5. Beauchamp TL, Childress JF: *Principles of biomedical ethics,* New York, 1983, Oxford University Press.
6. Beauchamp TL, Walters L: *Contemporary issues in bioethics,* Belmont, Calif, 1978, Wadsworth.
7. Bok S: *The tools of bioethics.* In Reiser SJ, Dyck AJ, Curran WJ, editors: *Ethics in medicine,* Cambridge, Mass, 1977, Massachusetts Institute of Technology Press.
8. Brody H: *Ethical decisions in medicine,* Boston, 1981, Little, Brown.
9. Commonwealth of Massachusetts, Revision of 234 CMR 200, vol 10, p 312, May 29, 1981.
10. Harron F, Burnside J, Beauchamp TL: *Health and human values,* New Haven, 1983, Yale University Press.
11. Stimmel B: *Pain, analgesia, and addiction: the pharmacological treatment of pain,* New York, 1983, Raven Press.
12. Stock F: Professional advertising, *Am J Public Health* 68:1207, 1978.

16 Risk Management in Dental Practice

Licensed health providers occupy a special place in society. The license granted them by the community enables them to pursue their profession in a virtual monopoly. Only those who are specially trained and who meet rigid qualifications and standards may hold themselves out to the community as providers of care and engage in practice defined by law. However, once having accepted the license, licensees are subjected to lifelong regulation by society as a whole and by individual patients whom they treat. The risks in practice are many. This chapter examines the risks in health practice and presents methods that enable practitioners to reduce and control them. The process is called *risk management*.

Following the crisis in medical and hospital malpractice in the early 1970s, risk management concepts borrowed from industry were adapted to the health field—particularly to hospitals. Lately, risk management principles have been applied to individual practice settings. They are designed primarily to protect the financial resources of an industry (e.g., hospital, private practitioner) from losses resulting from legal action. An effective risk management program includes the following:

1. Loss identification (exposure to legal claims)
2. Loss analysis (evaluation of loss experience)
3. Loss avoidance or reduction
4. Loss financing (financing claims exposure)

The following three activities are associated with risk management:

1. Identifying areas of legal vulnerability
2. Instituting corrective or preventive measures
3. Purchasing liability insurance

This chapter provides information related to the first two of these activities. It is based on a thorough review of cases brought against dentists and opinions of courts deciding medical and dental malpractice suits. The text summarizes the areas of legal vulnerability associated with the practice of dentistry. The italicized risk management rules (i.e., recommendations, suggestions) represent corrective or preventive measures associated with the subject matter of the text. The amount of liability insurance purchased (the third listed activity) is a personal matter; practitioners must consider cost, scope of coverage, and amount of indemnification of losses that are desired based on their ability to afford premium cost.

Risk management principles are applied to professional and general liability. General liability relates to negligence associated with injuries that result from the physical structures within the office. Professional liability relates to injuries that result from the treatment of patients. For example, if a patient falls in the waiting room as a result of tripping over an electric cord, the incident comes under the general liability category. If the patient's tongue is lacerated by a disk during a crown preparation, the incident becomes one of professional liability. This chapter deals solely with professional liability.

An effective risk management program does much to control the cost of malpractice insurance and to protect the reputation and resources of the practitioner.

This chapter also provides dentists, hygienists, dental assistants, and other office personnel with information about the legal risks of practice and methods designed to eliminate or reduce them. The goal is to enable the health practitioner to practice in a worry- and claims-free environment.

Because so much of risk management relates to law and the legal system, it is necessary to describe how the system works in the regulation of health professional practice to fully understand both the risks in practice and the methods recommended to reduce or eliminate them.

CAVEATS IN RISK MANAGEMENT AND THE LAW

There are 51 jurisdictions in the United States: 50 states and the federal government. Each of the 50 states has exercised its right to regulate the health professions, including dentistry. In addition, Puerto Rico, the Virgin Islands, and the District of Columbia regulate health practices. The federal government also regulates some elements of health practice. Therefore 54 separate jurisdictions regulate the practice of dentistry. Except for federal regulations that apply to practitioners in all states, each jurisdiction has independent regulations. Except for some federal laws, there is no generic law in the United States. There are, however, legal principles that apply nationwide. For example, the legal principle of the statute of limitations is the same in all jurisdictions, but the statute may operate at different times and for different lengths of time in each individual jurisdiction.

The caveat is that for practitioners to know the specifics of the regulation of dental practice, they must know local law. The same act may be legal in one state and illegal in another. As an example, in New York it is legal for a dental laboratory to select a shade for a crown. In Massachusetts it is illegal for a dentist to refer a patient to a laboratory for the purpose of selecting a shade. Therefore a dentist in New York who sends a patient to a dental laboratory for the selection of a shade is not in violation of the law, nor is the laboratory in violation of the state law. The same act performed by a dentist in Massachusetts would be in violation of the law.

Except for the purpose of presenting examples, this chapter describes generic legal principles. Local attorneys, government agencies, or a local dental society should be of assistance in determining the law of the jurisdiction in which you conduct your practice.

Levels of legal risk

This artificial legal concept of "levels of legal risk" relates to the degree to which a dentist is willing to take a risk in the performance of a professional act. Clearly, refusing to treat a patient who does not follow the advice of a dentist presents the lowest level of legal risk to the dentist. However, if the dentist agrees to treat the patient despite the

fact that the patient did not comply with the dentist's advice, the risk is great. A good example of the concept relates to a dentist's advice that the patient have a thorough radiograph examination before treatment is begun. If the patient refuses and the dentist proceeds with the care, there is a risk that because radiographs were not taken, an important pathologic condition was not discovered, and as a result the patient suffered an injury. The dentist may lose a suit should the patient allege that the dentist was negligent in not discovering the pathology. The dentist's defense is that the patient refused to have radiographs taken. Given the uncertainty of the outcome of jury trials, the dentist may lose the case. Therefore the lowest level of legal risk is to refuse to treat the patient. The highest level of legal risk is to treat a patient who refuses to follow your advice. Under some circumstances, you may be willing to take the risk after assessing the benefits of continuing to treat the patient.

While you review the risk management rules, you should keep the concept of levels of legal risk in mind. Prudent dentists make certain that they are aware of the risks attached to any professional decision before acting. That is what this chapter is all about: describing the risks.

Loss without fault

Another artificial legal concept is "loss without fault." It evolved from a study conducted by the author in the early 1980s during the crisis in dental malpractice litigation. Four hundred cases in which a dentist was accused of malpractice were tracked from the initial service of suit papers to the closing of the case. The results were that in 80% of 400 cases brought against dentists the insurance company, on the advice of a panel of dental experts and an attorney experienced in dental malpractice litigation, sought settlement before trial because it was apparent that the case could not successfully be defended. In only 20% of the cases the panel felt that the dentist was guilty of malpractice. In 60% of the cases where settlement was sought the dental experts were of the opinion that no negligence was present. The 60% represents "loss without fault"—no malpractice, but little or no chance of successfully defending the suit. Looking at the data from another perspective, of

400 cases brought against dentists alleging malpractice, in 80% there was no evidence of malpractice, but according to the expert panel, in only 20% could the suit be successfully defended. Loss without fault is the foundation of much of risk management.

REGULATION OF DENTAL PRACTICE

As stated previously, each of the jurisdictions has exercised its right to regulate dental practice. Except for federal regulation, the mechanism for regulation is similar. The elected body, the legislature, enacts legislation designed to regulate dental practice. Because the members of the electorate have neither the time nor the expertise to exercise control over the daily activities of the profession and the details of practice, they enact additional legislation (enabling legislation or statutory authority) establishing an administrative agency to further regulate the profession and grant to that agency the power to adopt administrative laws (rules and regulations) to carry out its mission.

Each state may vary the name of the administrative body and adopt any organizational structure to accomplish the goal of regulating the health profession, but the general regulatory structure is the same. In New York, for example, two administrative agencies regulate dentists and other health professionals: the State Education Department and the Board of Regents. The commissioner of education is empowered by legislative act to adopt regulations; the Board of Regents, to adopt rules. In New York the State Board for Dentistry is not authorized to adopt rules or regulations for the purpose of regulating dental practice. It serves as an examining body, recommends licensure, advises the commissioner and the Board of Regents on dental matters, and serves as an administrative body to hear violations of the rules and regulations. In Massachusetts one administrative agency regulates the practice of dentistry: the Massachusetts Board of Registration in Dentistry. It combines all the functions assigned to the three agencies in New York. Most other states also have only one administrative agency.

A combination of the statutes and the rules and regulations make up the body of dental black letter law, commonly referred to as the Dental Practice Act. However, in all jurisdictions there are many other laws that affect the practice of dentistry. These may be found in the public health law, the sanitary code, the education law, and others. The practitioner should be aware that the laws regulating dental practice are spread throughout the statutes and administrative laws of the state. In addition, a multitude of federal laws exercise control over dental practice. The old adage that ignorance of the law is no excuse should not be ignored.

The risk management principle is: learn the laws of the jurisdiction in which you practice and federal laws that apply to the practice of dentistry, and remain current on changes in the laws.

LEGAL VULNERABILITY IN DENTAL PRACTICE

Legal vulnerability in dental practice may be divided into two broad categories: criminal and civil. Each broad category has subcategories as shown in Figure 16-1. The intentional torts listed on the chart are those most frequently associated with dental practice. False imprisonment, abuse of process, trespass to real property, conversion, interference with performance of a contract, and others are recognized in law but have little relevance in dental practice.

CRIMINAL AND QUASI-CRIMINAL VULNERABILITY

Violations of statutory law are termed *crimes*. They constitute acts that are deemed by the government to be against the public interest. They may be defined as misdemeanors or felonies. Violations of that part of the Dental Practice Act that is statutory are classified as crimes and may include penalties such as loss or suspension of license, mandatory psychiatric counseling, drug rehabilitation, mandatory continuing education, fines, or even jail. If the legislature declares the violation a misdemeanor, the jail sentence may be less than if it classifies the violation a felony. In New York, for instance, aiding or abetting an unlicensed person to perform a service that requires a license is classified a class E felony, punishable by up to 3 years in jail. In other jurisdictions it is classified as a misdemeanor.

Violations of administrative laws (rules or regulations of administrative agencies, e.g., the state

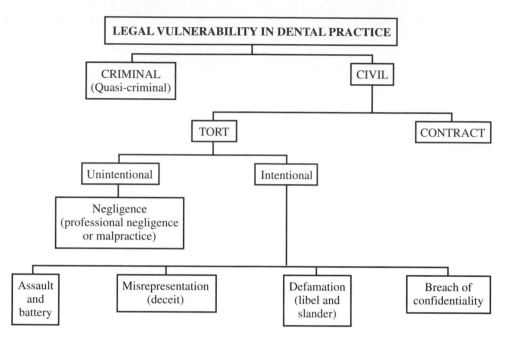

Fig. 16-1 Legal vulnerability in dental practice.

board, the state education department, the board of regents), are termed *quasi-crimes*. Penalties may include all actions that are possible under crimes, except loss of personal freedom (jail). Because members of administrative boards and agencies are appointed rather than elected, the framers of the constitution felt that appointed individuals should not be granted the power to deprive anyone of his or her liberty.

One of the major differences between a violation of a statute and that of an administrative law is the degree of evidence necessary to convict. In allegations of criminal behavior the state must prove "beyond a reasonable doubt" that the law was violated. For violations of administrative law the proof necessary is considerably less. (In civil actions the burden on the plaintiff is to prove by a "fair preponderance of the evidence" [more than 50%] that the defendant is guilty.)

In all dental practice acts there is authority granted to an administrative agency to impose punitive sanctions against a dentist who is found guilty of a violation. Therefore a dentist who is found guilty of violating the law regulating the prescription or the administration of controlled sub-

stances may have an additional action taken by the dental board, or if the violation occurs in New York, by the Board of Regents, against the license of the offender.

Professional liability insurance does not provide protection against either criminal or quasi-criminal allegations. However, if there is an allegation of negligence attached to a violation of the law, either criminal or quasi-criminal, the defense of a civil suit based on an injury resulting from the alleged illegal act becomes more difficult because of trial practice procedures.

The risk management admonition is: don't break the law!

DOCTOR-PATIENT CONTRACT
When the doctor-patient relationship begins

The legal foundation of the doctor-patient relationship is contract law. At the moment a dentist expresses a professional opinion to an individual who has reason to rely on the opinion, the doctor-patient relationship begins, and the doctor is burdened with implied warranties (duties). The fact that no fee is involved does not affect the relationship that attaches to the contract or the duties.

The example best demonstrating the moment the relationship begins and the duties that attach is a situation where a dentist gives a fellow party-goer dental advice at a social gathering. If the advice results in an injury, the dentist may be held liable for negligence. It is not a defense that no fee was charged or expected. The dentist would be held to the standard that patients should not be given dental advice unless an examination and a history are completed.

The risk management principle is: in social settings, never provide anyone, unless he or she is a bona fide patient, with advice regarding dental problems.

Must you accept anyone who presents to you for care? The answer is a qualified *no*. You may refuse to treat a patient for any reason except race, creed, color, or national origin. With the effective date of the federal Americans with Disabilities Act of 1990, refusal to accept a patient based upon a person's disability may be in violation of the law. Patients suffering from acquired immunodeficiency syndrome (AIDS), or who test positive for HIV, fall into the category of disabled persons and may not be refused care if the refusal is based solely on the presence of AIDS or their HIV-positive status. The law declares that all health providers' offices are "places of public accommodation" and therefore subject to antidiscrimination laws. Local jurisdictions have followed the same course as Congress. Therefore in many jurisdictions a dentist's office is subject to the jurisdiction of the local Human Rights Commission and the antidiscrimination policies that it enforces.

As long as the person is not a patient of record, you may even refuse to provide emergency care, subject to the limitations stated previously. It may be unethical, but it is not illegal and cannot form the basis of a civil suit. However, remember that just as soon as you express a professional judgment, or perform a professional act, the doctor-patient relationship begins, and duties begin to attach.

When the doctor-patient relationship ends

The relationship ends when any of the following happens:
1. Both parties agree to end it.
2. Either the patient or the dentist dies.
3. The patient ends it by act or statement.
4. The patient is cured.
5. The dentist unilaterally decides to terminate the care.

The dentist's unilaterally terminating the relationship may support an abandonment claim by the patient unless the dentist follows a procedure acceptable to the courts. In some jurisdictions, abandoning a patient is a violation of the law. In all jurisdictions, abandonment may lead to a civil suit.

The risk management rule to prevent findings of abandonment when you wish to discontinue treatment of a patient is to: (1) give the patient sufficient time to find alternate care, (2) assure the patient that you will cooperate by making copies of the patient's records, radiographs, and other diagnostic aids and reports available to the succeeding dentist, and (3) inform the patient that you will be available to provide emergency care for a reasonable period of time or until the patient locates another practitioner.

It is best to have the patient select the substitute dentist.

The major causes that contribute to a decision to terminate treatment before it is complete are: (1) the patient has not fulfilled the payment agreement, (2) the patient has not cooperated in keeping appointments, (3) the patient has not complied with home care instructions, and (4) there has been a breakdown in interpersonal relationships. Any of these is ample justification for the dentist to terminate treatment.

A risk management rule is: discontinue treatment of patients who do not cooperate in their care, become antagonistic, or exhibit a litigious attitude.

The procedure recommended to discontinue care begins with a discussion of the problem with the patient. Advise the patient that it is in his or her best interest to seek care elsewhere. Assure the patient that you will cooperate by making copies of the records available. Note the conversation on the patient's record. Follow up the conversation with a certified letter stating these facts, signed receipt requested. A risk management caveat is: do not discontinue treatment at a time when the patient's health may be compromised. The decision is professional rather than legal.

EXPRESS TERMS

An *express term* is one in which both parties are in agreement. Putting the term in writing is not required to make it enforceable, although to prevent misunderstandings a written agreement is always preferred. Usually, the express terms define items such as the fee, the treatment, and the manner in which payments are to be made. The risk management principle is: when in doubt, write it out. It may be done on separate forms or entered into the record of the patient. It is best done on a separate form because the treatment record should contain only treatment notes and patient reactions to treatment.

GUARANTEES

Guarantees made by the dentist or an employee constitute an express term in the agreement. In some jurisdictions, guarantees attached to health care are illegal. They are also in violation of the Principle of Ethics and Code of Professional Conduct of the American Dental Association (ADA). You may be held to a guarantee even if the treatment meets acceptable standards of care. A statement made by a dentist to the patient that he or she will be satisfied with the treatment is a guarantee. If the patient is not satisfied, the dentist has breached the contract despite the excellent quality of the service.

Therapeutic reassurances—statements whose purpose is to induce patients to accept care that is clearly in their best interest—are rare in dentistry, except in unusual situations and usually when related to oral surgery. Courts generally do not consider therapeutic reassurances guarantees.

Risk management rule: never guarantee a result!

IMPLIED WARRANTIES (DUTIES) OWED BY THE DOCTOR

Attached to the doctor-patient relationship are additional duties that are implied, unless the express terms serve to void them. They are enforceable although not written or stated. Over the years the courts have identified many of these implied duties. Some of the more important ones are included in the following list. In accepting a patient for care the dentist warrants that he or she will do the following:

1. Use reasonable care in the provision of services as measured against acceptable standards set by other practitioners with similar training in a similar community.
2. Be properly licensed and registered and meet all other legal requirements to engage in the practice of dentistry.
3. Employ competent personnel and provide for their proper supervision.
4. Maintain a level of knowledge in keeping with current advances in the profession.
5. Use methods that are acceptable to at least a respectable minority of similar practitioners in the community.
6. Not use experimental procedures.
7. Obtain informed consent from the patient before instituting an examination or treatment.
8. Not abandon the patient.
9. Ensure that care is available in emergency situations.
10. Charge a reasonable fee for services based on community standards.
11. Not exceed the scope of practice authorized by the license or permit any person acting under his or her direction to engage in unlawful acts.
12. Keep the patient informed of her or his progress.
13. Not undertake any procedure for which the practitioner is not qualified.
14. Complete the care in a timely manner.
15. Keep accurate records of the treatment rendered to the patient.
16. Maintain confidentiality of information.
17. Inform the patient of any untoward occurrences in the course of treatment.
18. Make appropriate referrals and request necessary consultations.
19. Comply with all laws regulating the practice of dentistry.
20. Practice in a manner consistent with the code of ethics of the profession.

The list generates a host of risk management rules. They are all important to the defense of an allegation of malpractice.

IMPLIED DUTIES OWED BY THE PATIENT

In accepting care the patient warrants the following:

1. Home care instructions will be followed.

2. Appointments will be kept.
3. Bills for services will be paid in a reasonable time.
4. That the patient will cooperate in the care.
5. That the patient will notify the dentist of a change in health status.

It is best to make the last duty part of the express terms of the agreement. This can be done by placing the statement at the end of the history form and reminding the patient of the need to notify the office of a change in health status.

If the patient breaches any of these duties, notes to that effect should be made in the patient's record.

RISK REDUCTION IN THE TRANSMISSION OF BLOOD-BORNE INFECTIOUS DISEASES:
Use of barrier techniques

The legal issue of the dentist's right to refuse to treat patients in high-risk groups for AIDS or those patients who suffer from AIDS or ARC has not been decided by any court to give positive direction to practitioners. However, as stated previously, with the passage of the Americans with Disabilities Act of 1990, Congress has imposed its will on the courts, and by declaring a health provider's office a "place of public accommodation" a dentist who refuses to treat a patient who is suffering from AIDS or is HIV positive is in violation of the law and subject to extreme penalties. Not all patients are aware of their HIV status or know if they suffer from other blood-borne contagious diseases; therefore the use of barrier techniques in the treatment of all patients becomes increasingly important. In addition, many high-risk patients who are in need of dental care may not disclose any information to their health history relating to the presence of AIDS or ARC, or their presence in a high-risk group, for fear of being refused care. The result is that all patients must be treated as high-risk patients. It is clear that the provider of care is at greater risk of contracting AIDS from an infected patient than the healthy patient is of contracting AIDS from an infected health care worker.

The fact that the risk of contracting and transmitting AIDS in the dental office is low does not change the responsibility of the dentist to use appropriate barrier techniques. Hepatitis B represents a greater risk in dental practice, and to ensure protection from transmission in the treatment of patients suffering from hepatitis, barrier techniques must be employed.

As a further complication, it is virtually impossible for the dentist to identify, with any high degree of accuracy, patients who may be in a high-risk category for either AIDS or ARC, HIV carriers, or suffering from hepatitis. Therefore appropriate measures should be taken in the treatment of all patients to prevent the transmission of a blood-borne disease to other patients, to the staff in the office, or to the dentist and his or her family. As these measures relate to the use of barrier techniques, the legal issue is: "To what standard will the dentist be held?" During the past several years the standard has seen dramatic changes.

Currently, dentists must employ six basic infection control procedures to meet an acceptable standard of office practice

1. All office personnel involved in the treatment of patients must wear protective eye shields.
2. All office personnel involved in the treatment of patients must wear surgical gloves.
3. All office personnel involved in the treatment of patients must wear surgical masks, as well as splash shields when aerosol sprays are used, or blood or saliva may splatter.
4. All instruments used in or near the oral cavity in the treatment of patients must be sterilized in a heat or heat-pressure sterilizer.
5. All touch or splash surfaces must be disinfected with an EPA-registered hospital-grade disinfectant.
6. All contaminated, hazardous, and medical wastes must be disposed of in a manner consistent with local law.

In addition, some states have mandated the use of these and other barrier techniques in the treatment of all patients. Some have addressed the issue of hepatitis B carrier testing and regular monitoring of sterilizing equipment.

Dentists should remain current with the latest Centers for Disease Control (CDC) recommendations, OSHA standards, ADA recommendations, and local law to determine what measures must be taken to prevent transmission of blood-borne diseases. Failure to meet the standards exposes the dentist to legal risk of action by a government agency for violation of the law and civil action by an individual (i.e., patient, staff), who contracted a blood-borne disease traced to the dentist's office.

Following are contact agencies from which information and their rules may be obtained:

ADA contact: Council of Dental Therapeutics, 211 E. Chicago Avenue, Chicago, IL 60611. Telephone 800-621-8099, ext. 2522.

CDC contact: Centers for Disease Control, 1644 Freeway Park, Atlanta, GA 30333. Telephone 404-639-1830.

Local law contact: Either the state dental board, the department of health, or a local attorney.

OSHA contact (by regional office):

Region I (CT,* MA, ME, NH, RI, VT*). 16-18 North Street 1 Dock Square Building, 4th Floor, Boston, MA 02109. Telephone: 617-565-1161.

Region II (NJ, NY,* PR*). 201 Varick Street, 6th Floor, New York, NY 10014. Telephone: 212-337-2325.

Region III (DC, DE, MD,* PA, VA,* WV). Gateway Building, Suite 2100, 3535 Market Street, Philadelphia, PA 19104. Telephone: 215-596-1201.

Region IV (AL, FL, GA, KY,* MS, NC,* SC,* TN*). 1375 Peachtree Street, N.E., Suite 587, Atlanta, GA 30367. Telephone: 404-347-3573.

Region V (IL, IN,* MI,* MN,* OH, WI). 230 South Dearborn Street 32d Floor, Room 3244, Chicago, IL 60604. Telephone: 312-353-2200.

Region VI (AR, LA, NM,* OK, TX). 525 Griffin Street, Room 602, Dallas, TX 75202. Telephone: 214-767-3731.

Region VII (IA,* KS, MO, NE). 911 Walnut Street, Room 406, Kansas City, MO 64106. Telephone: 816-374-5861.

Region VIII (CO, MT, ND, SD, UT,* WY*). Federal Building, Room 1576, 1961 Stout Street, Denver, CO 80294. Telephone: 303-844-3061.

Region IX (AZ,* CA,* HI,* NV*). 71

Stevenson Street, 4th Floor, San Francisco, CA 94105. Telephone: 415-995-5672.

Region X (AK,* ID, OR,* WA*). Federal Office Building, Room 6003, 909 First Avenue, Seattle, WA 98174. Telephone: 206-442-5930.

TORTS

A *tort* is a civil wrong or injury, independent of a contract, that results from a breach of a duty. The tort may be unintentional or intentional. An unintentional tort is one in which harm was not intended, as is the case in the tort of negligence. As the name implies, the intentional torts contain the element of intended harm.

Negligence is an unintentional tort. If the negligence involves an act that is performed in a professional capacity, it is termed *professional negligence,* or *malpractice.* Thus if a dentist is accused of negligence in the performance of dental treatment, the allegation is one of malpractice.

The intentional torts of major concern to the dentist include trespass to the person (better known as *assault and battery*), defamation, breach of confidentiality, and misrepresentation (deceit).

Malpractice (professional negligence) and the standard of care

Only malpractice related to dentistry is presented here. The New York courts have provided the most comprehensive definition of malpractice as it relates to physicians and dentists. Included are some editorial changes and updating; important risk management concerns are italicized.[†]

A doctor's responsibilities are the same whether or not he/she is paid for the services. By undertaking to perform a medical (dental) service, he/she does not—nor does the law require him/her to—guarantee a good result. He/She is liable only for negligence.

A doctor who renders a medical (dental) service is obligated to have that reasonable degree of knowledge and ability expected of doctors (or specialists) who do that particular (oper-

---

*These states and territories operate their own OSHA-approved job safety and health programs (except Connecticut and New York, whose plans cover public employees only).

†Modified from *New York Pattern Jury Instructions—Civil,* vol 1, ed 2, Rochester, NY, 1974, Lawyers Co-operative Publishing.

ation, examination) treatment in the community where he/she practices, or a similar community. (The trend in some jurisdictions, the most recent being New York for some of its appellate jurisdictions, is to apply a national standard.)

The law recognizes that there are differences in the abilities of doctors, just as there are differences in the abilities of people engaged in other activities. To practice his/her profession a doctor is not required to be possessed of the extraordinary knowledge and ability that belongs to a few people of rare endowments, but *he/she is required to keep abreast of the times and to practice in accordance with the approved methods and means of treatment in general use.* The standard to which he/she is held is measured by the degree of knowledge and ability of the average doctor (or specialist) in good standing in the community where he/she practices (or in a similar community).

In the performance of medical (dental) services the doctor is obligated to use his/her best judgment and to use reasonable care in the exercise of his/her knowledge and ability. The rule requiring him/her to use his/her best judgment does not make him/her liable for a mere error in judgment, provided he/she does what he/she thinks is best after careful examination. The rule of reasonable care does not require the exercise of the highest possible degree of care; it requires only that he/she exercise that degree of care that a reasonably prudent doctor (or specialist) would exercise under the same circumstances.

If a patient should sustain an injury while undergoing medical (dental) care and that injury results from the doctor's lack of knowledge or ability, or from his/her failure to exercise reasonable care or to use his/her best judgment, then he/she is responsible for the injuries that are the result of his/her acts.

Courts do not require that all dentists use the same modality of treatment. The standard can be met if a "respectable minority" of practitioners use the same treatment method. Therefore the Sargenti method in endodontic treatment and the Keyes technique in periodontal therapy may be acceptable to the courts as meeting the standard of rea-

sonable care. It should be noted that the standard to which a dentist is held is the standard set by other dentists, not what a text, article, or a guideline from a professional organization recommends. These are hearsay, not available for cross-examination, and therefore may not be directly entered into evidence.

Additional risk management principles applied to malpractice prevention are the following:

1. *Do not undertake treatment beyond your ability and training, even if the patient insists that you provide the care.*

2. *If, in your professional judgment, you believe that specialty care is required prior to the care you intend, do not undertake your treatment unless the patient follows your recommendation to obtain specialty care.* This is of importance when the patient needs to receive periodontal therapy prior to the fabrication of crowns or fixed bridges.

3. *If you recommend to the patient that specialty care is necessary, and the patient refuses to follow your recommendation, the legal risk is increased if you undertake the care that, by your own admission, should have been provided by a specialist.*

4. *If you believe that certain tests or diagnostic procedures should be completed before you undertake treatment and the patient refuses, as in the case of the need for radiographs, the legal risk is markedly increased if you treat the patient without the diagnostic aid you recommend.*

In the last three paragraphs above, you have established for yourself a standard of acceptable care. If you accede to the patient's refusal to follow your recommendations and treat the patient, even at the patient's request, you have departed from your own standard. This action presents a situation that is difficult to defend. Having the patient sign a statement to the effect that he or she is aware of the risk of noncompliance somewhat reduces the risk but does not eliminate it. A court might declare the statement exculpatory and void as against public policy. An exculpatory statement excuses an individual from liability for negligence. Agreements entered into by patients that relieve health practitioners from responsibility for negligent acts have not been enforced by the courts.

When having to address the issue, courts have declared exculpatory clauses in doctor-patient agreements against public policy and therefore void.

Trespass to the person (assault and battery)

The civil counterpart of the criminal act of assault and battery is trespass to the person. It constitutes a threat to harm (assault) and unauthorized touching (battery). Traditionally, lack of informed consent to care was treated as assault and battery. Recent decisions classify lack of informed consent as negligence. The change resulted in part from the recognition by the courts that, except in the most unusual cases, doctors do not intend to harm their patients, even though the touching was not authorized by the patients. In some jurisdictions if the consent is present, but faulty, the rules of malpractice will apply. If there is a total absence of consent, the case will be treated as assault and battery.

Assault and battery cases not associated with lack of consent have occurred in dentistry. The use of force or unnecessary physical restraints in the treatment of uncooperative children has led to allegations of criminal assault and battery and civil trespass to the person. Dentists should be aware that if the allegation is criminal, professional liability insurance will not provide coverage. In some older professional liability policies, civil actions of assault and battery are covered. However, recent professional liability policies limit coverage to professional negligence.

The risk management principle applied to trespass to the person is: avoid the use of physical force or unnecessary restraints in the treatment of children. If you feel that such measures are necessary, discuss the matter with the parents and have them present in the operatory.

Risk management as it applies to consent is discussed later in the chapter.

Misrepresentation (deceit)

Patients must be kept informed of their treatment status. This is one of the implied duties that the courts have attached to the doctor-patient relationship. If information is withheld that places a patient's health in jeopardy or deprives the patient of the legal right to bring suit against the practitioner, a legal action in deceit or fraudulent concealment may result. In the civil action of deceit

and fraudulent concealment, the statute of limitations may be extended, and professional liability insurance may not provide coverage. In addition, a criminal action of fraud may also be alleged. The problems in dentistry most frequently associated with deceit and fraudulent concealment include the failure to inform the patient when an instrument breaks off in a root canal, when a root is fractured and the tip remains in the jaw, and when the dentist is aware that the success of the treatment will be compromised because of lack of cooperation by the patient. Informing the patient of an untoward event at the time it occurs defeats any future attempt by the patient to extend or toll (delay the beginning of) the statute of limitations. A note on the patient's record of the event and of the fact that the patient was informed should be made; if possible, the patient should be asked to initial or sign the entry.

The risk management rules are: never lie to patients about their treatment, and keep them informed about their health status while in your care.

Third-party payment coverage has led to many allegations of deceit. It is usually associated with passing off one metal for another in the fabrication of prosthetic appliances by substituting nonprecious for precious metals, with not collecting copayment fees from the patient, or with substituting an approved-for-payment treatment for one that is not covered by the third party. Actions in criminal fraud also may result. Insurance companies are alert to such activities and are relentless in their pursuit of suspected dentists. The patient may also institute an action for the same act against the errant practitioner. Actions in fraudulent misrepresentation overlap actions in breach of contract. The choice is left to the plaintiff's attorney, and the one most damaging to the dentist's interests or most favorable to the success of the lawsuit will be selected.

The risk management rule is worth repeating: *never lie to or deceive a patient or an insurance company.*

Defamation

The intentional tort of defamation is not of major concern in dentistry because most dentists are aware of the problem and its consequences.

The risk management admonition is: keep your

opinions about your patients to yourself unless they are essential to their successful treatment. Expressions about the mental health of a patient are particularly risky.

Breach of confidentiality

Breach of confidentiality was not known as a tort under English Common Law. It is a product of recent case law and black letter law.

Information obtained from the patient in the course of diagnosis or treatment must remain confidential. Unless the patient waives confidentiality, a breach may lead to a suit. Patients may waive confidentiality by their actions or words. It may also be waived by action of law, as in the case of the requirement to report certain communicable diseases to government (health) agencies. When a patient visits a specialist or another health practitioner at your request, you are expected to inform that practitioner of the health status of the patient. In going to the specialist the patient, by his or her action, has waived confidentiality. A patient who seeks care from a group practice and is aware that the practitioners practice as associates has waived confidentiality. There are many other situations in which confidentiality is waived. However, there are many situations that a practitioner should be aware of when a specific waiver is required.

The risk management rule is: never reveal any information about a patient to anyone without first obtaining permission from the patient—preferably in writing (see the following section on Patient Records).

In some jurisdictions, information related to sexual activity obtained from a minor must not be revealed to the parent without the minor's consent. Both criminal and civil actions may result from this specific form of breach of confidentiality.

Patient records. The patient's dental record is a legal document. It serves many purposes in the judicial process. It contains information about the patient's complaint, health history, and basis for the diagnosis, and it reports all treatment rendered, the patient's reaction to treatment, and the results of the treatment. Case law (law as stated by courts in deciding cases) requires that health practitioners keep accurate records of the diagnosis and treatment of their patients. They constitute an essential part of patient care. Treating a patient without maintaining accurate records represents a serious

departure from an acceptable level of care as defined by the courts. Some jurisdictions require that accurate records be kept as part of the rules and regulations of administrative health or licensing agencies.

The outcome of many suits against dentists are decided on the content and quality of patient records. For the treating doctor the record is the only documentation of the course of treatment of the patient and the patient's reactions to the treatment. Memory alone is often viewed as self-serving and, as stated in one court decision, "the shortest written word lasts longer than the longest memory." In cases in which the doctor and patient disagree on what took place and there is no written documentation of the event, the question of how much weight will be given to the oral statements may be determined in court by who makes the most credible witness. It can become a risky situation for the doctor.

In summary, failure to keep accurate records may constitute negligence and, in some jurisdictions, a violation of law. In addition, failure to keep accurate records markedly increases the risk of losing a malpractice suit.

The risk management rule is: accurate and complete records must be maintained for each patient you treat or examine.

Record ownership. The right to ownership of the patient's treatment record has undergone considerable change during the past several decades. Courts have separated the physical record from the right of the patient to its contents. At one time, doctors had the exclusive right to the possession of the record and its contents. Today, after many suits, the law has evolved so that the doctor is considered the custodian of the record and the patient has a property right in its contents. Some jurisdictions have codified court decisions.

If the patient demands in writing to be sent a copy of the treatment record or demands that a copy be sent to another practitioner or to any other person or agency, you should comply with the request (in some jurisdictions, you *must* comply with the request), but, in either case, supply only copies. The term *record* includes the treatment record, radiographs, casts, results of tests, and consultation reports.

If you believe that the patient intends litigation against you, report the request to your insurance carrier after complying with the request. If there is no local law that you must comply with the request for copies of the record, do not comply unless the carrier approves in writing.

The risk management rules that are generated by the new view of the courts about the patients' rights to record ownership are: *on the patients' written request for their records, comply, but supply only copies. If you believe a patient intends to sue, before you comply, contact your insurance carrier for advice.*

The risk management rule that you retain the original of all patient records is underscored by what a California court said about a doctor's not producing the originals: "The inability of the physician to produce the original of the clinical record concerning his treatment of the plaintiff creates a strong inference of consciousness of guilt."

Form and content. The changing law on ownership of patient records has had a profound effect on the form and content of the record. Keeping in mind that what you write on the record may be seen by the patient will serve as a guide to what should be entered on the record.

Records serve as documentation of the care the patient has received. They are essential to your defense if you are accused of negligence. Patient records are considered legal documents and must be treated as such.

One of the legal authorities in the field of medical malpractice and editor of a major text on the subject had the following to say about dental records: "Dentists seem to be among the worst record keepers. It is not unusual for the complete dental records to consist mainly or solely of a billing chart. Such scant records should be considered malpractice in and of themselves."

Financial information has no place on the treatment record. Separate records should be kept to record charges and payments.

The treatment record should be written in black ink or black ballpoint pen. It should be neat, well organized, and easily read. A sloppy record implies a sloppy dentist and has a negative effect upon the jury and judge. Patient records, as all legal documents, should be legible and complete. There should be no blank spaces where information is supposed to be inserted. A decision by a New York court stated: "a patient record so sparse as to be accurate and meaningful only to the re-

cording physician fails to meet the intent of the requirement to maintain records which 'accurately reflect the evaluation and treatment of the patient.'"

A later section of this chapter provides suggestions on the form and content of record keeping.

How long should you retain your patient records? In many jurisdictions, laws specify the minimum time period for retention of patient treatment records. Failure to comply brings with it risk of allegations by a state agency of a violation of the law.

On the civil side, practitioners are advised to keep the original treatment records for as long as possible. Although the statute of limitations runs for a specific period, the exceptions suggest that the records be kept for a period considerably longer than the statute. For example, in New York, an occurrence state (where the statute of limitations begins to run from the time of the occurrence of the negligent incident), if you are accused of withholding information from a patient about a mishap in treatment, the courts may extend the statute based upon your fraudulent concealment. In Massachusetts, a discovery state (where the statute does not begin to run until the patient discovered, or should have discovered, the act that produced the injury), the suit may begin many years after the patient completed treatment. Two thirds of the states have the discovery rule. The rest have the time-of-injury rule. But even in those, there are exceptions that may include fraudulent concealment (noted previously), foreign body exception, and an exception for continuous treatment.

Without records, it is virtually impossible to succeed in defending a suit.

In the case of minors, in many jurisdictions, the statute on retention of records does not begin to run until the minor reaches majority. Therefore the records of minors must be kept for an extended period of time.

The risk management rule is: you should retain your original patient treatment records, including radiographs and all other documents related to the diagnosis and treatment of the patient, for as long as possible.

Record keeping rules
1. Entries should be legible, written in black ink or ballpoint pen.
2. In offices where more than one person is mak-

ing entries, they should be signed or initialed.

3. Entries that are in error should not be blocked out so that they cannot be read. Instead, a single line should be drawn through the entry, and a note made above it stating "error in entry, see correction below." The correction should be dated at the time it is made.

4. Entries should be uniformly spaced on the form. There should be no unusual or irregular blank spaces.

5. On health information forms, there should be no blank spaces in the answers to health questions. If the question is inappropriate, draw a single line through the question, or record "not applicable" (NA) in the box. If the response is normal, write "within normal limits" (WNL).

6. Record all cancellations, late arrivals, and changes of appointments.

7. Document consents, including all risks and alternative treatments presented to the patient. Include any remarks made by the patient.

8. It is important to inform the patient of any adverse occurrences or untoward events that take place during the course of treatment and to note on the record that the patient was informed.

9. Record all requests for consultations and responses.

10. Document all conversations held with other health practitioners relating to the care of the patient.

11. All patient records should be retained forever.

12. If the practice is discontinued, local law should be checked to determine the requirements on how, where, and in what form the records must retained.

13. Guard confidentiality of information contained on the record.

14. *Never* surrender the original record to *anyone,* except by order of a court or to your own attorney.

15. *Never* tamper with a record once there is some indication that legal action is contemplated by the patient.

What not to put on the treatment record

1. Financial information should not be kept on the treatment record. Use a separate financial form.

2. Do not record subjective evaluations, such as your opinion about the patient's mental health, on the treatment record unless you are qualified and licensed to make such evaluation. Record such observations on a separate sheet marked "Confidential—Personal notes."

3. Do not record any correspondence with your professional liability insurance company, your attorney, or the attorney representing a patient on the treatment record. Record all such notes and any conversations with the above on a separate sheet marked "Confidential—Personal notes."

Histories

THE MEDICAL HISTORY. An area of growing concern for dentists in malpractice liability relates to the health history. There have been major financial and professional losses caused by the dentist's failure to discover information about the patient's past medical history. The primary cause of the problem is the design of the typical self-administered health history form and the manner in which the dentist deals with the completed form. The form used by most dentists has led to considerable difficulties. The most common has two columns in which patients may indicate whether they have a particular health problem. They are asked to place a check mark in a "yes" or "no" box or to circle a "yes" or "no" word. In many cases there have been disputes at trial about who placed the check mark or circle, notwithstanding the fact that the patient signed the form. Facts in dispute lead to problems for the defense attorney in the trial of a case.

The risk management rule is: if you use a self-administered health history form in which the patient is to respond by marking a box, have them initial the appropriate box, rather than using a check mark.

Other problems have arisen with the self-administered health history form. Did the patient understand the questions? Did the patient know the answer at the time the form was completed? Was the patient aware of the importance of the question to his or her care? If the answer to any of these questions is no, the patient may leave a blank in place of an answer or may provide an answer that is not accurate. Blanks left on a completed history form may lead to difficulties; was the question ignored or was the answer negative?

If a self-administered health form is used, there should be four columns instead of two, to avoid a possibility of blanks. The column headings should be "Yes," "No," "Don't Know," and "Don't Understand the Question."

Another problem is related to the manner in which the dentist follows up the self-administered health history. It is usual for the dentist to question the patient further, but limiting the questioning to the positive answers on the form. Most forms are designed to alert the dentist solely to the positive answers. This process may lead to major errors. The patient may have misinterpreted or not understood the question and incorrectly answered in the negative. This has resulted in large malpractice losses. Several cases have been reported where the dentist, using a "Yes-No" form, failed to discover that the patient had a history of rheumatic fever and thus took no precautions in treatment.

Risk management rule: if you use a self-administered health history form and the choices to the patient are two—"yes" or "no"—follow up on the "no" answers as well as the "yes" answers to make certain the patient understood the questions, their importance in treatment, and the reason the questions were being asked.

Do not leave it to patients to decide if the answers to the questions on the health history are important to the success and safety of their care.

The best policy for the use of a self-administered health history form is not to use it. It leaves too much to chance in discovering medical problems that may compromise the successful and safe treatment of the patient. There is much more at stake than legal liability. When a history of rheumatic fever is not discovered, no matter who is at fault, the consequences to the patient and the dentist may be disastrous.

A more effective way to determine past medical history is to have someone take the history who has been trained in the procedure and who has the background to interpret the responses—preferably, the treating dentist. If the history is elicited by someone other than the treating dentist, the dentist should review the history with the patient prior to treatment.

Another type of history-taking form is simple to design. Use a blank sheet of paper with a reminder list of the questions to be asked in the left margin. It is better to spend the extra time this takes than to have a patient suffer permanent injury because

of your negligence as a result of the use of an inadequately designed form.

UPDATING THE MEDICAL HISTORY. Good dental practice requires that the patient's health history be updated at regular intervals. The frequency at which it should be done is a professional, not a legal, decision. The process is simple and effective: allow the patient to review the documented health history that was obtained at the last history-taking visit and ask if there are any changes. Make notes of the procedure and the patient's responses in the patient's record. An abbreviated history update form is simple to design. For example, one may state the following: "I have reviewed the health history form completed on _____, and I report the following: _____." If there has been no change, the patient writes, "No change." If there is a change, the patient so indicates on the form. At times, depending on the nature of the change, the dentist may ask the patient to complete another full health history form.

The risk management rule is: update the health history at appropriate intervals and document the process and responses.

If you continue to use a self-administered health history form, place the following statement before the space for the patient's signature: "I understand and agree that in the event there is any change in my health status, I will notify your office at the earliest possible time." As an express term in the doctor-patient contract it places some of the burden on the patient but will not relieve the doctor of the responsibility for updating the health status of the patient.

FOLLOW UP ON POSITIVE FINDINGS. It is essential to good patient care and to risk management concerns that positive findings in the medical history be followed up by consulting the patient's physician or another appropriate health provider or health facility. It is best to have consultant reports in writing. If this is inconvenient, information received by telephone should be noted on the patient's record.

The risk management rule is: document all conversations with other health practitioners and health facilities that are or were involved in the treatment of your patient and from whom you received information. If you receive a written report, it should be placed in the patient's treatment folder.

THE DENTAL HISTORY. The dental history presents few problems to the dentist. However, one issue not as yet addressed by the courts deserves attention. Dental disease is chronic and almost everyone suffers from it. It does not begin when the patient presents to the dentist. Most patients change dentists several times throughout their lives. To have a complete picture of the etiology of the patient's current dental problem and the history of their treatment, it is essential that, in addition to the history obtained from the patient, the treating dentist should make every effort to obtain the records of the previous dentist(s). It is possible that the previous dentist's notes may assist you in your treatment of the patient in areas such as an abnormal reaction to the administration of a drug, the level of patient cooperation, breaking of appointments, and delinquencies in the payment of fees. Not obtaining information that is available and may be essential in the treatment of the patient may constitute malpractice.

A good risk management practice is: obtain the records and radiographs of prior dentists and other health care providers who have treated your patient. Determine if there is some law in the state that enables patients to secure copies of their records and radiographs.

Examining the patient and completing a treatment plan. "Failure to diagnose" represents a growing area of legal vulnerability. A thorough clinical examination and radiographic review should be completed on each patient. The results should be recorded on the patient's record.

It is difficult to defend a case successfully when many of the questions on the form used to record the dental examination have been left blank. It is impossible to determine if the blank indicates that the question was mistakenly omitted in the examination or if the result was within normal limits. If the form you use has questions that are not germane to your practice habits, or seldom answered, design your own form or purchase one that is more suited to your particular needs and habits of practice.

Many recent cases involve failure to diagnose periodontal disease. Periodontal issues present a major problem if there is no evidence that the patient was examined to determine periodontal needs, for example, pocket depth, plaque scores,

bleeding points, mobility, or oral hygiene index. The answers to the following questions may become important if a suit alleging periodontal neglect is brought against the dentist: If periodontal disease was diagnosed, was the patient informed? Was the need for periodontal care neglected? Was a recommendation made for the patient to seek the services of a periodontist? In summary, was there failure to diagnose, failure to inform, failure to make a timely referral, or failure to treat? If the answer to any part of the question is positive, the dentist is at risk of an allegation of malpractice and is likely to lose the suit.

Issues related to the temporomandibular joint and surrounding tissues have become a target of litigation. The same questions raised about periodontal neglect apply equally to the joint, and the same risks in practice apply. The area of the joint should be examined and monitored during treatment. Problems may arise during orthodontic care, following the extraction of lower molars, and following procedures that require the jaws to open for long periods of time, such as the use of a rubber dam for an extended period of time during endodontic procedures.

Acceptable dental practice includes completing both a recommended treatment plan and a reasonable alternative. Either have the patient sign or initial the accepted plan, or make a note of the patient's acceptance in the record.

Good risk management practice includes completing a thorough dental examination and treatment plan before treatment is begun. The results should be accurately recorded, and all questions on the dental examination form should be answered. There should be documentation that the treatment plan was accepted by the patient.

Consent

Legal entanglements of consent to care. Legal problems related to lack of informed consent to dental care began to surface as a result of the explosion in medical malpractice in the early 1970s. The general principle that a doctor who treats a patient without the patient's express consent is guilty of an unauthorized touching, for which the doctor can be held liable to the patient in damages, began early in the century. The fact that the patient needed the treatment and benefited as a result of the treatment did not relieve the doctor of liability. In the early years the civil claim was that the doctor was guilty of trespass to the person or assault and battery. Today the courts feel that the legal action of malpractice is more appropriate, given the lack of intent to harm by the doctor. The legal procedure is quite different if the action is brought in trespass as compared with actions brought in malpractice. In addition, many courts opined that the failure to obtain the consent of the patient prior to initiating treatment was a breach of the doctor-patient contract. Actions in contract law differ in procedure from both trespass actions and malpractice actions. The modern view is that if *no* consent was obtained the action may be in contract. However, if the consent was obtained, but was faulty, as most of them are, the action in malpractice is more appropriate. The defendant dentist benefits if the action is in malpractice rather than in trespass or contract. In trespass and contract actions the patient-plaintiff is not required to produce an expert witness relating to the standard of professional care and whether the dentist-defendant departed from the standard. In malpractice actions an expert testifying on behalf of the patient-plaintiff is required.

Content of consent: what and how much to tell. Having discussed the legal form of action, we now turn our attention to the content of the consent. As the years progressed since the first major case dealing with the consent to medical care, the courts turned their attention to the issue of whether the consent was informed: was the patient given enough information upon which to make an intelligent decision? The modern view is that the patient must be informed of all the following:

1. A description of the proposed treatment
2. The material or foreseeable risks (described further next)
3. The benefits and prognosis of the proposed treatment
4. All reasonable alternatives to the proposed treatment
5. The risks, benefits, and prognosis of the alternative treatments

All these factors must be described to the patient in language the patient understands, and the patient must be given an opportunity to ask questions about the treatment and alternatives and have the questions answered.

What of the description of the risks? How much of the risk must be told to the patient for consent to meet the test of being informed? There is no agreement among state courts on which to present a bottom-line rule. In most states the patient must be given enough information about the risks to make an intelligent decision about whether to proceed with the proposed treatment. It is called the "subjective prudent person rule." Another standard is whether a reasonable person in the patient's situation was given enough information to make an intelligent decision. It is called the "objective reasonable person rule." In both rules the risks are called "material" because they are material either to the patient or to the reasonable person. The third standard is the "professional community standard"; that is, what do other practitioners tell their patients about the risks when the same condition exists? These risks are termed "foreseeable." As an example, in a state that follows the "professional community standard," a dentist would not have to explain the risk of breaking an instrument in a canal during an endodontic procedure if it can be shown that few, if any, dentists in the community warn their patients of the possibility. In a "reasonable person" state, whether objective or subjective, a dentist may not be required to inform an 80-year-old retiree of the possibility of permanent paresthesia following the extraction of an impacted lower third molar because the risk is not material to the patient or to any reasonable person in the same situation as the patient; the risk is not material. However, if the same dental situation is present where the patient is a trial lawyer, the risk becomes material, and should be told to the patient before treatment is begun.

In the "material risks" states the patient-plaintiff is not required to present the evidence of an expert dentist.

In the "foreseeable risk" states the patient-plaintiff is required to produce an expert witness for the judge and/or jury to determine the standard of disclosure of the professional community. Thus the burden on the patient-plaintiff in the "professional community (foreseeable risk)" states is greater than that in the "reasonable person (material risk)" states.

Superimposed upon court decisions, many states have adopted statutes, administrative rules, or court procedural rules that may have modified their courts' decisions. However, all fall in with the standards described previously.

The prudent dentist will tell each patient both the foreseeable and material risks. This approach will satisfy all court-imposed and black letter law (i.e., statutes, administrative rules and regulations) standards. Thus you are advised to inform each patient faced with the extraction of an impacted lower third molar the risk of permanent paresthesia regardless of who the patient is, their educational level, age, occupation, or whatever, no matter what you believe other dentists tell their patients.

Another issue relating to what the patient should be told is the "common knowledge" doctrine. There are certain risks of which the patient should be aware, by common knowledge, without having to be told by the dentist. All reasonable adults are expected to know that following the extraction of a tooth they will experience some bleeding and, when the anesthetic wears off, some pain. By contrast, no reasonable person would expect that following the extraction of an impacted lower wisdom tooth they would permanently lose sensation of the lower lip. However, the admonition is not to rely on common knowledge in describing the risks of the proposed procedure.

Form of consent: written or oral? Consent to health care, like all agreements between parties, may be written or oral, and it may be expressed or implied. An expressed consent is one in which both parties agree, either orally or in written form. An implied consent is present either by the action of the parties or by law. Expressed and implied consents will be discussed in the next section. Here we will examine written and oral consents.

As long as there is no dispute between the parties as to the details of the agreement, an oral agreement is effective and enforceable. Only when the parties disagree as to the details of the agreement does a written document become important. In general, laws that require agreements (contracts) to be written do not directly affect dental care. These include agreements relating to real property, contracts of sale over a specified amount, and contracts that cannot be completed within a year. They fall into a legal category called "the statute of frauds."

In a few situations the law requires that consent to health care be in writing and signed by the patient. Health facilities, such as hospitals, may require that the consent to treatment be written and signed by each patient. If you work in such a facility, you should comply with the rules and obtain the written and signed consent of each patient you treat in the facility. Failure to do so may compromise your legal position, and that of the institution, if a patient claims that you proceeded with treatment absent a valid consent. Other than institutional rules, few regulations require written consent to health care. Most refer to abortions, donation of human organs, in New York to acupuncture, in some jurisdictions to HIV testing, and in others to surgical procedures. You should check the local law to determine if any require that for the treatment you propose consent must be written and signed. Also, you should check if local law requires that you include specific information in informing the patient about the treatment you propose.

As a general rule, despite the absence of any law requiring that consent be written, you should have documentation that a valid consent was obtained for a procedure that has high risks or is invasive. The best documentation is to have a written and signed consent to care that contains all the elements required for it to be valid. The problem is that absent a written document there may be conflicting testimony as to exactly what the dentist informed the patient about the procedure and its attendant risks, and exactly to what the patient agreed. In nonemergent situations it is best to allow patients to take consent forms home before signing to allow them time to discuss the matter with family or friends. Your records should indicate that this was done and that the consent was discussed before treatment was begun.

Form of consent: implied or expressed? In some dental practice situations implied consent may serve as an effective defense for the dentist. In simple, common, and noninvasive procedures, implied consent is likely to be supported by the courts. A routine dental examination is a good example of one in which the dentist does not have to rely on a written signed consent. Another situation is one in which the patient understands what is being done and makes no attempt to interrupt the procedure. In both situations consent is implied by the action of the party. However, as stated before, if the procedure is invasive or the risks are great and likely to occur, written consent may prepare the patient for the possible consequences and serve to defuse a lawsuit.

In an emergency situation in which care must be rendered at once and consent of the patient could not be obtained, consent is implied by law, as compared with the previous situation in which consent is implied by the action of the party. Courts have applied the following test to support consent implied by law in an emergency situation: (1) consent would have been granted had the patient been able to do so, (2) a reasonable person in the patient's condition would have granted consent, and (3) an emergency was present where treatment was necessary and time was of the essence to preserve the life or health of the victim. This legal theory is present in Good Samaritan situations; consent is implied by law.

Who should obtain consent? As a general rule the health provider is the person charged with obtaining consent to care. However, in practice, others associated with the office or institution in which the care is provided are assigned the responsibility to obtain consent. Two recent court cases, one in Pennsylvania and the other in New York, stated that anyone designated and trained by the provider may obtain a valid consent to care. Despite the rulings, you are advised to review the consent document with the patient; offer to answer any questions concerning the procedure, its risks, benefits, and alternatives, and note on the patient's record that this was done.

Who may grant consent? As a general rule, only the recipient of care may grant a valid consent. As with all general rules, there are exceptions. The most obvious is that minors cannot grant valid consent for their health care. Only a minor's parent or legal guardian can grant a valid consent for the care of the minor—not the minor's adult sibling, not a neighbor, not even a grandparent who supports and pays for the care of the grandchild, and not the child's schoolteacher. However, the parent may grant to any of these people authority to consent to health care for the minor child. The authorization should be written and signed by the parent for the dentist to rely on the authorization.

The obvious question is, When does a minor become an adult? Most states set the majority age at 18. There are exceptions. The age at which a minor may grant a valid consent to health care may be established by state statute. It may be as low as 14 years of age. In addition, many states have defined an "emancipated minor" in contract law and extended it to include consent to health care. In general, an "emancipated minor" is no longer dependent upon parents for support. In addition, pregnant minors are emancipated, as are married minors. The net result is that emancipated minors may grant a valid consent to health care independent of parental consent. Who pays for the service has no effect on the consent to care. Payment for it is a separate issue; the parent may consent to the payment, but the emancipated minor must consent to the care.

In the case of divorced or separated parents, either may consent to the care of the child. Again, payment is a separate issue.

Keeping in mind that only the patient can grant a valid consent to his or her health care, a husband cannot grant a valid consent to the care of his wife despite her inability to do so, nor can an adult for an aged parent. In either case the spouse or adult child of the aged parent must be appointed the legal guardian of the patient.

Telephone consent. Telephone consent, properly executed, is acceptable to the courts. It must, however, contain all the elements that constitute a valid consent. In addition, it must be properly documented. In the case of a minor, the parent or guardian should be contacted by phone and told that a third party is listening on an extension. The parent should be told of the situation and the need for treatment, including all the facts that would be required to meet a valid consent. After the consent is obtained, appropriate notes should be made on the patient's chart, signed by the one who obtained the consent and countersigned by the third party.

Summary. For a summary of consent as it relates to risk management, see the box on p. 325.

Informed refusal

A new legal concept appears to be developing in the arena of malpractice litigation as an outgrowth of informed consent: informed refusal. In a medical malpractice case a woman was advised to undergo a PAP smear test. She refused. Later she developed cervical cancer and died. The physician

---

CONSENT: A RISK MANAGEMENT GUIDE

1. In general, the more invasive the procedure or the greater the risk, the more the requirements of a valid consent must be met; documentation that consent was obtained becomes important. For example, to obtain consent for an examination in which no invasive procedure is to be performed, it might be that implied consent by the actions of the patient is sufficient, with little or no documentation on the patient's record. By contrast, in a situation where an invasive procedure is to be performed, all the requirements of a valid consent should be met, and documentation in the patient's record is essential.
2. The better the documentation, the less the legal risk. Written forms may be used, provided that the delivery of the form is linked to the patient's awareness by sufficient notes made on the patient's record, such as "Patient given handout number x to read, the proposed treatment and alternatives were discussed, and all the patient's questions were answered."
3. Make certain that the one from whom consent is obtained has legal standing to grant consent.
4. When consent for the treatment of a minor is obtained by telephone, it is best to follow up on the telephone conversation by sending a written consent in the mail to be signed by the parent or guardian and returned to the office.
5. Check the local law to determine if written consent is required in situations related to specific treatment.
6. If you delegate to anyone in your office the responsibility to obtain consent from a patient, document that the person was trained in obtaining consent and that you reviewed the consent, discussed it with the patient, and answered all the patient's questions about the procedure.
7. Make certain that in obtaining the consent, all elements to make the consent valid are included: a description of the procedure, why it is necessary, an estimate of the anticipated success, the prognosis if it is not done, the foreseeable and material risks in having it done, and alternatives to the recommended procedure, including their risks, benefits, and prognoses. Present this in language the patient understands (use lay terms), and give the patient an opportunity to discuss all these topics with you. By describing the material risks, as well as the foreseeable risks, all bases are covered to satisfy any local law or court decision.
8. When the treatment includes an invasive procedure, it is best to allow the patient to take the consent form home before signing it.

---

was sued for failing to sufficiently inform the patient of the consequences of her refusal. Several members of the court agreed that the patient must be told of the possible consequences of refusal to make an intelligent decision in refusing a recommended course of treatment. Thus the concept of informed refusal is gradually emerging.

If you recommend to a patient that surgery is the best course of treatment, you must inform the patient of the consequences of refusal. If the patient refuses the care and later suffers an injury because of not having the surgery performed, you may be liable to the patient in damages because you did not inform the patient of the consequences of the refusal.

Having now been informed of this modification to the informed consent concept, you must not only incorporate it into your practice but also remember to document that the patient has been told of the risks of refusal.

The risk management rule relating to the refusal of a patient to follow professional advice is to document that the patient was informed about the best course of action to take to preserve or improve his or her oral health and about the likely consequences if the advice is not followed.

Emergencies and the Good Samaritan law

The Good Samaritan law, enacted in all states, provides immunity from suit for specified health practitioners who render emergency aid to victims of accidents. Generally the statutes require that the aid is provided with no expectation of financial remuneration. Should an injury result from negligence, the victim is precluded by law from instituting a suit, provided there was no evidence of gross negligence. *Gross negligence* is defined as a wanton disregard for another's safety or the failure to exercise slight care.

Immunity does not extend to acts performed in the office or in any health facility.

The standard to which the Good Samaritan is held is based on his or her education and experience. Therefore an act performed by an oral and maxillofacial surgeon may constitute gross negligence, whereas the same act performed by a general practitioner may not be considered negligence at all.

Not all states include dentists in their Good Samaritan law.

The risk management rule is: determine if the jurisdiction in which you practice includes dentists in the Good Samaritan law. Be guided by the answer in rendering emergency aid at the scene of an accident.

An *emergency* is defined as any situation when care must be provided at once to preserve the life or health of the patient. Because the interpretation is broad in most states, dental care may fall within the definition. In cases where a dental emergency exists, and consent cannot be obtained because of a time constraint, consent to care is implied by operation of law.

The risk management rule in dealing with emergencies in which a minor is involved and brought to the office by someone other than a parent is: efforts should be made to obtain the consent of the parent before treatment is begun.

One of the duties owed by the dentist to patients of record, by case law, and in some jurisdictions by black letter law is to make care available to patients in emergency situations. Generally the patient determines what constitutes an emergency.

The risk management rule in emergency situations for patients of record is: the availability of care is a 24-hour-a-day, 7-day-a-week responsibility. If you are on vacation, someone must cover for you.

MISCELLANEOUS ISSUES
Package inserts

Inserts in drug packaging have been accepted into evidence in malpractice cases. Dentists and physi-

cians have been found guilty of negligence for not following the warnings contained on the package inserts. Statements contained in the *Physicians' Desk Reference* (PDR) have also been admitted into evidence.

The risk management rule is: read all drug package inserts and the PDR before administering or prescribing a drug. Because inserts and the PDR are updated frequently, they should be consulted regularly.

What to do when doctors disagree

Situations may arise when the treating dentist and the patient's physician disagree on what prophylactic measures should be taken with a cardiac-compromised patient. The physician may recommend that no preventive measures be taken or that measures be taken that are not consistent with those the dentist feels are appropriate. If the physician's advice is followed and an injury results, it is difficult for the dentist to claim immunity based on the physician's recommendation. The patient is a patient of the dentist, and the dentist operates on his or her own license. Dentists are not employees of physicians or required to carry out a physician's orders if they believe the orders are not consistent with the patient's needs. Whatever care is rendered by a dentist to the patient is interpreted as what the dentist, in her or his best judgment, thinks should be done.

If the dentist does not follow the advice of the physician and an injury occurs, the dentist will be judged on what other dentists in the community would do under similar circumstances and not on what the physician recommended. If the dentist's care meets acceptable community standards, there may be no liability.

If the patient demands that the physician's advice be followed by the dentist and the dentist feels that the advice is not in the best interests of the patient's health, the best course for the dentist to follow is to refuse to treat the patient.

The risk management rule is: exercise your own judgment when deciding on the dental care of the patient. Use advice by others, including physicians, as recommendations that you may either accept or reject. The final decision as to what is done is yours and the patient's.

Associates and employees

There are several important legal issues involved with associates and employees of the dentist. Those with an impact on legal vulnerability are discussed in this section. It is important for dentists to be aware that the more complex the arrangements of practice, the more exposure there is to legal entanglements.

Associations in practice may take many forms, some of which increase legal risk. The employer-employee relationship between dentists makes the employer-dentist individually or jointly liable for the negligent acts of the employee dentist. The legal doctrine for this transfer of liability to the employer, an innocent party, is known as *respondeat superior* (the person in the superior position, the employer, must answer for the acts of the one in an inferior position, the employee, to injured third parties). It is a form of vicarious liability (the substitution of an innocent party for a guilty one in the matter of liability to third parties). However, the employer may sue the employee for indemnification of the employer's losses. If both are insured by the same professional liability insurance company, complications may be avoided.

The same principle of respondeat superior applies to all employees of the dentist, including hygienists, dental assistants, receptionists, and others. The employer-dentist is held liable for all acts performed by an employee in the course of conducting the business of the employer-dentist, even if the acts are specifically prohibited or illegal.

Another form of associate practice among dentists is the partnership. All partners are individually liable for the negligent acts of one partner. The choice of whom to sue is exercised by the plaintiff or the plaintiff's attorney. If a generalist, who is low risk, has a partner who practices oral and maxillofacial surgery, which is high risk, the generalist may be held liable for the negligent acts of the surgeon. It is not unusual for all partners to be joined in the suit. Vicarious liability is supported by the legal theory that all partners are united in interest (each benefits from the acts of others). To avoid serious complications all should be covered by the same professional liability insurance company. From the standpoint of legal liability for negligent acts, practicing in a partnership agreement brings with it serious risks. In several cases,

courts have stated that if the patient considers the practice to be a partnership, the courts will treat it as such. Even if the agreement among a group of dentists is to practice as solo and independent practitioners, if they engage in sharing to the extent that the arrangement appears to be a partnership, they may take on the risks of a partnership.

The third form of associateship is the professional corporation. This relationship represents the lowest level of the transfer or sharing of legal risk. Except in unusual circumstances, innocent shareholders are not liable for the negligent acts of other shareholders. Only the guilty practitioner and the corporation are liable. However, all shareholders and the corporation should be insured by the same professional liability insurance company.

The independent contractor (IC) is the final form of associateship to be considered. With this arrangement, the principal hopes to avoid liability for the negligent acts of the IC. The courts examine, in detail, the arrangement between the parties before determining if the principal is free from liability for the negligent acts of the IC. The matter of control of the ICs, who sets the hours for the IC, whose patients are they, who hires and pays auxiliary personnel, and who provides the equipment and supplies used by the IC are all questions that determine if the IC is truly an IC or simply an employee in determining the liability of the principal (employee). Having the same professional liability insurance company prevents many complications.

The lowest level of legal risk in associateship practice is to practice as a professional corporation and, in any form of joint practice, for all parties to be insured by the same professional liability insurance carrier.

The acts or statements made by nondentist employees present forms of legal risks to the employer-dentist other than those described previously. An employee of a dentist is treated by the courts as an agent of the dentist when the employee is serving in the capacity for which he or she was employed. Thus if a receptionist, hygienist, or assistant assures a patient that following treatment the patient will be satisfied with the result, an express guarantee has been made to which the dentist may be held.

The risk management advice is: educate your

employees to the precise role they are to play in communicating and dealing with patients. Supervise them carefully and monitor their activities at regular intervals. Remain current on changes in the law that affect dental auxiliaries.

Interpersonal relationships

A deterioration in good interpersonal relations between patient and dentist or between patient and staff still ranks as one of the leading causes of malpractice allegations.

When a patient becomes angry, upset, or frustrated, instituting a lawsuit is one of the methods available for retaliation against the dentist or the dentist's staff. The resulting annoyance to the dentist may be reason enough to sue, regardless of the merits of the claim. For the patient, it works. For the dentist, it becomes a real problem involving time, effort, and emotional distress. Too often, efforts of the auxiliary staff made in the interest of shielding the dentist from complaints of difficult patients or patients with annoying problems result in a patient seeking redress through the courts. Most of these situations can be defused by an understanding and compassionate staff. The dentist must be accessible to patients, particularly to those with perceived problems. The judgment of the staff as to what is important to the patient should not be substituted for the patient's judgment of what is important.

The risk management advice is: monitor the staff in their interpersonal relationships with patients. Listen to your patients. Make certain that patients with problems have access to you. Don't hide from your patients. Arrange for substitute care when absent for extended periods. If all efforts fail to restore a cordial relationship with a difficult patient, the safest course to follow is to discontinue treatment.

Return of a fee and suing to collect one

At one time, courts viewed the return of a fee by a doctor as an admission of wrongdoing. Today, it is viewed as an expression of good faith. If you feel that the return of a fee, or part of it, will appease a hostile patient and defuse a difficult situation, it is best to do so. With a patient who threatens to sue unless the fee is returned, and you decide to return the fee, it is best to have the patient execute a release from liability form with accep-

tance of the returned fee. You should weigh the refusal to return the fee with the trauma and loss of time in defending a claim of malpractice; you might even lose the case.

One of the major causes of malpractice allegations is response to an attempt by a doctor to collect a fee. Patients who are delinquent or refuse to pay are inclined to claim poor quality of care as the reason. Should the doctor press to collect, especially through the courts, the patient is likely to countersue for malpractice. Weighing the risk of a countersuit in malpractice should guide you before suing to collect the fee.

If you use a collection agency to act on your behalf for fee collection, review all correspondence sent to a patient. Usually there is more at stake for the practitioner than the fee.

The risk management advice is: think of what might be prevented if a fee is returned and of the possible consequences if a suit is instituted to collect a fee. Do not let pride and principle interfere with making a practical decision. If you return a fee, insist that the patient execute a release-from-liability form.

Current targets in malpractice litagation

The traditional problems leading to allegations of malpractice are still with us: the ill-fitting dentures and the extraction of wrong teeth. The ill-fitting denture problem is often linked with statements made by the dentist that constitute guarantees of satisfaction or serviceability (see the previous section, Guarantees). Most wrong-tooth extraction cases are the result of poor office management and, in situations that involve oral and maxillofacial surgeons, inadequate communication with the referring dentist.

Over the past several years, new grounds of vulnerability have been discovered by patients and their attorneys. In addition, risks have increased because of the introduction of new and more sophisticated techniques into dental practice. New fertile grounds of litigation include the following:

1. Failures in treating problems related to the temporomandibular joint (TMJ)
2. Failures associated with implants
3. Failure to diagnose, monitor, treat, and/or refer (particularly, periodontal disease and TMJ dysfunctions)
4. Failure to obtain the informed consent of

the patient by not informing him or her of the risk of failure and its consequences (particularly endodontics and orthodontics)

5. Failure to take necessary precautions (rubber dam, use of assistants, etc.) to prevent mechanical injury to the patient, such as aspiration of foreign bodies (crowns and instruments) and lacerated soft tissues
6. Continuing to treat when the dentist is aware that the result will not be satisfactory, for example, in orthodontics when the patient is not cooperating in home care
7. Failure to identify a patient with a compromised medical history, such as rheumatic fever, heart murmur, or allergies
8. Failure to take precautions to protect a patient having a compromised medical condition, for example, to prevent subacute bacterial endocarditis
9. Performing a service at the insistence of the patient that is not in the best interest of the patient and will not produce acceptable results, such as treating periodontal disease that should be treated by a specialist; the same holds true in oral surgical cases
10. Not performing a service, at the insistence of the patient, that should be performed before certain treatment is undertaken, for example, radiographs prior to any treatment and periodontal care by a specialist prior to fabrication of fixed prostheses
11. Failure to inform the patient about the risk of paresthesia following surgical procedures
12. Failure to provide follow-up care after surgery, for example, abandonment
13. Failure to consult the patient's physician when the patient's health is compromised

The risks are significantly increased for failure to maintain adequate records or remain current with new advances in the profession. Deteriorating interpersonal relationships between patient and doctor or patient and office staff and attempts by the dentist to collect the fee may be causes of the patient seeking redress in the courts.

What to do and what not to do if you are sued

If a patient threatens you in writing with a suit, if you receive a letter threatening suit from an attorney representing a patient, or if you receive a summons, the following apply.

Things to do
1. At the earliest time after receiving the letter or summons, report it to your insurance carrier by telephone.
2. Make a copy of the papers and send the originals to your carrier; use certified mail, signed receipt requested. Include a copy of any envelope that contained the papers.
3. Write a summary of the treatment of the patient using the treatment record to refresh your memory. Include all you recall, even if it is not on the record. Sign and date the summary.
4. Make a copy of the records, including radiographs, reports, and the summary. Lock the originals in a safe place.
5. Tell your staff about the suit and instruct them not to talk to anyone asking questions about the case without obtaining your permission.
6. Cooperate with your insurance carrier and the attorney assigned by it to your case.

Don't do the following
1. Tell the patient or her or his representative that you are insured
2. Agree to or offer a settlement
3. Agree to or offer to pay for a specialist's services without first consulting with your carrier or the attorney assigned to your case
4. Alter your records in any way
5. Lose or misplace any of your records
6. Discuss the case, or the treatment of the patient, with anyone except representatives of your insurance company or the attorney assigned to your case
7. Admit fault or guilt to anyone
8. Contact any other practitioner about the case even if the practitioner has written a report
9. Agree to or treat the patient-plaintiff during the course of the action

SUMMARY STATEMENT ON RISK MANAGEMENT

Data indicate that a majority of cases brought against doctors are decided in favor of the doctor. If a judge and jury are convinced that the doctor acted in the best interest of the patient, they will be likely to decide that the doctor was free of culpability.

The best advice that an attorney can give to

health practitioners to enable them to enjoy professional life free from litigation brought by patients is to be careful and caring in all they do. It is advice that is simple and short but goes a long way to prevent legal entanglements with patients and courts, should a lawsuit become a reality.

REFERENCES

1. PJ1 2:150. Malpractice—Physician, *Pattern jury instructions-civil, vol 1,* ed 2, Rochester, NY, The Lawyers Cooperative Publishing Co.
2. Louisell, Williams: *Medical Malpractice,* New York, 1988, Matthew Bender.
3. *Schwartz v Board of Regents,* 453 NYS 2d 836.
4. *Thor v Boska,* 38 Cal App 3rd 558, 11 Cal Rptr 296.

Index

A

AAP; *see* American Academy of Pediatrics
Abandonment, 311
Acceptable care, 315
Accidents, preventive services for, 162
Acidulated phosphate fluoride
  for applied aqueous solutions, 174-175
  in topical gels, 184
Acquired immunodeficiency syndrome
  epidemiology and, 141
  in medically compromised patients, 48-56
ACT; *see* Action for Children's Television
Action for Children's Television, 202
Actuarial analysis for dental insurers, 123
ADA; *see* American Dental Association
ADC; *see* Advanced developing countries
Adequacy of instrument, 262
ADHA; *see* American Dental Hygienists Association
Administered health history form, 320
Administrative research in community health, 270
Advanced developing countries, 80
Age distribution, 85
Agency for Health Care Policy and Research, 9
Agency for Toxic Substances and Disease Registry, 9
Agent factors in epidemiology, 153-154
Aging
  changes in geriatric health, 108
  process of, and disease, 108
  of United States population, 105
AIDS; *see* Acquired immunodeficiency syndrome
Alzheimer, 114
American Academy of Pediatrics
  community dental programs and, 202, 203
  and fluoride supplementation, 168
American Association for Dental Research, 99
American Association of Public Health Dentists, 214
American Board of Dental Public Health, 4
American Dental Association, 5
  and ethical issues, 299
  and fluoride supplementation, 168
  plan standards and, 129
  school-based programs and, 205-207
American Dental Association Directory, 280
American Dental Hygienists Association
  and ethical issues, 299
  health education and, 197-198
  and International Dental Hygienists Federation, 99
Americans with Disabilities Act of 1990
  doctor-patient relationship and, 311
  reduction of infectious disease and, 313
Analysis
  cost-benefit, 261-262
  in decision making, 302

Analysis—cont'd
  observations, quantification, and; *see* Indices in epidemiology
  in planning for community programs, 226, 230, 232-235
  steps in, 246
  of variance, 255
Analytical epidemiology, 143-144
ANOVA; *see* Analysis, of variance
Anticalculus ingredients, 182
Anticoagulant therapy, 114
Antimicrobials, 112
APF; *see* Acidulated phosphate fluoride
Applied research, 268
Approaches to health education, 205-218
Appropriateness of health program, 6
Artificial salivas, 113
Aspartame, 179
Aspirin in elderly, 112, 114
Assault and battery, 316
Assessment
  in decision making, 302
  of program, 6
Associates and risk management, 327-328
Association of School Dentists, 90
Author reputation in research literature, 281
Authority to consent, 324
Autocratic decision making, 291
Autonomy
  ethical issues and, 300
  in team management, 286
Auxiliary, 63-76
  in community, 235
  dental assistant as, 64-66
  dental hygienist as, 66-67
  as educator, 73-74
  factors influencing, 67-72
    external, 71-72
    internal, 68-70
    role of, 72-75
  in private practice, 118
  in United Kingdom, 93

B

Bar graph, 248
Barrier technique, 313
Baseline data in questionnaire survey, 280
Basic concepts of health education, 199-204
Basic model plan, 129
Basic research, 268
Bates and O'Steen v. State Bar of Arizona, 305
Battery, assault and, 316
Behavior, in public health, 4

Behavior of learner, 199-201
Behavioral learning model, 199-201
Behavioral research in community health, 270
Beneficence, 300
Benefit package, 127
Benzethonium chloride, 186
Benzophenanthradine alkaloids, 186
Bias in sampling, 246
Biomedical research, 268
Biostatistics, 245-256
    descriptive data display in, 246-252
    inferential statistics and, 252-256
    sampling in, 245-246
Blood-borne disease, 313
Board of Regents, 309, 310
Brain-related symptoms in elderly, 108
Breach of confidentiality, 317-321
British Fluoridation Society, 93
Budget of Pan American Health Organization, 96
Bureau of Dental Health, 207

C

Capitation, 128, 129
Care
    consent to, 321
    delivery systems, 80-94
    social and financial aspects of, 77-138
Care for the Homebound Patient, 198
Care provider, 74-75
Caries
    activity tests, 180
    characteristics of, 7
    in epidemiology, 148-150, 153-154
    global measures of, 79
    as market force, 121
    in nonfluoridated areas, 122
    prevalence of, 102, 156
        in elderly, 109
        in selected countries, 87
    preventive services and, 159
    reduction of, 123
Case control study, 144
Case law, 317
Causal theory for periodontal disease, 143, 144
Cause of death, 112
Caveats in risk management, 308-309
CDC; *see* Centers for Disease Control
CDEP; *see* Commission on Dental Education and Practice
CDFDS; *see* Commission on Defense Forces Dental Services
CDP; *see* Commission of Dental Products
CEJ; *see* Cervico-enamel junction
Center for Science in the Public Interest, 202

Centers for Disease Control, 313
Central tendency, 249-250
Cervico-enamel junction, 152-153
Cetylpyridinium chloride, 186
Changes
    in behavior of learner, 199-201
    in marketplace, 127
    in tissues of mouth, drug-induced, 113
Cherry v. Board of Regents of the State of New York, 125
Chewing gum, 179
Chi-square test, 253-255
Child Health Act of 1967, 11
Child health services, 10-11
Children's Television Act of 1990, 203
China, care delivery system of, 83-89
Chronic ailments in geriatric health, 106
Classical studies in indexing, 148
Climate of team, 292
Clinical effectiveness, 269
Clinical research, 268
Clinical trial
    in community health, 269
    in research design, 274-277
Closed plan, 135, 136
CODA, 17
Code of ethics, 304-305
Cognitive impairment in elderly, 107
Cognitive model, 199, 200, 206
Cohort study, 144
Collaborating Center in Oral Health of Pan American Health
        Organization, 97
Collection
    of data in preventive dentistry, 188
    of fee, 327-328
Collection agency, 328
Commission of Dental Products, 98
Commission on Defense Forces Dental Services, 98
Commission on Dental Education and Practice, 98
Commission on Oral Health, Research, and Epidemiology,
        98
Common knowledge doctrine, 323
Communication
    of team, 292
    in team management, 287-289
Community
    health model of, 201-204
    and migrant health centers, 11-12
    organization of, 202
    primary preventive services in, 158-173
    standards and doctor disagreement, 326
Community-based dental hygienists, 215, 216-218
Community-based preventive procedures, 269
Community dental health, 268-282
Community dental health advocate, 73

Community dental program, 195-242
  alternative strategies in, 239
  compared with private patient programs, 226
  definition of, 227-228, 229
  ecological approach to, 238
  evaluation of, 240-241
  goals and objectives of, 236-239
  identifying constraints in, 238-239
  implementation of, 227, 229, 239-240
  individual patient education and, 198
  monitoring of, 240-241
  needs assessment in, 228-235
  priorities in, 235-236
  reasoning for, 225-227
  revision of, 240-241
  supervision of, 240
Community Health Center, 11
Community Periodontal Index of Treatment Needs, 98, 147, 153
Compatibility of data, 262
Complex service, 129
Comprehensive health planning, 238
Computer literature search, 232
Confidentiality, 301, 317-321
Conflict in team management, 295-296
Confounding variables, 278
Confrontation in supervising, 294
Confrontation meeting, 295, 296
Consensus decision making, 291
Consent
  to care, 321-325
  informed, 272, 300
Consultation and coordination of program, 6
Consultative decision making, 291
Consumer
  demand for services, 123
  influence on auxiliaries, 71-72
  response to, 241
Contact agencies, 314
Contact International, 100
Contemporary community health model, 201-204
Continuous equal interval measures, 256
Contract research, 271
Contracting for Services in Alternative Practice Settings, 198
Convenience sample, 246
Cooperation of team, 296
Coordination of program, 6
CORE; *see* Commission on Oral Health, Research, and Epidemiology
Core area objectives of questionnaire survey, 278
Correlation and inferential statistics, 253-256
Cost
  in community health, 268, 269
  of fluoridation, 164-165

Cost—cont'd
  of fluoride mouthrinse program, 170
  of health services in United Kingdom, 92
  personal, 131
  of pit and fissure sealant, 178
  of sealant program, 173
  of service in geriatric health, 107
Cost-benefit analysis, 261-262
Coumadin, 112
Council, on Dental Health, 15
CPITN; *see* Community Periodontal Index of Treatment Needs
Criminal and quasi-criminal vulnerability, 309-310
Crippled children, 11
Criteria for decision making, 291
CSPI; *see* Center for Science in the Public Interest
Cumulative frequency distribution, 247
Curve, normal, 251-252

D

Data
  collection and evaluation, 246
    of community programs, 226, 230, 232-235
    in preventive dentistry, 188
    and questionnaire survey, 280
  cost and availability of, 262
Date of publication of research literature, 281
De facto rationing, 15
Debriefing, 287-288
Decay in China's care delivery system, 88
Decayed, missing, or filled surfaces, 122, 146, 148
Deceit, 316
Decision making
  ethical reasoning in, 302-304
  informational needs of, 265
  in team management, 290-292
Defamation, 316-317
DEFS; *see* Decayed, missing, or filled surfaces
DEFT; *see* Decayed, missing, or filled surfaces
Degrees of freedom, 253
Delivery of services, 15-17, 158
Demand side of market forces in financing care, 121-124
Dementia in evaluation of elderly, 114
Demographic data and questionnaire survey, 280
Demographics, affect on dentistry, 20
Dental assistant, 64-66
Dental Benefits Advisory Committee, 91
Dental care payments, 125
Dental Health Consultant in Community Based Programs The, 198
Dental history and breach of confidentiality, 320
Dental Hygiene Care of the Special Needs Patient, 198

Dental hygienist, 66-67
  in China, 88
  community-based, 215, 216-218
  emergencies and, 117
  in international health, 102
  and mobile care, 116-117
  tasks for, 118
  in United Kingdom, 93
Dental index; *see* Indices in epidemiology
Dental Knowledge and Attitude Survey, 207
Dental nurse in China, 88
Dental Practice Act, 309
Dental professionals, 79
Dental resins, as sealants, 176-177
Dental schools in Japan, 89
Dental service providers, 1-76
Dentifrices, fluoride, 182
Dentist-to-population ratio
  of China, 88
  of Japan, 86, 90
  of New Zealand, 86, 91
  of United Kingdom, 86, 92
  of Venezuela, 86, 94
Dentists, number of in community, 235
Department of Defense and Veterans Administration, 14
Department of Health and Human Services, 8-9, 203, 272
  expenditures in 1988 of, 10
  Texas preventive program and, 207
Dependence level of geriatric patient, 106
Description of risks and consent, 322
Descriptive data display, 246-252
Descriptive feedback, 288
Design of research in community health, 273-280
df; *see* Degrees of freedom
DHHS; *see* Department of Health and Human Services
Diagnostic-preventive service, 129
Dichotomous-response question, 278
Diet
  counseling in professional primary preventive services, 178-180
  fluoride supplements in, 169
Differences in supervising, 294
Dipyridamole, 114
Director-general candidate of World Health Organization, 95
Disease, 7-8
  and aging process, 108
  consequences of, 200
  in elderly, 109-110
  hypothetical causal theory for periodontal, 143, 144
  patterns of, 141-142
  prevalence and prevention of, 139-194
  and public health practitioners, 5
Distribution, parametric tests and, 256

Division of Dental Health in North Carolina Department of Environment, Health, and Natural Resources, 212
DMF as index; *see* Decayed, missing, or filled surfaces
DMFS; *see* Decayed, missing, or filled surfaces
DMFT; *see* Decayed, missing, or filled surfaces
Doctor
  disagreement and risk management, 326
  implied duties of, 312-313
Doctor-patient contract and risk management, 310-311
Doctor-patient relationship, 124, 125
Donabedian's framework for evaluation, 258
Drafting plan in implementation of program, 6
Drops in fluoride treatment program, 97
Drug-induced change in tissues of mouth, 113
Duties
  of doctor, 312
  of patient, 312-313
Dynamics of group process, 292

E

Ecological approach to comprehensive health planning, 238
Economics
  medical, 127
  problem in team management, 289
Education
  approaches to health, 205-218
  community dental programs and, 198
  concepts of health, 199-204
  model of, 200
Educational research in community health, 270
Educator, auxiliary as, 73-74
Efficiency in evaluation of health program, 6
Elderly; *see* Geriatric patient
Electronic mail system of project HOPE, 101
Emancipated minor, 324
Employees
  benefit package for, 121
  and risk management, 327-328
Enamel fluorosis, 163
Environment
  affect on dentistry, 57-59, 60
  in epidemiology, 153-154
  and public health, 4
Epidemiology, 141-155
  analytical, 143-144
  caries and, 153-154
  definition of, 142-145
  of disease, 7-8
  experimental, 144-145
  indices in, 143-154
    caries, 148-150
    periodontal health, 152-153

Epidemiology—cont'd
  indices in—cont'd
    plaque and oral hygiene, 150-151
    selection of, 145-148
Epidemiology and Oral Disease Prevention Program in
      National Institute of Dental Research, 100
Ethical issues, 299-306
  codes of, 304-305
  principles of, 299-302
  professional responsibility and, 299
  reasoning in decision-making and, 302-304
  of research in community health, 271-273
Ethics, in care, 283-330
Evaluation
  in care, 243-282
  of community dental program, 238, 239-241
  in decision making, 302
  of elderly patient, 111-115
  formative, 258-259
  instrument for, 262
  in preventive dentistry, 188
  of program, 6-7
  reasons for undertaking, 265
  summative, 259
Evaluative research, 270
Examiners, reliability of, 145
Executive board of World Health Organization, 95
Expanded-duty auxiliary program, 102
Expanded model plan, 129
Expected frequencies, 254
Expenditures
  for dental care, 16-17
  of general practice, 122
Experimental epidemiology, 144-145
Experimental subject, consent of, 272
Express term, 312
Expressed form of consent, 323-324
Extended-care facilities in geriatric health, 106
External factors influencing auxiliaries, 71-72
External validity, 264
Extramural Program in National Institute of Dental Research,
      100
Extramural research in community dentistry, 271

F

Fédération Dentaire Internationale, 98-99
Facilities for community programs, 231, 235
Factors affecting dentistry, 20-62
  demographics, 20
  elderly, 20-26
  environmental, 57-59, 60
  infection control, 56-57, 58

Factors affecting dentistry—cont'd
  malpractice, 30-32
  medically compromised patients, 32-56
    acquired immunodeficiency syndrome in, 48-56
    hepatitis B in, 47-48
    herpes in, 56
    systemic diseases in, 33-47, 48, 49
  personnel, 26-30
Factors influencing auxiliaries, 67-72
Failure to diagnose, 321
FCC; see Federal Communication Commission
FDI; see Fédération Dentaire Internationale
FDI News, 99
FDI-WHO Joint Working Group 10, 99
Feasibility, adequacy of instrument and, 262
Federal Communication Commission, 203
Federal government
  dental activities of, 9-14
  influence on auxiliaries, 71
  in public health, 8-14
Federal Trade Commission, 203
  and ethical issues, 305
Fee-for-service, 127-128
Fee-for-service-spectrum, 128
Feedback in team management, 287, 288
FFS; see Fee-for-service
FGM; see Free gingival margin
Financial aspects of care, 77-138
Financial support in research literature, 281
Financing care, 121-137
  demand in market forces in, 121-124
  plan standards in, 129
  provider reimbursement structure in, 127-129
  supply in market forces in, 124-127
First National Symposium on Dental Health Education in
      Schools, 206
First world country, 80
Five City Project, 202
Flossing, 184-185
Fluoridated water
  in United Kingdom, 93
  in Venezuela, 93-94
Fluoridation
  adults and, 164
  caries before and after, 149
  in community programs, 231
  community support of, 166-167
  costs of, 164-165
  opposition to, 217-218
  recommended level of, 165
  status of selected countries, 83
Fluoride, 20
  acidulated phosphate
    applied aqueous solutions and, 174-175

Fluoride—cont'd
  acidulated phosphate—cont'd
    topical gels and, 184
  dentifrices, 181-182
  gel, 183-184
  mouthrinse program, 169-170, 171
  supplement, 167-169
    prenatal, 274-277
  topical, 175-176
Fluorosis, 163
  increase in prevalence of, 156
Follow-up in community program, 226-227
Follow-up study, 144
Form and content and breach of confidentiality, 318
Formal contract in team role negotiations, 293
Formative evaluation, 258-259
Forms of health services, 15-16
Forseeable risk, 322
"Framework for Dental Health Education," 212
Free gingival margin, 152-153
Frequency, expected, 254
Frequency curve, normal, 252
Frequency distribution, 246-247
  of service use, 111
Frequency polygon, 248
FTC; *see* Federal Trade Commission
Funding
  for activities, 9-10
  for community programs, 230-231
  for project HOPE, 101
The Future of Public Health, 4
Future programming direction, 265

G

Games, health-related, 205
General Assembly of Fédération Dentaire Internationale, 98
General practice, 122
Geriatric patient, 105-120
  affect on dentistry, 20-26
  ailments of, 106
  dependence level of, 106
  programs for, 210
  services for, 106-107
  treatment of, 107-119
    aging changes and disease in, 108
    disease in, 109-110
    evaluation for, 111-115
    mobile, 116-118
    payment in, 115-116
    private practice in, 118-119
    socioeconomic factors in, 115

GI; *see* Gingival index
Gingival index, 147, 152
Global Oral Data Bank
  in Japan, 89
  in New Zealand, 91
  in Venezuela, 94
  in World Health Organization, 95
GNP; *see* Gross national product
Goal
  assessment of, in preventive dentistry, 188
  of community program, 236-239
  of program, 259, 260
  of questionnaire survey, 278
Goldfarb v. Virginia State Bar, 305
Good Samaritan law, 325-326
Government
  in community research, 271
  of Japan, 89
  of New Zealand, 90
  of United Kingdom, 91
  of Venezuela, 93
Government agencies
  and community health information, 232
  community programs and, 202-203
Grant in extramural research, 271
Graphing techniques, 247-249
Gross national product, 81
Gross negligence, 326
Grouped frequency distribution, 247
Guarantees in risk management, 312
Guidelines for oral health promotion programs, 80

H

Handbook for Improving High Blood Pressure Control in the Community, 240
Handicapped, private practice and, 118
HCFA; *see* Health Care Financing Administration
Head Start program, 12
Health care consumers, 241
Health care delivery, 158
  in developed nations, 79
Health Care Financing Administration, 9
Health-disease continuum, 157
Health education, 197-224
  approaches to, 205-218
  basic concepts of, 199-204
  changes affecting, 221
  definition of, 197
  model of, 200
  programs in, 216-217
  research in, 218-220
  in transition, 204-205

Health educators in school-based programs, 205
Health history form, 319-320
Health maintenance organization, 125
Health Policy Agenda, 129
Health policy and public health practitioners, 5
Health program
    adequacy of, 6
    and systems in public health, 4
Health program development area of Pan American Health
        Organization, 96
Health-related games, 205
Health Resources and Services Administration, 9
Health services, 15-16
Health statistics of selected countries, 83
Health system
    components of, 262, 263
    infrastructure area of Pan American Health Organization,
        96
Health system agency, 232
Healthy Communities 2000: Model Standards, 10
Healthy People 2000, 10
Hepatitis B, 47-48
Herpes, 56
High-risk needs in community programs, 236
High-risk procedure in elderly, 114
Hippocratic oath, 301
Histogram, 248
HMO; *see* Health maintenance organization
Host factors, 153-154
HRSA; *see* Health Resources and Services Administration
HSA; *see* Health system agency
Human biology in public health, 4
Human Rights Commission, 311
Hydrogen peroxide in mouthrinse, 186
Hygiene
    education program in China, 88
    performances index modified, 146, 150, 151
Hyperthyroidism and treatment of elderly, 108
Hypothetical causal theory, 143, 144

I

IADR; *see* International Association for Dental Research
IADReports, 99
Iatrogenic disease, 300
IC; *see* Independent contractor
ICS I; *see* International Collaborative Study of Dental
        Manpower Systems in Relation to Oral Health Status
        Part I
ICS II; *see* International Collaborative Study Part II
IDHF; *see* International Dental Hygienists' Federation
IDP; *see* International Oral Health Development Program

Immune-mediated disease, 108
Implementation
    of community program, 238, 239-241
    of program, 6-7
Implied duties of doctor and patient, 312-313
Implied form of consent, 323-324
Incidence, 142, 143
IND; *see* Investigative exemption for new drug
Independent contractor, 327
Independent practice association model, 129
Index to Dental Literature, 281
Indices in epidemiology, 143-154
Individual
    in China's care delivery system, 88
    patient education, 198
    plan products, 129
    primary preventive services of, 180-186
Infant mortality
    in Physical Quality of Life Index, 81
    rate of China, 88
Infection control, 56-57, 58
    risk reduction and, 313
Infectious diseases
    in medically compromised patients, 47-56
    transmission of, 313-314
Inferential statistics and biostatistics, 252-256
Information
    difficulties in obtaining, for evaluation, 261-262
    gathering and analysis of, in community programs, 226,
        230
        case study in, 232-235
    importance of, 262
Informational needs of decision makers, 265
Informed consent, 272, 300
Informed refusal, 324-325
Institutional Review Board for Studies Involving Human
        Subjects, 270
Institutionalized patients in geriatric health, 106
Instrument, assessment
    ease of use and interpretation of, 262
    reliability and validity of, 261
Insurable risk, 127
Insurance
    as market force, 121
    medical economics and, 127
    option, 126
    payments, 121
Interexaminer reliability, 145
Internal factors influencing auxiliaries, 68-70
Internal validity, 264
International Association for Dental Research, 80, 99
International Code of Medical Ethics, 301
International Collaborative Study of Dental Manpower
        Systems in Relation to Oral Health Status Part I, 79

International Collaborative Study Part II, 80
International Dental Care Delivery Systems, 80
International Dental Hygienists' Federation, 99-100
International Dental Journal, 99
International health, 79-104
  care delivery system in, 80-94
    China's, 83-89
    Japan's, 89-90
    New Zealand's, 90-91
    terminology of, 80-82
    United Kingdom's, 91-93
    Venezuela's, 93-94
  Fédération Dentaire Internationale in, 98-99
  International Association for Dental Research in, 99
  International Dental Hygienists' Federation in, 99-100
  National Institute of Dental Research in, 100-101
  Pan American Health Organization in, 95-98
  Project HOPE in, 101
  World Health Organization in, 94-95
International Oral Health Development Program, 98
Intervention in group process, 292
Interviewing patient in evaluation of elderly, 111
Intramural research in community, 271
Intramural Research Program in National Institute of Dental
    Research, 100
Investigative exemption for new drug, 270
IPA; *see* Independent practice association
IRB; *see* Institutional Review Board for Studies Involving
    Human Subjects
Ischemic heart disease in evaluation of elderly, 114

J

Japan, care delivery system of, 89-90
Japanese Dental Association, 90
*John R. Bates and Van O'Steen Appellants v. The State Bar
    of Arizona,* 125
Joint prosthesis infection in elderly, 114
Journal of Dental Research of International Association for
    Dental Research, 99
Judgment sample, 246
Justice and ethical issues, 301
Justification in decision making, 302
JWG 10; *see* FDI-WHO Joint Working Group 10

L

Labor for community programs, 231, 235
Laboratory research, 268
Law and consent, 324
LDC; *see* Less developed countries

Leadership
  continuum of, 290, 291
  in team management, 290-292
Learner
  educational process and, 200-201
  level of knowledge of, 199
"Learning about Your Oral Health," 205-207
Learning process, 200-201
Legal problems and consent for care, 321
Legal risk, 308
Legal vulnerability in practice, 309, 310
Legislature in regulation of practice, 309
Less developed countries, 81
Life expectancy in Physical Quality of Life Index, 81
Life-style in public health, 4
Literacy in Physical Quality of Life Index, 81
Literature
  on research in community health, 280-281
  sources for indexing, 148
Loe and Silness gingival index, 147, 152
Longitudinal results of toothpaste study, 264
"Looking to the Future: Exploring Community Approaches to
    Dental Health," 212
Loss
  of organs in elderly, 107
  without fault, 308-309
Loss of attachment index, 147

M

Major insurer, 128
Malocclusion, 162
Malpractice, 314-316
  affect on dentistry, 30-32
  litigation in risk management, 328-329
Management and ethics in care, 283-330
Manpower statistics for selected countries, 86
Market forces
  in financing care, 121-127
  interplay of, 122-124
Marketplace, changes in, 127
Massachusetts Board of Registration in Dentistry, 309
Massachusetts Public Employees Health and Welfare Fund,
    130-136
Material risk and consent, 322
Materials technology, 123
Maternal and child health services, 10-11
Matrix format question, 279
MDC; *see* Middle developing countries
Mean in measures of central tendency, 250
Means test, 110
Measures
  of central tendency, 249-250

Measures—cont'd
objective versus subjective, 261
obtaining necessary information for, 261-262
of outcomes, 260
Media, community programs and, 202-203
Median in measures of central tendency, 250
Medicaid
expenditures for care, 16-17
in geriatric health, 105, 115
and public health, 12-13
Medical considerations of elderly, 111-113
Medical economics and insurance, 127
Medical history, 320
Medically compromised patients, 32-56
Medicare
end expenditures for care, 16-17
and ethical issues, 301
in geriatric health, 105, 115
and public health, 13-14
MEDLINE, 232
Member states of Pan American Health Organization, 96
Membership guidelines in team management, 296
Mental status of elderly, 114-115
Middle developing countries, 80
Migrant health centers, 11-12
Ministry of Health and Social Welfare, 93
Ministry of Health in New Zealand, 91
Minority groups in team management, 286
Misrepresentation, 316
Mobile dental care and geriatric patient, 116-118
Mode in measures of central tendency, 249
Model
behavioral learning, 199-201
cognitive, 199, 200
evaluation of, 206
contemporary community health, 201-204
of health education process, 200
plans of America Dental Association, 129
public health, 201-204
self-care motivation, 200
Moderate-risk procedure in elderly, 114
"Mom It's Up to You! Your Baby Depends on You!," 210
"Mom It's Up to You! Your Health Depends on You!," 210
"Mom It's Up to You! Your Toddler Depends on You!," 210
Monitoring performance, 293
Mottling, 269
Mouth, drug-induced change in tissues of, 113
Mouthrinse, 185-186
in multiple fluoride treatment program, 97
self-applied, 182
Multiple-choice question, 279
Multiple fluoride treatment program, 97
Myocardial infarction, 108

N

NaF; *see* Sodium fluoride
National Caries Program of National Institute of Dental
Research, 218-220
National Children's Dental Health Week, 204
National Congress of Parents and Teachers, 202, 203
National Health Service Corps, 14
National Health Service of United Kingdom, 92
National Health Surveys, 232
National Heart, Lung, and Blood Institute, 240
National Institute of Dental Research, 100-101, 142
budget of, 271
disease indexing and, 147, 152
in geriatric health, 106
National Caries Program of, research and, 218-220
national survey by, 7, 156
National Institutes of Health, 9
Sealant Consensus Panel, 171
National Library of Medicine, 232
National member associations of International Dental
Hygienists' Federation, 100
National Preventive Dentistry Demonstration Program, 219
National PTA; *see* National Congress of Parents and
Teachers
National Survey of Adult Oral Health of U.S. Adults, 142,
152
National Survey of Oral Health in U.S. Schoolchildren, 153
Necessary and sufficient causes, 143
Needs assessment in community program, 226, 228-235
New Zealand, care delivery system of, 90-91
New Zealand Dental Nurse Program, 90
NHS; *see* National Health Service
NHSC; *see* National Health Service Corps
NIDR; *see* National Institute of Dental Research
NIH; *see* National Institutes of Health
1976 Supreme Court decision, 124
Noncompliance and malpractice, 315
Nonmaleficence, 300
Nonparametric test, 256
Normal continuous equal interval measures, 256
Normal curve in graphing data, 251-252
Normal distribution, parametric tests and, 256
North Carolina Citizens for Public Health, Inc., 212
North Carolina program, 210-213, 214-215
NPDDP; *see* National Preventive Dentistry Demonstration
Program
Nuremberg Code of Ethics for Medical Research, 271-272
Nursing facilities, 10
Nursing home
and dental hygienist, 117
in geriatric health, 106, 110
and mobile dental care, 116

Nursing home—cont'd
    and public health, 10-14

O

Objective feedback in team management, 288
Objective reasonable person rule, 322
Objectives
    of community program, 236-239
    of International Dental Hygienists' Federation, 100
    program outcomes and inputs and, 259, 260
    of World Health Organization, 94
OBRA 89; see Omnibus Reconciliation Act of 1989
OBRA 90; see Omnibus Reconciliation Act of 1990
Observations, quantification, analysis, and understanding of;
        see Indices in epidemiology
Occupational Safety and Health Administration, 299
Office personnel, 123
OHI-S; see Oral Hygiene Index Simplified
Omnibus Reconciliation Act of 1989, 13
Omnibus Reconciliation Act of 1990, 13
OPEC; see Organization, of Petroleum Exporting Countries
Open panel, fee-for-service, 127-128
Open plan, in Massachusetts care program, 134, 135
Openness in team management, 288
Operating budget of National Institute of Dental Research,
        271
Operatories, 235
Oral cancer, 161
Oral Data Bank
    in China, 88
    in United Kingdom, 93
Oral examinations of elderly, 109
Oral form of consent, 323
Oral health
    and dental professionals, 79
    promotion programs, 80
    and public health practitioners, 5
Oral Health Unit of Pan American Health Organization, 96
Oral hygiene
    indices, 150-151
    in individual primary preventive services, 184-186
Oral Hygiene Index Simplified, 146, 150-151
Oral prophylaxis in elderly, 110
Organization
    in community, 202
    of Health Services Based on Primary Health Care, 96
    of Petroleum Exporting Countries, 80
Orientation in team development, 296
Orofacial defects, 162
Orthodontic service, 129
OSHA; see Occupational Safety and Health Administration

Outcomes of program evaluation in health care, 259-262
Owned feedback in team management, 288

P

Pacemakers in elderly, 112
Package inserts, 326
PAHO; see Pan American Health Organization
Paid claim, 133
Pan American Health Organization, 95-98
    and Venezuela, 93
Pan American Sanitary Bureau, 96
Paradental program, 89
Parametric test, 256
Parents, community programs and, 203, 210
Participating provider, fee-for-service, 128
Partnership, 327
PASB; see Pan American Sanitary Bureau
Paternalistic practice, 300
Patient
    contact with, 123
    diversity of, in elderly, 111
    duties of, 312-313
    education of, community programs and, 198
    medical history of, 319, 320
    provided services for, 132
    records of, 317
Payment
    for care of geriatric patient, 115-116
    dental care, 125
PDR; see Physicians' Desk Reference
People-to-People Health Foundation, Inc., 101
People v. Duben, 125
Percent expenditure by service, 124
Periodontal disease
    and breach of confidentiality, 321
    characteristics of, 7
    global measures of, 79
    hypothetical causal theory for, 143, 144
    preventive services and, 160
Periodontal health indices in epidemiology, 152-153
Permanent dentition, 88
Persantine; see Dipyridamole
Personal cost, 131
Personal social services of United Kingdom, 92
Personal hygiene performances index modified, 146, 150,
        151
Personnel
    in office, 123
    status of dental, 26-30
Phenolic compounds, 186
Phenothiazines in elderly, 113
PHP-M; see Hygiene, performances index modified

PHS; *see* Public Health Service
Physical Quality of Life Index, 81
Physicians' Desk Reference and package inserts, 326
Physiologic change and disease in elderly, 108
PI; *see* Russell's periodontal disease index
Pit and fissure sealants, 176-178
Placebos in research, 273
Plan standards in financing care, 129
Planning for community program; *see* Community dental
    program
Plaque
    control of
        and elderly, 109
        in professional primary preventive services, 180
    indices for, 150-151
Platelet aggregation in elderly, 114
Political repression in developing countries, 82
Population
    of China, 83, 84
    defined, 245
    distribution by age, 106
    distribution by sex, 105
    growth, as world problem, 81
    of Japan, 84, 89
    of New Zealand, 84, 90
    statistics for selected countries, 84
    of United Kingdom, 84, 91-92
    of Venezuela, 84, 93
Postnatal dental programs, 210
Practitioners of public health, 5
Pregnancy, fluoride supplements and, 169
Premature goal statement, 289
Prenatal dental program, 210
Prenatal fluoride supplements, 274-277
Prepaid care plan, 127
Pretesting and questionnaire survey, 280
Prevalence, 142-143
    of caries, 102, 149
    and prevention of disease, 139-194
Prevention
    of disease, 139-194
    health-disease continuum and, 157
    and hygienist, 117
    procedures for, 269
    services for, 157, 158-163
Prevention Block Grant, 15
Preventive dentistry, 156-193
    definition of, 156-157
    primary services of, 157, 158-186
        community, 163-173
        individual, 180-186
        professional, 173-180
    services of, 157-158, 159-162
    treatment planning in, 186-189

Price elasticity, 123
Primary dentition, 88
Primary health care in United Kingdom, 92
Primary preventive services; *see* Preventive dentistry, primary
    services of
Principles of ethics, 299-302
Principles of Ethics and Code of Professional Conduct, 304,
    312
Priorities
    in community program, 235-236
    in implementation of program, 6
    of Oral Health Unit, 98
    of program, 259-260
Private practice and handicapped and elderly, 118
Problem solving
    model for, 290
    in team management, 289-290
Problems
    recognition of, in preventive dentistry, 187-188
    in team management, 285
Procedures per patient per year, 134
Process observation in team management, 292-293
Productivity in team development, 296
Professional
    community standards and, 322
    corporation in risk management and, 327
    liability insurance and, 311
    negligence and, 314-316
    primary preventive services of, 173-180
    responsibility of, 299
Program
    design of, 260, 262-264
    direction for future, 265
    evaluation of, 257-267
        components of health system and, 262, 263
        constraints on results of, 265
        focus of, 258-259
        outcomes and inputs of, 259-262
        purpose of, 257
        study designs in, 262-264
    management of, 5
    of public health, 6
    structure of, 258
"Programs for the Mass Control of Plaque: An Appraisal,"
    214
Project HOPE, 101
Prospective study, 144
Protectionism, 82
Provider-patient ratio, 86
Providers of service, 1-76
Psychological problem in team management, 289
PTA; *see* National Congress of Parents and Teachers
Public health, 3-19
    definition of, 3-7, 198

Public health—cont'd
  disease in, 7-8
  government and, 8-14
    department of health and human services, 8-9
    funding for activities, 9-10
    nursing homes and, 10-14
  model of, 201-204
  state agencies of, 14-15
  use and delivery of services in, 15-17
Public health report, 4
Public Health Service, 9
Publication date of research literature, 281

Q

Quantifiable item of questionnaire survey, 279
Quantification, analysis, and understanding of observations;
    see Indices in epidemiology
Quasi-criminal vulnerability, 309-310
Quaternary ammonium compounds, 186
Questionnaire survey
  in community health, 270
  in research design, 277-280
Questions in team role negotiations, 293

R

Random sampling, 245-246
Rationing in health services, 15
RCI; *see* Root caries
Reasoning in decision-making, 302-304
Recall, community programs and, 225
Record keeping, 318-319
Refereed journal, 281
Regional offices of World Health Organization, 95
Regulation of practice, 309
Regulatory agencies, 202-203
Reliability, of instrument, 262
Replacement services in loss of function, 157
Reputation of research literature, 281
Request for application or proposal, 271
Requirements of professionals, 299
Research
  in community health, 268-282
    design of, 273-280
    ethics of, 271-273
    literature on, 280-281
    types of, 268-271
  and evaluation in care, 243-282
  in health education, 218-220
  priorities for, in community dentistry, 271
  and public health practitioners, 5

Research Committee of the American Association of Public
    Health Dentists, 214
Resins as sealants, 176-177
Resource identification, 226-227, 230-231, 237
Respondeat superior, 327
Responsibilities of World Health Organization, 94
Retrospective study, 144
Return of fee in risk management, 327-328
Revenue
  in general practice, 122
  shifts of, 124
Review in research literature, 281
Revision of community program, 238, 239-241
Risk management, 307-330
  associates and employees in, 327-328
  caveats in, 308-309
  criminal and quasi-criminal vulnerability and, 309-310
  of doctor, 312
  doctor-patient contract and, 310-311
  express term in, 312
  fee in, 327-328
  guarantees in, 312
  guide and consent, 325
  infectious diseases in, 313-314
  legal vulnerability and, 309
  malpractice litigation in, 328-329
  package inserts in, 326
  of patient, 312-313
  regulation of practice and, 309
  tort in, 314-326
Risk-sharing option, 128
Roles in team management, 292, 293
Root caries, 109, 146, 149-150
Russell's periodontal disease index, 146, 152

S

Saccharin, 179
Salt fluoridation, 97
Sample
  defined, 245
  size of, 261
Sampling in biostatistics, 245-246
Sanguinarine, 186
Scatter diagram, 255
School-based programs, 198, 203, 204-207
  fluoride mouthrinse in, 169-170, 171
  National Preventive Dentistry Demonstration Program and,
    219
  sealant in, 172-173
School Health Education Evaluation, 203-204, 207
School sealant program, 170-173

Second world country, 80
Secondary decay in elderly, 109
Secondary preventive services, 157, 158-163
Secretariat of World Health Organization, 95
Selection
    in decision making, 302
    of indices, 145-148
Self-administered health history form, 319-320
Self-administration, 126
Self-care motivation model, 200
Self-indemnification, 126
Senile dementia, 114
Senior citizen program, 210
Sensitivity, statistical adequacy and, 262
Service lines, 123
Services
    consumer demand for, 123
    for geriatric patient, 106-107, 110, 111
    percent expenditure by, 124
    of preventive dentistry, 157-158, 159-162
SHEE; *see* School Health Education Evaluation
Significance, of inferential statistics, 252-253
Skilled nursing facilities, 10
SnF$_2$; *see* Stannous fluoride
Social aspects of care, 77-138
Social health insurance system, 89
Social Security
    affect on elderly, 115
    of United Kingdom, 92
Social Security Administration, 9
Social welfare system, 92
Socioeconomic factors affecting elderly, 115
Sodium fluoride
    for applied aqueous solutions, 174
    in mouthrinse, 182, 183
    in topical gels, 184
Solution finding in team management, 289
Sorbitol, 179
Special Committee on the Future of Dentistry, 5-6
SSA; *see* Social Security Administration
Staff development, 293
Staff model group, 129
Staining, 269
Standard deviation, 251
Standards
    of acceptable care, 315
    ethical, 299
Stanford Five City Project, 202
Stannous fluoride
    for applied aqueous solutions, 174
    in topical gels, 183, 184
State Board for Dentistry and regulation of practice, 309
State Education Department and regulation of practice, 309

State government
    auxiliaries and, 71-72
    in public health, 8-14
    restrictions on advertising, 124
State public health agencies, 14-15
Statistic, defined, 245
Statistical adequacy of assessment instrument, 262
Statistical significance, 253
Statute of frauds, 323
Steps in team role negotiations, 293
Stomatitis, 112
Stomatologist, 89
Strategies in community program, 239
Strategy flow chart, 229
Stratified sampling, 246
Student's *t*-test, 253, 255-256
Study designs
    in program evaluation in health care, 262-264
    and research literature, 281
Study population in questionnaire survey, 278
Subgoal, 278
Subjective prudent person rule, 322
Subjectivity, 145
Sugar consumption, 179
Suing to collect fee, 327-328
Summative evaluation, 259
Supervision
    of community program, 238, 239-241
    in team management, 293-295
Supply side of market forces in financing care, 124-127
Supreme Court decision of 1976, 124
Survey instrument in community health, 270
Systemic diseases in medically compromised patients, 33-47, 48, 49
Systemic sampling, 246

T

t distribution, 255-256
t-test, 253
Tables, 248-249
Tablets in multiple fluoride treatment program, 97
Target
    as group in community programs, 236
    in implementation of program, 6
    in malpractice litigation, 328-329
    as population of Pan American Health Organization, 96
"Tattletooth II, A New Generation," 207-210
Team management, 285-298
    communication in, 287-289
    conflict utilization in, 295-296
    definition of, 285-286
    development of, 296-297

Team management—cont'd
  leadership and decision making in, 290-292
  membership guidelines in, 296
  problem solving in, 289-290
  process observation in, 292-293
  roles in, 293
  supervisory function in, 293-295
  theories of, 286-287
Techniques, clinical trials of, 269
Teenagers, periodontal health of, 156
Telephone consent, 324
Television, community programs and, 202-203
Temporomandibular joint, 321
Terminology of care delivery systems, 80-82
Tertiary preventive services, 157, 158-163
Texas preventive program, 207-210
Theories of team management, 286-287
Theory X
  in decision making, 290
  of management, 286-287
Theory Y
  in decision making, 290
  of management, 287
Therapeutic agents, 269
Therapeutic reassurances in risk management, 312
Third party
  as administrator, 126-127
  intervention by, in conflict, 295, 296
  misrepresentation by, 316
  in payment for care, 121, 125, 316
Third world country, 80
Timed feedback in team management, 288
Timing, evaluation results and, 265
Tissues of mouth, drug-induced change in, 113
Toothbrush modifications, 110
Toothbrushing, 184
  studies of, 262-264
  summary of methods for, 185-186
Toothpaste study, 264
Topical fluoride, 173-176
  in preventive services, 182-184
Tort, 314-326
TPA; see Third party, as administrator
Trauma, 162
Treatment
  of geriatric patient, 107-119
  record of, 318-319
  termination of, 311
Treatment plan
  and breach of confidentiality, 321
  in preventive dentistry, 188
Treatment planning
  community dental programs and; see Community dental
    program

Treatment planning—cont'd
  in preventive dentistry, 186-189
Trespass to person, 316
Truth and ethical issues, 301
TSCMM; see Self-care motivation model
Two-party conflict, 295

U

United Kingdom, care delivery system of, 91-93
U.S. Census Bureau, 232
U.S. Public Health Service, 164
U.S. Surgeon General, 203
University of the West Indies Distance Teaching Experiment,
    101
Unmet restorative treatment needs index, 148-149
UTN index; see Unmet restorative treatment needs index
UWIDITE; see University of the West Indies Distance
    Teaching Experiment

V

VA; see Veterans Administration
Validity of research instrument, 261, 262, 264
Variability, 250-251
Variables in questionnaire survey, 278
Variance, 250-251, 255
Venezuela, care delivery system of, 93-94
Veracity and ethical issues, 301
Veterans Administration, 14
Vicarious liability, 327
*Virginia State Board of Pharmacy v. Virginia Citizens
    Consumer Council,* 305
Vulnerability
  criminal and quasi-criminal, 309-310
  and malpractice litigation, 328

W

Water fluoridation
  in community primary preventive services, 163-167
  in Japan, 89
  in New Zealand, 91
Water source of community, 231
WHO; see World Health Organization
Worksheet for resource identification, 237
World Health Assembly, 94-95
World Health Organization, 94-95, 202
  definition of public health, 3
  in international health, 79
World studies in epidemiology, 153-154

Writing style and research literature, 281
Written form of consent, 323
Written response, on questionnaire survey, 279

X

X^2 test; *see* Chi-square test

Y

Yes-No form in medical history, 320

Z

Zero variance, 250